Neurology and Psychiatry of Women

Mary Angela O'Neal
Editor

Leena Mittal
Guest Editor

Neurology and Psychiatry of Women

A Guide to Gender-based Issues in
Evaluation, Diagnosis, and Treatment

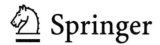 Springer

Editor
Mary Angela O'Neal
Department of Neurology
Brigham and Women's Hospital
Boston, MA
USA

Guest Editor
Leena Mittal
Department of Psychiatry
Brigham and Women's Hospital
Boston, MA
USA

ISBN 978-3-030-04244-8   ISBN 978-3-030-04245-5   (eBook)
https://doi.org/10.1007/978-3-030-04245-5

Library of Congress Control Number: 2019930963

This Springer imprint is published by the registered company Springer Nature Switzerland AG
The registered company address is: Gewerbestrasse 11, 6330 Cham, Switzerland

Preface

The need to understand how neurologic and psychiatric disorders are different in women is important to appropriately care for female patients. There is a vast amount of knowledge about how sex affects disease incidence, course, and treatment, as well as how drugs and disease interact with reproductive health, pregnancy, and menopause. Yet many practitioners only have a limited understanding of these important concerns. Further, there is no single text which provides this critical information. This book was written for all providers who take care of women with these conditions to provide sex-appropriate care guidelines.

Many providers think that women's issues in medicine only relate to pregnancy. In fact, gender concerns are important throughout a woman's life. Of course, the factors important to consider vary as to where patients are in their life cycle. For example, to understand stroke risk in women, a history regarding pregnancy-related disorders such as preeclampsia/eclampsia and gestational diabetes is essential.

I wanted to assemble a comprehensive textbook that reflects the significant issues as regards both neurologic and psychiatric disorders spanning a woman's life including reproductive health, pregnancy, and healthy aging. Each chapter is written by experts in their field to give practical up-to-date advice about some of the considerations to best address our female patients' health. I hope you enjoy reading the book.

Boston, MA, USA   Mary Angela O'Neal, MD

Contents

Part I Issues in Women During Their Reproductive Years

Women and Migraine 3
Regina Krel and Paul G. Mathew

Connective Tissue Disorders in Women 7
Sophia L. Ryan, Shamik Bhattacharyya, and Mary Angela O'Neal

Functional Neurological Disorder and Dissociative Disorders in Women 15
Geoffrey Raynor and Gaston Baslet

Contraception in Neurologic and Psychiatric Disorders 27
Caryn Dutton, Andrea Hsu Roe, and Deborah Bartz

Neuroendocrine Disorders in Women 37
Alexandra J. Lovett and Whitney W. Woodmansee

Somatoform Disorders 47
Timothy M. Scarella

Anxiety Disorders 69
Madeleine A. Becker, Nazanin E. Silver, Ann Chandy, and Subani Maheshwari

Neuro-inflammatory Disorders in Women 77
Ivana Vodopivec

Catamenial Epilepsy 85
P. Emanuela Voinescu

Neuro-oncological Disorders in Women 95
Na Tosha N. Gatson and Erika N. Leese

Substance Use Disorders in Women 103
Whitney Peters, Connie Guille, and Leena Mittal

Part II Pregnancy

Neurologic Imaging in Pregnancy 117
Jesse M. Thon, Robert Regenhardt, and Joshua P. Klein

The Normal Physiology of Pregnancy: Neurological Implications 121
Cesar R. Padilla and Nicole A. Smith

Epilepsy and Pregnancy 125
Mariel Velez and Kimford J. Meador

Headaches in Pregnancy and Postpartum 131
Mary Angela O'Neal

Stroke in Pregnancy 139
Steven K. Feske

Demyelinating Disease and Pregnancy 145
Tamara B. Kaplan and Riley Bove

Mood Disorders in Pregnancy 157
Kara Brown and Dylan Kathol

Postpartum Neuropathy 173
Janet F. R. Waters

Myasthenia Gravis and Pregnancy 177
Christyn Edmundson and Mohammad Kian Salajegheh

Ethical Decisions in Pregnancy 183
Thomas I. Cochrane

Part III   Women's Health and Aging

Menopausal Hot Flashes, Sleep and Mood Disturbances 191
Geena Athappilly and Margo Nathan

Stroke Risk Factors in Women 205
Emer R. McGrath and Kathryn M. Rexrode

Gender Differences in Parkinson's Disease 213
Michael T. Hayes

Sex-Related Differences in Alzheimer's Disease 219
Diler Acar and Carolyn Jane King

Successful Aging 227
Marie Pasinski

Index 233

Contributors

Diler Acar, MD Brigham and Women's Hospital, Boston, MA, USA

Geena Athappilly, MD Harvard Medical School, Boston, MA, USA

Edith Nourse Rogers Memorial Veterans Hospital, Bedford, MA, USA

Site Director for Boston University Family Medicine Residency at Edith Nourse Rogers Memorial Veteran Affairs Hospital, Boston, MA, USA

Deborah Bartz, MD, MPH Department of Obstetrics and Gynecology, Brigham and Women's Hospital, Boston, MA, USA

Harvard Medical School, Boston, MA, USA

Gaston Baslet, MD Department of Psychiatry, Brigham and Women's Hospital, Boston, MA, USA

Harvard Medical School, Boston, MA, USA

Madeleine A. Becker, MD, FACLP Department of Psychiatry and Human Behavior, Thomas Jefferson University Hospital, Philadelphia, PA, USA

Shamik Bhattacharyya, MD, MS Department of Neurology, Brigham and Women's Hospital, Boston, MA, USA

Harvard Medical School, Boston, MA, USA

Riley Bove, MD, MMSc Department of Neurology, Weill Institute for the Neurosciences, University of California, San Francisco, CA, USA

Kara Brown, MD Southeast Louisiana Verterans Health Care System, New Orleans, LA, USA

Ann Chandy, MD Department of Psychiatry and Human Behavior, Thomas Jefferson University Hospital, Philadelphia, PA, USA

Thomas I. Cochrane, MD, MBA Brigham and Women's Hospital, Center for Bioethics, Harvard Medical School, Boston, MA, USA

Caryn Dutton, MD, MS Department of Obstetrics and Gynecology, Brigham and Women's Hospital, Boston, MA, USA

Harvard Medical School, Boston, MA, USA

Christyn Edmundson, MD Division of Neuromuscular Medicine, Department of Neurology, Hospital of the University of Pennsylvania, Philadelphia, PA, USA

Steven K. Feske, MD Harvard Medical School, Division of Stroke and Cerebrovascular Disease, Neurology Department, Brigham and Women's Hospital, Boston, MA, USA

Na Tosha N. Gatson, MD, PhD Geisinger Neuroscience Institute, Danville, PA, USA

Geisinger Cancer Institute, Danville, PA, USA

Connie Guille, MD Medical University of South Carolina, Institute of Psychiatry, Charleston, SC, USA

Michael T. Hayes, MD Department of Neurology, Brigham and Women's Hospital, Boston, MA, USA

South Shore Hospital, Weymouth, MA, USA

Harvard Medical School, Boston, MA, USA

Tamara B. Kaplan, MD Department of Neurology, Harvard Medical School, Brigham and Women's Hospital, Boston, MA, USA

Dylan Kathol, MD Department of Psychiatry, NorthShore University Health System, Evanston, IL, USA

Carolyn Jane King, BA Brigham and Women's Hospital, Boston, MA, USA

Joshua P. Klein, MD, PhD Department of Neurology, Brigham and Women's Hospital, Boston, MA, USA

Regina Krel, MD Hackensack Meridian School of Medicine at Seton Hall University, Nutley, NJ, USA

Neuroscience Institute, Hackensack University Medical Center, Hackensack, NJ, USA

Brigham & Women's Hospital, Department of Neurology, John R. Graham Headache Center, Boston, MA, USA

Harvard Vanguard Medical Associates, Department of Neurology, Braintree, MA, USA

Cambridge Health Alliance, Division of Neurology, Cambridge, MA, USA

Harvard Medical School, Boston, MA, USA

Erika N. Leese, PA-C Geisinger Neuroscience Institute, Danville, PA, USA

Alexandra J. Lovett, MD Massachusetts General Hospital, Boston, MA, USA

Subani Maheshwari, MD Department of Psychiatry, Wilmington Hospital, Christiana Care Health System, Wilmington, DE, USA

Paul G. Mathew, MD, DNBPAS, FAAN, FAHS Hackensack University Medical Center, Hackensack, NJ, USA

Seton Hall University, Nutley, NJ, USA

Brigham & Women's Hospital, Department of Neurology, John R. Graham Headache Center, Boston, MA, USA

Harvard Vanguard Medical Associates, Department of Neurology, Braintree, MA, USA

Emer R. McGrath, MB, PhD Department of Neurology, Brigham and Women's Hospital and Harvard Medical School, Boston, MA, USA

Kimford J. Meador, MD Department of Neurology and Neurological Sciences, Stanford University, Palo Alto, CA, USA

Leena Mittal, MD Department of Psychiatry, Brigham and Women's Hospital, Boston, MA, USA

Margo Nathan, MD Division of Women's Mental Health and Department of Psychiatry, Harvard Medical School, Brigham and Women's Hospital, Boston, MA, USA

Mary Angela O'Neal, MD Department of Neurology, Brigham and Women's Hospital, Boston, MA, USA

Cesar R. Padilla, MD Brigham and Women's Hospital, Boston, MA, USA

Marie Pasinski, MD Harvard Medical School, Nahant, MA, USA

Whitney Peters, MD Department of Psychiatry, Beth Israel Deaconess Medical Center, Boston, MA, USA

Geoffrey Raynor, MD Department of Psychiatry, Brigham and Women's Hospital, Boston, MA, USA

Robert Regenhardt, MD, PhD Partners Neurology Residency Program, Brigham and Women's Hospital, Massachusetts General Hospital, Boston, MA, USA

Kathryn M. Rexrode, MD, MPH Division of Women's Health, Department of Medicine, Brigham and Women's Hospital and Harvard Medical School, Boston, MA, USA

Andrea Hsu Roe, MD, MPH Department of Obstetrics and Gynecology, Hospital of the University of Pennsylvania, Philadelphia, PA, USA

Perelman School of Medicine, University of Pennsylvania, Philadelphia, PA, USA

Sophia L. Ryan, MD Department of Neurology, Brigham and Women's Hospital, Boston, MA, USA

Department of Neurology, Massachusetts General Hospital, Boston, MA, USA

Harvard Medical School, Boston, MA, USA

Mohammad Kian Salajegheh, MD Neuromuscular Center & EMG Laboratory, Department of Neurology, VA Boston Healthcare System, Harvard Medical School, Boston, MA, USA

Timothy M. Scarella, MD Department of Psychiatry, Beth Israel Deaconess Medical Center/Harvard Medical School, Boston, MA, USA

Nazanin E. Silver, MD, MPH, FACOG Division of Women's Behavioral Health, Department of Obstetrics and Gynecology, University of Pittsburg Medical Center Pinnacle, Camp Hill, PA, USA

Nicole A. Smith, MD, MPH Maternal Fetal Medicine, Brigham and Women's Hospital, Boston, MA, USA

Department of ob/gyn, Brigham and Women's Hospital, Boston, MA, USA

Jesse M. Thon, MD Department of Neurology, Massachusetts General Hospital, Boston, MA, USA

Mariel Velez, MD, PhD California Pacific Medical Center, California Pacific Neurosciences Institute, San Francisco, CA, USA

Ivana Vodopivec, MD, PhD Department of Neurology, Brigham and Women's Hospital, Harvard Medical School, Boston, MA, USA

P. Emanuela Voinescu, MD, PhD Brigham and Women's Hospital, Harvard Medical School, Boston, MA, USA

Janet F.R. Waters, MD, MBA University of Pittsburgh Medical Center, Pittsburgh, PA, USA

Whitney W. Woodmansee, MD Division of Endocrinology, Diabetes and Metabolism, University of Florida, Gainesville, FL, USA

Part I

Issues in Women During Their Reproductive Years

Women and Migraine

Regina Krel and Paul G. Mathew

Women and Migraine

Migraine is a condition which affects over 36 million people in the United States alone [1]. These vast numbers make migraine the third most common condition and sixth most disabling condition worldwide [2]. Up until puberty, the ratio of female-to-male sufferers is approximately equal, however this ratio significantly shifts at the onset of menarche, at which time the ratio increases to a nearly 3:1 female-to-male ratio. A diagnosis of migraine is established through taking a thorough history, performing a physical examination, and by ruling out secondary causes of headache with additional testing based on clinical suspicion, such as neuroimaging. The diagnostic criteria for migraine is established in the The International Classification of Headache Disorders Third Edition (ICHD) (Table 1) [3]. An estimated 11% of women who suffer from migraines have headache onset at the time of menarche. This population

R. Krel
Hackensack Meridian School of Medicine at Seton Hall University, Nutley, NJ, USA

Neuroscience Institute, Hackensack University Medical Center, Hackensack, NJ, USA

Brigham & Women's Hospital, Department of Neurology, John R. Graham Headache Center, Boston, MA, USA

Harvard Vanguard Medical Associates, Department of Neurology, Braintree, MA, USA

Cambridge Health Alliance, Division of Neurology, Cambridge, MA, USA

Harvard Medical School, Boston, MA, USA

P. G. Mathew (✉)
Hackensack University Medical Center, Hackensack, NJ, USA

Seton Hall University, Nutley, NJ, USA

Brigham & Women's Hospital, Department of Neurology, John R. Graham Headache Center, Boston, MA, USA

Harvard Vanguard Medical Associates, Department of Neurology, Braintree, MA, USA
e-mail: PMATHEW@PARTNERS.ORG

subset is more likely to develop menstrual migraine [4]. Migraines which have a close menstrual association are further classified by ICHD into pure menstrual migraine without aura or menstrually related migraine without aura (Table 2). Studies demonstrate that menstrually related migraine is far more common than pure menstrual migraine, and can be present in 20–60% of women compared to pure menstrual migraine which occurs in <10% [5].

Table 1 ICHD 3 diagnostic criteria for migraine with and without aura

Migraine without Aura
A. At least five attacks fulfilling criteria B–D
B. Headache attacks lasting 4–72 h
C. Headache has at least two of the following four characteristics:
  1. Unilateral location
  2. Pulsating quality
  3. Moderate or severe pain intensity
  4. Aggravation by or causing avoidance of routine physical activity
D. During headache at least one of the following:
  1. Nausea and/or vomiting
  2. Photophobia and phonophobia
E. Not better accounted for by another ICHD-3 diagnosis

Migraine with Aura
A. At least two attacks fulfilling criteria B and C
B. One or more of the following fully reversible aura symptoms:
  1. Visual
  2. Sensory
  3. Speech and/or language
  4. Motor
  5. Brainstem
  6. Retinal
C. At least two of the following four characteristics:
  1. At least one aura symptoms spreads gradually over ≥5 min, and/or two or more symptoms occur in succession
  2. Each individual aura symptom lasts 5–60 min
  3. At least one aura symptom is unilateral
  4. The aura is accompanied, or followed within 60 min, by headache
D. Not better accounted for by another ICHD-3 diagnosis, and transient ischaemic attack has been excluded

© Springer Nature Switzerland AG 2019
M. A. O'Neal (ed.), *Neurology and Psychiatry of Women*, https://doi.org/10.1007/978-3-030-04245-5_1

Table 2 ICHD 3 diagnostic criteria for menstrual migraine

Pure menstrual migraine without aura

A. Attacks, in a menstruating woman, fulfilling criteria for Migraine without aura and criterion B below

B. Documented and prospectively recorded evidence over at least three consecutive cycles has confirmed that attacks occur exclusively on day 1 ± 2 (i.e. days -2 to $+3$) of menstruation in at least two out of three menstrual cycles and at no other times of the cycle

Menstrually related migraine without aura

A. Attacks, in a menstruating woman, fulfilling criteria for Migraine without aura and criterion B below

B. Documented and prospectively recorded evidence over at least three consecutive cycles has confirmed that attacks occur on day 1 ± 2 (i.e. days -2 to $+3$) of menstruation in at least two out of three menstrual cycles, and additionally at other times of the cycle

Table 3 Short-term menstrual migraine prophylaxis options [5]

Drug class	Medication	Dose/directions
NSAID	Naproxen sodium	550 mg twice daily for 5–14 days starting the week before anticipated period onset
Triptan	Frovatriptan	Started 2 days before period onset with 5 mg taken twice daily on day 1, then 2.5 mg twice daily for 6 days
Triptan	Naratriptan	1 mg twice daily for 6 days to be started 3 days before period onset
Triptan	Zolmitriptan	2.5 mg twice or 3 times daily for 7 days starting 2 days before expected period onset

The diagnosis of menstrually related migraine is typically made based on a thorough history, and is confirmed by reviewing prospective headache diaries. Patient diaries should document migraine attacks and menstrual cycles over the course of at least three consecutive cycles. A diagnosis of menstrually related migraine can be established when at least two of three consecutive menstrual cycles correlate with migraine onset within -2 to $+3$ days of menses. Unlike in pure menstrual migraine, patients with menstrually related migraine will also have headache attacks at other points in their cycle. It should be noted that patients who have high frequency migraine or those with chronic migraine may not initially recognize a relationship between their migraine attacks and menstrual cycles. The connection becomes more obvious with the use of headache diaries and/or with the start of prophylactic migraine medication which reduces the frequency of non-menstrually related headaches [5].

The phenotype of menstrually related migraine tends to differ from migraine attacks not related to menstruation. The attacks tend be longer lasting, more severe and resistant to treatment. They typically are not associated with aura symptoms but tend to have higher rates of functional disability [6].

Research examining the correlation between migraine attacks and menstruation suggests that abrupt drops in serum estrogen, such as the one which occurs during the luteal phase of the menstrual cycle, can precipitate migraine attacks. It has also been demonstrated that trigeminal nerve activity can be influenced by sudden drops in estrogen and prolonged duration of elevated levels of estrogen by activating sensory nerve fibers. In addition to estrogen, prostaglandins may also play a role in menstrual migraine. Studies have demonstrated a significant increase in prostaglandin levels just prior to and within the first 48 h of menstruation, which typically corresponds to the timing of an attack [6]. As stated before, menstrual migraine tends to occur without aura. Higher levels of estrogen are associated with increased frequency of aura and since menstrually related migraine

attacks occur during the time of lowest estrogen concentrations, aura does not tend to occur [7].

Several treatment options exist for menstrual migraine and depend on consistency of menstrual cycle, predictability of attacks, and response to standard acute therapies. For those women who carry a diagnosis of menstrually related migraine and have regular cycles, short-term prophylaxis may be indicated. Prophylactic medication options include triptans, non-steroidal anti-inflammatories (NSAIDs), and hormonal options [8–11]. Naproxen sodium 550 mg twice daily, naratriptan 1 mg twice daily, zolmitriptan 2.5 mg twice daily, as well as frovatriptan 5 mg twice on day 1 and continued at 2.5 mg twice daily starting prior to onset of menstruation and continuing into menstruation are useful strategies for spot prophylaxis (Table 3). Estrogen supplementation can be used to maintain a steady estrogen level and thus prevent the abrupt decline which occurs during the luteal phase. Women who are on a combined contraceptive, and have migraine without aura, can forgo the placebo week and continue with estrogen supplementation. Estrogen based contraceptives are associated with an increased stroke risk and patients who suffer from migraine with aura also carry an increased risk of stroke. As such, The World Health Organization designates a medical eligibility criteria category for contraceptive use category 4 for combined hormonal contraceptive use in patients who suffer from migraine with aura. This means that the condition poses an unacceptable health risk if this method is used and thus it is advised that alternative contraceptives be considered [12].

Much of the data associating migraine with aura and the use of estrogen containing contraceptives with higher stroke risk is based on high dose estrogen formulations (150 μg of mestranol). In contrast, very low dose formulation (20–25 μg ethinyl estradiol) and ultra low-dose formulation (10–15 μg ethinyl estradiol) studies have demonstrated no significant increased risk, and may even reduce aura frequency, thereby potentially decreasing stroke risk [13]. Progestin-only oral formulations are generally considered a safer alternative, but it should be noted that such formulations prevent ovulation only half the time, and therefore may not be effective in reducing headache attacks. An alternative is an implanted progestin-only contraceptive, which is safer to use in patients with migraine aura, and may prevent ovulation with greater consistency [7].

That being said, it is important to recognize that migraine aura increases a patient's risk for stroke with some studies demonstrating a nearly twofold increase and this risk is higher in those with increased frequency of migraine aura attacks [14]. Future studies may further draw into question whether current hormonal therapy contraindications are warranted.

References

1. Lipton RB, Silberstein SD. Episodic and chronic migraine headache: breaking down barriers to optimal treatment and prevention. Headache: J Head Face Pain. 2015;55:103–22. https://doi.org/10.1111/head.12505_2.
2. WHO | Headache disorders. n.d. Retrieved from http://www.who.int/mediacentre/factsheets/fs277/en/.
3. Headache Classification Committee of the International Headache Society (IHS). The international classification of headache disorders, 3rd edition (beta version). Cephalalgia. 2013;33(9):629–808. https://doi.org/10.1177/0333102413485658.
4. Brandes JL. Migraine in women. Continuum: Lifelong Learn Neurol. 2012;18:835–52. https://doi.org/10.1212/01.con.0000418646.70149.71.
5. Macgregor EA. Migraine management during menstruation and menopause. Continuum: Lifelong Learn Neurol. 2015;21:990–1003. https://doi.org/10.1212/con.0000000000000196.
6. Mathew PG, Dun EC, Luo JJ. A cyclic pain. Obstet Gynecol Surv. 2013;68(2):130–40. https://doi.org/10.1097/ogx.0b013e31827f2496.
7. Combined hormonal contraceptives and migraine: update on evidence.
8. Macgregor EA, Frith A, Ellis J, Aspinall L, Hackshaw A. Prevention of menstrual attacks of migraine: a double-blind placebo-controlled crossover study. Neurology. 2006;67(12):2159–63. https://doi.org/10.1212/01.wnl.0000249114.52802.55.
9. Brandes J, Poole A, Kallela M, Schreiber C, Macgregor E, Silberstein S. Short-term frovatriptan for the prevention of difficult-to-treat menstrual migraine attacks. Cephalalgia. 2009;29(11):1133–1148. https://doi.org/10.1111/j.1468-2982.2009.01840.x.
10. Macgregor EA. Contraception and headache. Headache: J Head Face Pain. 2013;53(2):247–76. https://doi.org/10.1111/head.12035.
11. Krel R, Mathew PG. In: O'Neal MA, editor. Women's neurology. What do I do now? Oxford: Oxford University Press; 2017. p. 15–25.
12. Medical eligibility criteria for contraceptive use. 5th ed. 2015. 126.
13. Calhoun AH. Hormonal contraceptives and migraine with aura-is there still a risk? Headache. 2017;57(2):184–93.
14. Kurth T, Diener H. Migraine and stroke: perspectives for stroke physicians. Stroke. 2012;43(12):3421–6. https://doi.org/10.1161/strokeaha.112.656603.

Connective Tissue Disorders in Women

Sophia L. Ryan, Shamik Bhattacharyya,
and Mary Angela O'Neal

Introduction

Connective tissue disorders describe diseases affecting the fascia and are now understood to encompass both genetic and autoimmune causes. Although the diseases have divergent mechanisms, the term is still commonly used and found in the name of some diseases such as "mixed connective tissue disorder." Of the genetic disorders such as Marfan syndrome or Loeys-Dietz syndrome, some of the causative genes have been identified and mechanisms well explored. Other disorders such as fibromuscular dysplasia remain important clinically without clearly known genetic mechanisms. Depending on the mode of inheritance, each one of the genetic diseases has different proportion of women affected. Connective tissue disorders with autoimmune etiologies, i.e. autoimmune diseases, are common affecting millions of people within the United States and known to injure most organs in the body ranging from skin to kidney to heart to nervous system. Among the people affected, roughly 78% are women making autoimmunity a significant concern in women's health [1]. Why autoimmunity should be more prevalent in women, however, is not obvious and the subject of ongoing investigations. One observation is that while autoimmunity is generally more prevalent in women, the degree of sex disparity is disease specific. Some diseases such as Sjögren's syndrome, systemic lupus erythematosus, and scleroderma have an overwhelming female predominance of more than 80% of patients [2]. Diseases such as multiple sclerosis and myasthenia gravis have a more modest sex disparity ranging around 60–75% of patients. In diseases like sarcoidosis and inflammatory bowel diseases, the prevalence is more balanced. Finally, in some instances like ankylosing spondylitis and pulmonary fibrosis, there is *increased* disease burden in men suggesting that disease specific mechanisms vary in their sensitivity to sex differences.

The immune response to an antigen differs between males and females. In mouse models, female mice generate more antibodies after vaccination compared to males [3]. While antibodies are generally protective against infections, women are also consequently more likely to generate higher number of autoantibodies, which correlates with the risk of developing autoimmune diseases and often precedes clinical symptoms. For example, the risk of developing Type I diabetes within 5 years increases from 10% to about 60–80% when comparing children with one and three autoantibodies [4]. This model may explain why diseases associated with autoantibodies such as systemic lupus erythematosus are especially more prevalent in women compared to diseases associated primarily with cell mediated injury such as myocarditis or ankylosing spondylitis. This model, while appealing, is simplistic with significant limitations. One is that vaccination studies in human beings have yielded more inconclusive results regarding antibody production differences in males and females. Second is that common human diseases do not segregate neatly into antibody mediated and cell mediated mechanisms and likely have significant components of both in the final pathogenesis.

These differences in immune responsiveness are modulated by sex steroids of which the roles of estrogen, proges-

S. L. Ryan
Department of Neurology, Brigham and Women's Hospital, Boston, MA, USA

Department of Neurology, Massachusetts General Hospital, Boston, MA, USA

Harvard Medical School, Boston, MA, USA
e-mail: SRYAN9@PARTNERS.ORG

S. Bhattacharyya (✉)
Department of Neurology, Brigham and Women's Hospital, Boston, MA, USA

Harvard Medical School, Boston, MA, USA
e-mail: SBHATTACHARYYA3@PARTNERS.ORG

M. A. O'Neal
Department of Neurology, Brigham and Women's Hospital, Boston, MA, USA
e-mail: maoneal@bwh.harvard.edu

© Springer Nature Switzerland AG 2019
M. A. O'Neal (ed.), *Neurology and Psychiatry of Women*, https://doi.org/10.1007/978-3-030-04245-5_2

terone, and testosterone have been most studied. The importance of sex steroids in women is best illustrated by pregnancy, a time during which there is marked increase in the systemic levels of estrogen and progesterone. The effect of pregnancy is disease specific. In systemic lupus erythematosus, pregnancy increases disease activity. On the other hand, in multiple sclerosis and rheumatoid arthritis, there is generally attenuation of disease activity during pregnancy with increased risk of disease flare during the post-partum period. The differences in disease expression are likely from selective suppression of particular populations of immune cells (such as favoring T_H2 versus T_H1 response) mediated in part by sex steroids especially estrogen. In experimental mouse models of multiple sclerosis, the protective effects of pregnancy can be recreated by estrogen supplementation. On the other hand, supplementation with progesterone (the other hormone increased during pregnancy) does not have the same effect [5].

This apparent protective role of estrogen at first glance appears paradoxical since women have higher levels of estrogen compared to men but also have a higher burden of autoimmune disease rather than having less disease than men. The likely explanation is that estrogen has variable effects based on dose with lower levels enhancing immune reactivity and higher levels suppressing it [2]. Additionally, estrogen modulates the immune system at multiple levels making its interactions complex. Estrogens are known to regulate innate immunity, immune cell counts, chemokine/cytokine production, antigen presentation, and adaptive immunity including B cells and multiple subsets of T cells. Finally, the effects of sex steroids occur within the context of multiple other sex differences, and exclusive focus on estrogen is limiting. During pregnancy, immunomodulation is also affected, for example, by pregnancy associated glycoproteins and maternal-fetal microchimerism. In fact, efforts to treat multiple sclerosis with pregnancy level estrogen supplementation in human beings have not been successful suggesting that estrogen is one part of many immunobiological differences between men and women [6].

In this chapter, we will review three illustrative connective tissue disorders which act via different mechanisms and are all more prevalent in women – systemic lupus erythematosus, Sjogren syndrome, and fibromuscular dysplasia.

Systemic Lupus Erythematosus (SLE)

SLE is a chronic inflammatory disorder of unclear etiology more common in women compared to men becoming clinically manifest in the majority between the late teens and early 40s. SLE is a heterogenous disease with variable clinical severity ranging from minor disease requir-

ing symptomatic management to refractory disease unresponsive to immunosuppression. The American College of Rheumatology formulated classification criteria in 1987 for SLE and required four of the following eleven features [7]:

1. Facial erythema over the malar eminences and/or bridge of the nose (malar rash)
2. Erythematous raised patches with keratotic scaling and follicular plugging (discoid lupus)
3. Photosensitivity defined as any skin reaction from exposure to sunlight
4. Oral or nasopharyngeal ulcers (often painless)
5. Nonerosive arthritis characterized by tenderness, swelling, or effusion of 2 or more peripheral joints
6. Serositis typically pleuritis or pericarditis
7. Renal disorder manifesting as proteinuria or cellular casts
8. Neurologic disorder broadly characterized by seizures or psychosis
9. Hematologic disorder consisting of hemolytic anemia, leukopenia, lymphopenia, or thrombocytopenia
10. Presence of antidouble-strand DNA (dsDNA), anti-Smith (Sm), or antiphospholipid antibodies
11. Presence of antinuclear antibody

These criteria were developed to create an operational definition and not to diagnose individual patients. Thus, patients may have SLE and not have four of the above eleven features, especially in early disease.

The pathogenesis of SLE is unclear and likely multifactorial with contributions from genetic susceptibility, environmental factors such as infection with Epstein Barr virus, abnormalities in apoptosis, and hormonal factors [8]. SLE is associated with multiple autoantibodies frequently against intracellular components. The antinuclear antibody (ANA) is present in about 95% of patients, but the antibody is not specific and can be found in asymptomatic individuals or those with other autoimmune diseases. There have been more than 100 other autoantibodies described in SLE though only a smaller subset is clinically tested. The anti-dsDNA antibody is less sensitive but correlates with disease activity. There are other antibodies such as anti-Sm antibody which are highly specific but insensitive.

SLE can injure both the central and peripheral nervous system through a variety of mechanisms. There have been a series of neuropathological studies published regarding the neurological involvement of SLE. Most frequently, in the central nervous system, SLE is associated with injury to the small vessels causing microinfarcts from vasculopathy or in some cases from cardioembolism from Libman-Sacks endocarditis. Most importantly, although often invoked, "lupus vasculitis" is not a frequent cause of neurologic damage and rarely substantiated by pathology [9]. Other modes of injury include inflammatory causes such as encephalitis. Although many have been proposed, there is not yet an autoantibody that is sufficiently sensitive or specific for neuropsychiatric lupus to be clinically useful. Some proposed examples include anti-ribosomal P antibody and anti-NMDA receptor NR2 subunit antibody.

Historically, there have been many terms used to describe neurological impairment in the setting of SLE including neurolupus and lupus cerebritis. The current preferred term is neuropsychiatric SLE, which is agnostic of the mechanism of the injury (i.e. not necessarily inflammatory as implied by lupus cerebritis). The estimated prevalence of neuropsychiatric involvement in SLE is about 56%, though the range varies [10]. The most frequent associated syndrome is headache followed by mood disorder, cognitive dysfunction, seizures, and cerebrovascular disease.

A cautionary point is that just because a neurological syndrome occurs in the context of SLE does not imply a causal relationship. Even though headache is the most commonly associated neurological complaint, in epidemiological studies, headache in isolation is no more frequent in patients with SLE compared to the general population and does not correlate with SLE activity [11]. Neither tension type nor migraine headache is more prevalent in patients with SLE. Headache consequently is treated symptomatically. Importantly, headache in combination with other red flag symptoms such as neck stiffness or postural headache can indicate serious complications such as aseptic meningitis or cerebral venous sinus thrombosis. Like headache, mood disorder is also frequent but the causality is less clear. Depression is commonly reported in SLE, and in controlled epidemiological studies, elevated SLE disease activity increases the odds of major depression minimally, though contradictory results have also been reported [12]. On the other hand, psychosis is more closely related to disease activity and can be the presenting symptom of SLE. In patients with SLE and psychosis, an important secondary cause to exclude is steroid induced psychosis. A clinical clue is that steroid induced psychosis contains more prevalent auditory hallucinations while SLE psychosis has more prominent visual hallucinations. There is no clear biomarker for SLE associated psychosis. The syndrome responds to immunosuppression.

Stroke is a major cause of morbidity and mortality in patients with SLE. In a 10 year prospective series of 1000 patients with SLE, stroke accounted for 12% of deaths and, as an individual cause of death, ranked second only behind infectious complications [13]. Overall, across all age groups, patients with SLE have a roughly twofold increased risk of stroke compared to the general population [14]. This increased risk is especially significant in the younger age groups in which the general population baseline risk is low.

For example, in the 30–39 age group, there is a 21-fold increased risk of stroke in patients with SLE. The pathogenesis of stroke in the context of SLE is complex and likely involves multiple mechanisms including accelerated small vessel disease in the arterioles, embolic infarcts both from infective and Libman-Sacks endocarditis, antiphospholipid syndrome, and accelerated large vessel atherosclerosis. Cerebral vasculitis is a rare and likely minor contributor to stroke in SLE. Of the various mechanisms, antiphospholipid syndrome is a major cause, and antiphospholipid antibodies are found in the majority of patients with SLE who have an ischemic stroke.

Cognitive dysfunction is a less well recognized association with SLE. In neuropsychiatric testing, mild to severe cognitive impairment is detected in as many as 60–80% of patients with SLE. Most common deficits are in visuospatial processing as well as verbal and visual memory. The pathophysiology of how cognitive dysfunction develops is unclear but likely involves effects of vascular injury to the brain, effects of treatment, and inflammatory causes. Because of the lack of understanding of the pathophysiology of cognitive dysfunction, when to test for and what to do with cognitive complaints have remained unclear. Seizures occur in many patients with SLE estimates ranging around 10% [15]. Many patients have provoking causes such as electrolyte abnormalities, renal failure, prior strokes, or developmental abnormalities. However, a substantial number of patients with SLE experience seizures with no other explanation. Fortunately, in this subgroup, longitudinal studies show that more than 80% of seizures are single episodes and do not result in epilepsy. Consequently, patients with SLE with first seizure should be evaluated and managed similarly to other patients with first seizure including imaging with MRI of the brain and EEG. Whether to perform lumbar puncture and what to test for are unclear.

Myelitis is relatively rare with estimated prevalence of less than 1% and likely of heterogeneous etiology. Some have longitudinally extensive myelitis and test positive for anti-aquaporin 4 antibodies. These patients also respond to treatment for neuromyelitis optica. However, most patients will not test positive for NMO IgG, and the pathophysiology remains unclear (Fig. 1). Examination of CSF often shows inflammatory disease. Patients are generally treated with aggressive immunotherapy including with cyclophosphamide, plasmapheresis, intravenous immunoglobulin and rituximab.

Aside from these syndromes discussed, SLE has been associated with multiple neurological syndromes including different kinds of neuropathy, movement disorders, aseptic meningitis, posterior reversible encephalopathy syndrome, hypophysitis, and increased intracranial hypertension. As a field, we are still learning and describing the effects of SLE on the nervous system.

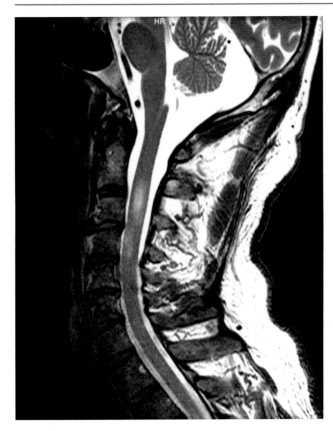

Fig. 1 MRI of the cervical spinal cord shows T2 hyperintense lesion in a patient with SLE associated myelitis

Sjogren Syndrome

Sjogren's Syndrome (SS) is a disease primarily of middle-aged, post-menopausal women affecting two to four million people in the US. The average age of diagnosis is 55 but there is a bimodal distribution with peaks at ages 30 (during childbearing years) and 55 (just after menopause) [16]. The female to male predominance is striking at somewhere between 9 and 20:1, higher than for any other connective tissue disorder, and only second to Hashimoto's Thyroiditis among autoimmune disorders [17]. Onset of SS is thought to be earlier in women than men, although this may be an artifact of delayed diagnosis in men given the lower prevalence in this population [18]. Furthermore, men appear to have a less robust autoimmune expression of the disease, further confounding early diagnosis [19]. Clinically, for primary SS, four of the following six criteria are required: (1) ocular symptoms (typically for more than 3 months); (2) oral symptoms (typically for more than 3 months); (3) evidence of ocular exocrine dysfunction (i.e. Positive Schirmer's test or Rose Bengal stain); (4) evidence of oral exocrine dysfunction (decreased whole salivary flow, abnormal parotid sialography or abnormal salivary scintigraphy); (5) histopathology (salivary gland showing lymphocytic foci); (6) serology pos-

itive for anti-Ro/SSA and/or anti-La/SSB. Other laboratory changes in SS include elevation of paraproteins, cryoglobulins, hypergammaglobulinemia and autoantibodies. Of the associated autoantibodies, both anti-SSA/Ro and anti-SSB/La are included in the most recent diagnostic criteria for SS, despite their relatively low sensitivity (40% and 50% for anti-Ro/SSA and 10–20% for anti-La/SSB). Other commonly observed autoantibodies are anti-nuclear antibodies (ANA) and rheumatoid factor (RF). Low complement (C3, C4) levels are also frequently observed in patients with SS. Notably, some of these serologic changes are thought to be directly related to SS itself, while others are more likely due to other comorbid autoimmunity.

Pathologically, SS is characterized by lymphocytic infiltration of the exocrine glands – the salivary and lacrimal glands. Thus, it frequently manifests as dry eyes and dry mouth, the so-called "sicca syndrome." In addition to the exocrine system, SS can involve many other organs including the brain, lungs, kidneys, thyroid, muscle and skin. As a result, it can give rise to a diverse set of extraglandular symptoms including depression, pain, cutaneous lesions and mild arthritis. The most common complaint, seen in 50% of patients with SS, is extreme fatigue [20]. It is more frequent in female than male patients and is a major contributor to decreased functional status in patients with SS. SS is often associated with thyroid dysfunction, present in approximately 45% of patients, and more common in women than men. It is thought that subclinical hypothyroidism may be an important contributor to the fatigue seen in SS [20].

Neurologically, SS affects both the central (CNS) and peripheral nervous system (PNS). Notably, neurologic manifestations frequently precede the onset of the more typical sicca symptoms, which can lead to a delay in diagnosis [21]. The PNS has traditionally been thought to be more commonly affected than the CNS with 10% of patients diagnosed with peripheral neuropathy. Of these, predominantly sensory manifestations are most commonly reported. If one looks for subclinical changes in nerve conduction or intraepidermal nerve fiber density, estimates of peripheral nerve involvement in SS patients increase to as high as 60% [22]. The range of neuropathies includes mixed polyneuropathy, axonal sensory neuropathy, sensory ataxic neuropathy, axon sensorimotor polyneuropathy, trigeminal or other cranial neuropathies, demyelinating polyradiculoneuropathy, autonomic neuropathy, pure sensory neuronopathy, mononeuritis multiplex and small-fiber neuropathy. Raynaud's phenomenon, which occurs in many connective tissue autoimmune diseases, including SS, is another symptom that may be a result of peripheral nerve dysfunction via dysregulation of autonomic and small nerve fibers resulting in prolonged vasoconstriction of peripheral vessels. This phenomenon may occur more frequently in women than men with SS.

The CNS is affected somewhere between 2% and 60% of the time depending on how involvement is defined (with clear structural changes at the low end and functional changes including fatigue and headache at the higher end). In the CNS, SS can present similarly to multiple sclerosis with numerous white matter lesions, as a neuromyelitis optica spectrum disorder (with 90% of these patients showing seropositivity for AQP4 antibodies) or with recurrent aseptic meningoencephalitis (fever, headache, meningismus, confusion paired with CSF pleocytosis) [17]. In addition to the more focal CNS manifestations, there is increasing evidence that SS can be accompanied by diffuse non-focal neuropsychiatric manifestations. Depression and fibromyalgia, for example are important CNS manifestations that affect women more commonly than men. Furthermore, on neuropsychiatric testing, patients often have frontal, executive and verbal memory dysfunction. It remains unclear whether this is a direct effect of the disease, a psychological reaction to it or a byproduct of treatment.

All treatment recommendations for the neurologic manifestations of SS are derived from small, retrospective case series. Possible disease modifying drugs include IV immunoglobulin (IVIg), corticosteroids, plasmapheresis, rituximab, and infliximab. IVIG and corticosteroids have been shown in a small case series to bring about a 30–40% improvement in neuropathy [23]. This was further broken down by the type of peripheral neuropathy with multiple mononeuropathies seeming to respond best to corticosteroids, and painful neuropathy responding best to IVIg. Infliximab, rituximab and plasmapheresis have also been used with anecdotal success. In addition to disease modifying drugs, the neurologic symptoms resulting from SS can be treated with a variety of medications such as gabapentin, pregabalin, tricyclic antidepressants, duloxetine, and topical lidocaine, all of which are frequently used for neuropathic pain. As with most conditions, treatment of SS in women during pregnancy is fraught with concerns about potential teratogenicity butting up against the need to control symptoms and the potential harmful effects of active disease itself. Furthermore, cost and drug availability are at the forefront of any treatment decisions, particularly given that no standard of care exists in SS due to the lack of randomized control trials.

There have been increasing pregnancies among women with SS in recent years. This is likely explained by the bimodal peaks of SS onset with one peak in the early 30s paired with trends toward women deferring pregnancy later and later. There has thus been increasing interest in the effect of SS on pregnancy and vice versa. While data is still scarce, it appears that the course of SS is likely to worsen during and after pregnancy. This is thought to be related to pulmonary hypertension as a complication of SS [24]. Additionally, obstetrical outcomes appear to be worse in women with SS, depending on the disease severity and antibody profile. Congenital heart block (CHB) as a manifestation of neonatal lupus is the best known and most severe complication observed in women with SS and is thought to be related to circulating maternal anti-Ro/SSA and anti-La/SSB antibodies. The occurrence rate of CHB is ~2% in infants born to women who are anti-Ro/SSA antibody positive and ~3% in infants born to women who are anti-La-SSB positive [25]. Outcomes in such infants with heart block are poor with higher rates of morbidity and mortality, and most surviving infants requiring early permanent pacemaker placement. Maternal treatment with fluorinated steroids during pregnancy can reduce the antibody-mediated damage to nodal tissue. In addition to the known association with CHB, women with SS have increased rates of spontaneous abortions, preterm deliveries, lower neonatal birth weights and increased frequency of cesarean deliveries. Some of these findings, however, appear to be confounded by advanced maternal age as compared to controls.

Fibromuscular Dysplasia

Fibromuscular dysplasia (FMD) is a nonatherosclerotic, noninflammatory vascular disease of small and medium-sized arteries. FMD is classified based on the arterial layer affected. Medial fibroplasia is the most common pathological manifestation (accounting for greater than 70% of patients with FMD), although any of the arterial layers can be affected (intimal, medial, adventitial) and, in fact, more than one layer is frequently involved [26]. The classic angiographic finding of FMD is the "string of beads," which seems to correlate with medial fibroplasia pathology and represents focal areas of stenosis with interspersed aneurysmal outpouchings (Fig. 2). FMD can cause stenosis, aneurysms, dissections and occlusion of involved vessels. FMD affects women about nine times as often as men [27]. Indeed, 91% of the more than 1000 patients with FMD from 14 different sites identified in a US FMD registry were female. The mean age at symptom onset was 47 years old with a mean age at diagnosis of 52 years. This is in contrast to the previously commonly held belief that FMD most often affects women in their 20s–30s. Overall, the mean delay in diagnosis is about 4 years, according to the US registry.

The prevalence of FMD in the general population is unknown. It is thought to be a rare disorder that is often asymptomatic. In data from potential kidney donors, estimates of asymptomatic renal FMD range from 3.8% to 6.6% on angiography [27]. It is important to note, however, that many of these patients had family members with chronic kidney disease and thus may not be representative of the general population. Figures from autopsy studies yield different

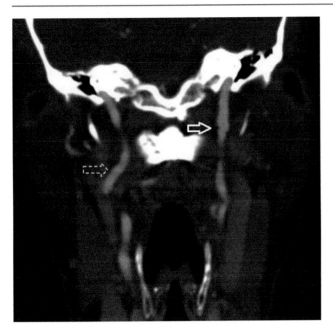

Fig. 2 Coronal view of CT angiogram of the internal carotid arteries of a 60 year old woman shows stenosis and dilation (solid arrow) and areas of luminal irregularity (dashed arrow)

numbers with one study of 819 consecutive autopsies suggesting a prevalence of only 1%. Symptomatic FMD is thought to be even less common, with some estimates placing it at 0.4% in the renal arteries [28]. It is not known whether the disease is more common in any racial, ethic or geographic distributions.

The etiology of FMD is unknown with outstanding questions regarding genetic, hormonal and environmental contributions. There is thought to be some genetic contribution to the development of FMD. More than one study has suggested an autosomal dominant pattern of inheritance with variable penetrance [29]. Concordance among first-degree relatives has ranged from 11% to 60% in different studies [30]. No gene has yet been identified. The strong female predominance has suggested a possible hormonal contribution, whether endogenous or exogenous. However, there is thus far no evidence to suggest that pregnancy, oral contraceptive use or hormone replacement therapy is associated with risk of FMD. An association with smoking has also been postulated but remains unproven.

Any vascular bed can be affected in FMD and the location of dysplasia determines the clinical presentation. FMD was previously thought to preferentially affect the renal arteries, followed by the extracranial internal carotid or vertebral vessels. Interestingly, however, the US FMD Registry, which was started in 2008, found approximately the same prevalence of FMD in the renal and extracranial cerebrovascular vessels. Additionally, the two vascular beds were frequently involved concurrently. Among patients with extracranial carotid or vertebral artery disease, renal FMD was present

64.5% of the time. The converse was true 64.8% of the time. Intracranial FMD, on the other hand, is thought to be much less common and was found in only 8% of patients in the US registry. Cerebrovascular vessels are usually affected bilaterally. Men are more likely to have renal FMD while women are more likely to have carotid FMD, according to the US FMD registry. Notably, FMD appears to be more aggressive in men with higher rates of dissection and aneurysms in men compared to women.

Renal FMD tends to present with medically refractory hypertension. Cerebrovascular FMD can present with Horner's syndrome, cranial neuropathies, pulsatile tinnitus, TIA/stroke or subarachnoid hemorrhage. However, patients may also present with nonspecific symptoms such as dizziness, headache, syncope or altered mental status. Symptoms are typically caused by thrombosis, embolization, aneurysmal rupture or severe stenosis leading to hypoperfusion. Among patients with spontaneous cervical artery dissections, a common cause of stroke in young adults, 15–20% are associated with FMD of the cervical artery [27].

Catheter-based angiography is the gold standard for diagnosis of FMD. However, several other less invasive methods of diagnosis are frequently utilized. In terms of extracranial imaging, 73% of patients in the US FMD Registry underwent ultrasound, 30% underwent magnetic resonance angiogram (MRA) and 28% had computed tomographic angiography (CTA). Only 28% underwent catheter-based angiography. Each modality has different strengths and weaknesses, which should be considered when deciding which to use for screening or diagnosis. For example, according to a study done at Cleveland Clinic, ultrasound, which detects not beading but increased peak systolic velocities, has a high positive predictive value (87.7% and 94.2% in the carotid and renal arteries, respectively). However, the negative predictive value is only 62%. Importantly, catheter-based angiography allows physicians to determine the hemodynamic significance of a lesion and is the only technique that has the option of simultaneous treatment.

Treatment of FMD depends on the vascular bed affected, as well as the associated complications (stenosis, dissection or aneurysm). There are no specific guidelines for patients with FMD as there is not enough data to drive such recommendations. In general, empiric antiplatelets are the treatment of choice for asymptomatic FMD, although there have been no adequately powered, randomized studies to evaluate effectiveness. Rather, this practice is based on physiologic understanding that this class of medications is likely to reduce adherence of platelets to intravascular webs that form in FMD. In patients with symptomatic cerebrovascular FMD, percutaneous angioplasty is generally first line with aneurysms often requiring coiling or stenting, stenosis requiring balloon angioplasty and dissection requiring stenting. Surgery is an alternative to this, especially for treatment of aneurysms. In the US registry, interventional procedures were used most commonly in renal FMD, however. They were used in only 16.5% of patients with disease in the extracranial carotids and even less commonly intracranially (in only 3.3% of patients). Symptomatic improvement was noted 50% of the time with a 7.6% complication rate, although this was not broken down by location of intervention [26]. Patients with FMD are recommended to get regular surveillance of looking for carotid artery involvement. Ultrasound is the recommended modality on a 6–12 month basis. Surveillance intervals looking for intracranial aneurysms is less clear.

Conclusion

Many connective tissue disorders are more common in women and include both genetic and autoimmune causes. The clinical expression of disease, the degree of sex disparity, and changes with pregnancy are specific for individual diseases.

References

1. Fairweather D, Rose NR. Women and autoimmune diseases. Emerg Infect Dis. 2004;10(11):2005–11.
2. Whitacre CC. Sex differences in autoimmune disease. Nat Immunol. 2001;2(9):777–80.
3. Eidinger D, Garrett TJ. Studies of the regulatory effects of the sex hormones on antibody formation and stem cell differentiation. J Exp Med. 1972;136(5):1098–116.
4. Fairweather D, Frisancho-Kiss S, Rose NR. Sex differences in autoimmune disease from a pathological perspective. Am J Pathol. 2008;173(3):600–9.
5. Kim S, Liva SM, Dalal MA, Verity MA, Voskuhl RR. Estriol ameliorates autoimmune demyelinating disease: implications for multiple sclerosis. Neurology. 1999;52(6):1230–8.
6. Langer-Gould A. Sex hormones and multiple sclerosis: another informative failure. Lancet Neurol. 2016;15(1):22–3.
7. Hochberg MC. Updating the American College of Rheumatology revised criteria for the classification of systemic lupus erythematosus. Arthritis Rheum. 1997;40(9):1725.
8. D'Cruz DP, Khamashta MA, Hughes GRV. Systemic lupus erythematosus. Lancet. 2007;369(9561):587–96.
9. Johnson RT, Richardson EP. The neurological manifestations of systemic lupus erythematosus. Medicine (Baltimore). 1968;47(4):337–69.
10. Unterman A, Nolte JES, Boaz M, Abady M, Shoenfeld Y, Zandman-Goddard G. Neuropsychiatric syndromes in systemic lupus erythematosus: a meta-analysis. Semin Arthritis Rheum. 2011;41(1):1–11.
11. Mitsikostas DD, Sfikakis PP, Goadsby PJ. A meta-analysis for headache in systemic lupus erythematosus: the evidence and the myth. Brain J Neurol. 2004;127(Pt 5):1200–9.
12. Palagini L, Mosca M, Tani C, Gemignani A, Mauri M, Bombardieri S. Depression and systemic lupus erythematosus: a systematic review. Lupus. 2013;22(5):409–16.
13. al CR et. Morbidity and mortality in systemic lupus erythematosus during a 10-year period: a comparison of early and late manifestations in a cohort of 1,000... – PubMed – NCBI [Internet]. [cited 2018 Feb 19]. Available from: https://www.ncbi.nlm.nih.gov/pubmed/14530779.
14. Schoenfeld SR, Kasturi S, Costenbader KH. The epidemiology of atherosclerotic cardiovascular disease among patients with SLE: a systematic review. Semin Arthritis Rheum. 2013;43(1):77–95.
15. Appenzeller S, Cendes F, Costallat LTL. Epileptic seizures in systemic lupus erythematosus. Neurology. 2004;63(10):1808–12.
16. Brandt JE, Priori R, Valesini G, Fairweather D. Sex differences in Sjögren's syndrome: a comprehensive review of immune mechanisms. Biol Sex Differ. 2015;6:19.
17. Bhattacharyya S, Helfgott SM. Neurologic complications of systemic lupus erythematosus, sjögren syndrome, and rheumatoid arthritis. Semin Neurol. 2014;34(4):425–36.
18. Horvath IF, Szodoray P, Zeher M. Primary Sjögren's syndrome in men: clinical and immunological characteristic based on a large cohort of Hungarian patients. Clin Rheumatol. 2008;27(12):1479–83.
19. Ramos-Casals M, Solans R, Rosas J, Camps MT, Gil A, Del Pino-Montes J, et al. Primary Sjögren syndrome in Spain: clinical and immunologic expression in 1010 patients. Medicine (Baltimore). 2008;87(4):210–9.
20. Kassan SS, Moutsopoulos HM. Clinical manifestations and early diagnosis of sjögren syndrome. Arch Intern Med. 2004;164(12):1275–84.
21. Delalande S, de Seze J, Fauchais A-L, Hachulla E, Stojkovic T, Ferriby D, et al. Neurologic manifestations in primary Sjögren syndrome: a study of 82 patients. Medicine (Baltimore). 2004;83(5):280–91.
22. Chai J, Logigian EL. Neurological manifestations of primary Sjögren's syndrome. Curr Opin Neurol. 2010;23(5):509–13.
23. Mori K, Iijima M, Koike H, Hattori N, Tanaka F, Watanabe H, et al. The wide spectrum of clinical manifestations in Sjögren's syndrome-associated neuropathy. Brain J Neurol. 2005;128(Pt 11):2518–34.
24. Gupta S, Gupta N. Sjögren syndrome and pregnancy: a literature review. Perm J. 2017;21:16–47.
25. De Carolis S, Salvi S, Botta A, Garofalo S, Garufi C, Ferrazzani S, et al. The impact of primary Sjogren's syndrome on pregnancy outcome: our series and review of the literature. Autoimmun Rev. 2014;13(2):103–7.
26. Sharma AM, Kline B. The United States registry for fibromuscular dysplasia: new findings and breaking myths. Tech Vasc Interv Radiol. 2014;17(4):258–63.
27. Olin JW, Gornik HL, Bacharach JM, Biller J, Fine LJ, Gray BH, et al. Fibromuscular dysplasia: state of the science and critical unanswered questions: a scientific statement from the American Heart Association. Circulation. 2014;129(9):1048–78.
28. Plouin P-F, Perdu J, La Batide-Alanore A, Boutouyrie P, Gimenez-Roqueplo A-P, Jeunemaitre X. Fibromuscular dysplasia. Orphanet J Rare Dis. 2007;2:28.
29. Olin JW, Sealove BA. Diagnosis, management, and future developments of fibromuscular dysplasia. J Vasc Surg. 2011;53(3):826–836.e1.
30. Rushton AR. The genetics of fibromuscular dysplasia. Arch Intern Med. 1980;140:233–6.

Functional Neurological Disorder and Dissociative Disorders in Women

Geoffrey Raynor and Gaston Baslet

Functional Neurological Disorder

Functional neurological disorder (abbreviated FND and also called conversion disorder or functional neurological symptom disorder) is included in the chapter of somatic symptom and related disorders in the fifth edition of the Diagnostic and Statistical Manual of Mental Disorders (DSM 5) [1]. FND is characterized by the presence of one or more symptoms of altered voluntary motor or sensory function which are not compatible with any recognized neurological condition [1]. Different subtypes of FND include, but are not limited to, functional weakness, functional abnormal movements, psychogenic nonepileptic seizures (PNES), functional gait, and functional sensory loss. The term "hysteria" was previously used to describe FND and it translates from Greek to mean "wandering uterus", reflecting what was once felt to be the cause of the symptoms. Later in the seventeenth century, hysteria was acknowledged as a disorder of the brain that men could also readily suffer from [2]. Disability and symptomatic outcomes in FND are poor based on long-term studies [3, 4]. Therefore, FND should be promptly recognized and treated to minimize such a negative impact.

Epidemiology

Although large epidemiological data are lacking in FND, a variety of studies places the estimated incidence between 4 and 12 per 100,000 population per year and the estimated prevalence in 50 per 100,000 population [5]. According to a study conducted in Scotland, in an outpatient neurological setting, 16% of 3781 new consults were diagnosed with a primary FND, making it the second most common condition seen by a neurologist (the first being headache) [6].

It is well-established that women outnumber men in FND in a ratio of 2–3:1. When comparing different subtypes of FND, PNES usually presents with a higher female-to-male ratio (3:1) than functional movement disorder (1.5–3:1) [7]. There is evidence that women present to ambulatory practices roughly 1.5 times more frequently than men for care [8] and report more somatic symptoms than men [9]. Clinicians may underreport a diagnosis of FND in general, and especially in men, due to a variety of reasons, including the fact that they may not feel certain about the diagnosis [10].

Although FND has been described in both sexes and occurring at any age, onset most commonly occurs between 35 and 50 years of age [5], with PNES presenting earlier (mid 20's) than other subtypes of FND [7]. PNES are uncommon under 6 years of age, and female preponderance is not present before puberty [11]. In late onset PNES (older than 55 years), men were found to be affected more often than women [12], with health-related trauma as a very common etiologic factor compared to sexual trauma in young women.

Clinical Phenomenology and Evaluation

According to DSM 5 criteria, to establish the diagnosis of FND the clinician must provide evidence of preserved physiological function despite the presence of a neurological symptom (for instance, in the case of functional limb weakness, the clinician needs to demonstrate through a neurological exam, that the affected limb has preserved strength when tested with specific maneuvers). The diagnosis is therefore based on positive findings demonstrating inconsistency with the presenting symptom. Table 1 lists positive signs in different functional neurological symptoms [13].

Criteria for diagnostic certainty has been proposed for psychogenic movement disorders, however, their reliance on

G. Raynor (✉)
Department of Psychiatry, Brigham and Women's Hospital, Boston, MA, USA
e-mail: graynor@bwh.harvard.edu

G. Baslet
Department of Psychiatry, Brigham and Women's Hospital, Boston, MA, USA

Harvard Medical School, Boston, MA, USA
e-mail: gbaslet@bwh.harvard.edu

© Springer Nature Switzerland AG 2019
M. A. O'Neal (ed.), *Neurology and Psychiatry of Women*, https://doi.org/10.1007/978-3-030-04245-5_3

Table 1 Examples of positive signs in FND (functional neurological disorder)

Sign	Positive finding
Motor symptoms	
Hoover's sign	Hip extension weakness that returns to normal with contralateral hip flexion against resistance
Hip abductor sign	Hip abduction weakness returns to normal with contralateral hip abduction against resistance
Inconsistency	E.g., weakness of ankle plantar flexion on the bed but patient able to walk on tiptoes
Global pattern of weakness	Global weakness affecting extensors and flexors equally
Movement disorder	
Tremor entrainment test	Patient with a unilateral tremor is asked to copy a rhythmical movement with their unaffected limb. The tremor in the affected hand either 'entrains' to the rhythm of the unaffected hand, stops completely or the patient is unable to copy the simple rhythmical movement
Fixed dystonic posture	A typical fixed dystonic posture, characteristically of the hand (with flexion of fingers, wrist and/or elbow) or ankle (with plantar and dorsiflexion)
Hemifacial over-contraction	Orbicularis oculis over-contraction especially when accompanied by jaw deviation and/or ipsilateral functional hemiparesis
Psychogenic seizures	
Prolonged episode of motionless unresponsiveness	Paroxysmal motionlessness and unresponsiveness lasting longer than a minute
Long duration	Episodes lasting longer than 2 min without any clear-cut features of focal or generalized epileptic seizures
Eye closure	Closed eyes during an attack, especially if there is resistance to eye opening
Ictal weeping	Crying either during or immediately after the episode
Memory recall	Ability to recall the experience of being in a generalized shaking episode
Visual symptoms	
Fogging test	Vision in the unaffected eye is progressively "fogged" using lenses of increasing dioptres while reading an acuity chart. A patient who still has good acuity at the end of the test must be seeing out of their affected eye
Tubular visual field	A patient is found to have a field defect, which has the same width at 1 m as it does at 2 m

some factors unrelated to the phenomenology of the movement (such as psychological factors) limit their inter-rater reliability [14]. There are proposed levels of diagnostic certainty for PNES supported by the International League Against Epilepsy, that take into account history, phenomenology, and electrophysiological findings (Table 2) [15]. When episodes are frequent and resources are readily available, the "gold standard" for establishing the diagnosis of PNES is to record typical events on video and synchronize with EEG demonstrating no epileptic correlate and that the event is atypical for any type of epileptic seizure. Prolactin levels drawn within 20 min of an episode have been used to help assess whether an event is epileptic or not, however, this test has a low negative predictive value and a high false positive rate [16, 17].

In a retrospective review of 100 outpatients with FND, the percentage of women presenting with each subtype of FND was: 82% in PNES, 79% in psychogenic movement disorder and 68% in functional weakness [18]. Another study comparing psychogenic movement disorder and PNES showed a significant difference in female distribution (86% in PNES, 67% in psychogenic movement disorder) [19]. This significant finding was not replicated in another study comparing the two FND subtypes [20]. Tremor and dystonia are the most common psychogenic movement disorders, irrespective of sex [14].

Table 2 Diagnostic levels of certainty for psychogenic nonepileptic seizures (PNES)

Diagnostic level	History	Witnessed event	EEG
Possible	+	By witness or self-report/description	No epileptiform activity in routine or sleep-deprived interictal EEG
Probable	+	By clinician who reviewed video recording or in person, showing semiology typical of PNES	No epileptiform activity in routine or sleep-deprived interictal EEG
Clinically established	+	By clinician experienced in diagnosis of seizure disorders (on video or in person), showing semiology typical of PNES, while not on EEG	No epileptiform activity in routine or ambulatory ictal EEG during a typical ictus/event in which the semiology would make ictal epileptiform EEG activity expectable during equivalent epileptic seizures
Documented	+	By clinician experienced in diagnosis of seizure disorders, showing semiology typical of PNES, while on video EEG	No epileptiform activity immediately before, during or after ictus captured on ictal video EEG with typical PNES semiology

In the case of PNES, semiological differences between sexes have been identified. One study showed that women were more likely to have non-motor events, while men were more likely to have convulsive events [21, 22]. Tremor is the commonest PNES manifestation in children, with girls having "atonic" falls and longer episodes, and boys having "tonic-clonic" like episodes [23]. Other studies have not shown significant differences in event semiology between men and women [24].

A detailed neuropsychiatric assessment is necessary to uncover predisposing, precipitating and perpetuating factors that need to be addressed in treatment. Some patients may initially resist an exploration of psychosocial factors, in which case, a delay in the assessment of such factors may be warranted [13]. Psychiatric comorbidities, including depression, anxiety, post-traumatic stress disorder (PTSD) and dissociative disorders are common. One study showed that anxiety was more common in women than men with FND [18]. Prior traumatic experiences occur in 14–100% of patients with FND, with many studies showing that these rates are significantly higher than in the general population [25]. Physical and sexual abuse are the most commonly reported type of trauma [25] and women consistently have higher rates of trauma than men [18, 26, 27]. PNES may be associated with a higher rate of sexual abuse compared to other subtypes of FND [20].

Other physical complaints (such as cognitive, pain and other medically unexplained symptoms) are usually over-represented in FND. The co-existence of prior well-established diagnoses of epilepsy, traumatic brain injury and other neurological or medical disorders should not bias the clinician towards an organic diagnosis, but rather provide a background for an objective evaluation based on the phenomenology of symptoms [28]. Personality traits and environmental factors (such as emotion processing and interpersonal styles, family dynamics, illness and health perception) should be noted, as they are usually relevant targets for treatment [29]. Figure 1 summarizes the many predisposing, precipitating and perpetuating factors that provide a biopsychosocial framework to help explain the development of a FND [29].

Psychological Theories and Pathophysiology

FND has classically been explained by different psychological theories. The classical Freudian theory postulates that intolerable affect is "converted" into neurological symptoms. Theories that focus on dissociative processes, originally postulated by Pierre Janet, conceptualize FND as a disorder arising from mechanisms such as compartmentalization and detachment that are originally adaptive, usually in the face of traumatic experiences, but become dysfunctional over time. Dissociative theories characterize FND as an "autosuggestive disorder", with symptoms being like those seen in hypnotic states. Finally, more modern cognitive models explain

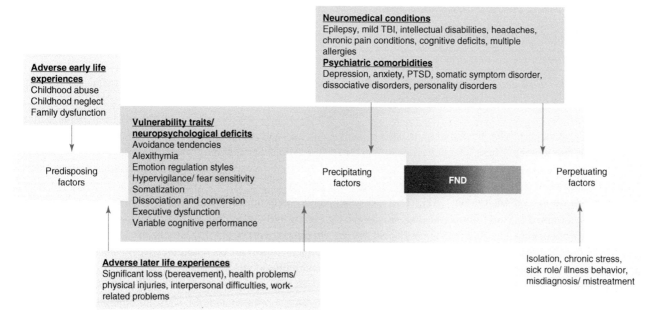

Fig. 1 Multiple factors are associated to functional neurological disorder (FND) including vulnerability traits/ neuropsychological deficits, adverse life experiences and psychiatric comorbidities and neuromedical conditions. These factors interact at different time points as predisposing, precipitating or perpetuating. (Reprinted from Baslet et al. [29] with permission from Elsevier. Copyright 2016. Elsevier.) FND Functional neurological disorder, TBI traumatic brain injury, PTSD post-traumatic stress disorder

FND as resulting from an alteration in the allocation of attentional resources on certain sensory states, leading to activation of dysfunctional hypotheses about sensory and motor function. Such dysfunctional hypotheses arise from prior experiences, cognitive interpretations, learning models, hardwired tendencies [30, 31].

Electromyography studies show normal function of the primary pathways (motor efferent and sensory afferent pathways), but alterations at the level of premotor and sensory association cortex processing. For instance, smaller motor evoked potentials were detected in functional motor disorder compared to healthy controls during motor imagery tasks [32].

Alterations in the autonomic nervous system in PNES include lower heart rate variability, which signals lower parasympathetic activity, compared to healthy controls [33], and variable sympathetic activity compared to epilepsy controls [34].

Changes in brain anatomy and function provide further insight about the neurobiological underpinnings of FND. Volumetric magnetic resonance imaging (MRI) studies show evidence of differences in the anatomy of both cortical and subcortical brain regions in patients with FND compared to healthy controls. Decreased volumes in subcortical nuclei (thalamic, lentiform, and caudate) have been demonstrated in functional motor disorder [35, 36]. At the cortical level, patients with functional motor disorders have shown bilateral increased thickness of the premotor cortex [37] whereas those with PNES showed cortical atrophy of the motor and premotor regions in the right hemisphere and bilateral cerebellar atrophy [38]. Functional MRI studies (fMRI) have demonstrated hypoactivation in motor pathway areas in functional motor disorders, and hypoactivation in visual cortical areas in functional visual disorders [39]. Additional studies point to dysfunction in sensorimotor integration along with hypoactivation of the right temporoparietal region possibly responsible for an altered sense of agency [39, 40].

Alterations in connectivity in response to stress differ between men and women. These changes are postulated to result from the interaction of sex chromosome genes with dynamic hormonal changes during vulnerable periods of brain reorganization and maturation [41]. The role that genetically-determined sex and hormonal fluctuations play in FND-specific connectivity alterations is not known at this point. Nonetheless, this link could hypothetically explain some of the female preponderance in FND from a neurobiological perspective.

Treatment

Communicating the diagnosis can by itself be therapeutic for a subset of FND patients, with improvement in symptom severity [42] and medical utilization [43, 44]. The most commonly emphasized communication strategies include: (1) reassure patients that the symptoms are genuine and not considered fake; (2) provide a name for the disorder; (3) highlight predisposing, precipitating and perpetuating factors, and a mechanism for the disease; (4) state that there are treatments that work [42]. Acceptance of the diagnosis and subsequent engagement in treatment are important goals of the diagnosis communication strategy. One study demonstrated that caregivers', but not patients' acceptance of the PNES diagnosis was higher for female patients [26].

Physical therapy (PT) is helpful to treat motor and gait manifestations of FND [45, 46]. A randomized cross over controlled study of 3-week inpatient PT, showed sustained benefit a year after the program was completed [47]. Other studies also demonstrate durable benefit from relatively short interventions [46]. PT demonstrates to patients their capacity for normal movement, educates them about their condition, and helps limit maladaptive motor responses. Both the intensity and educational component of the PT program appear to be important factors for success.

The evidence for antidepressant treatment in FND comes from few uncontrolled studies [48, 49]. No randomized placebo-controlled trials have demonstrated efficacy of any particular antidepressant in patients with sole FND. However, a few studies have demonstrated efficacy of newer-generation antidepressants against placebo in patients with a variety of somatic symptoms [50]. Choosing which antidepressant or anxiolytic medication is most appropriate, if any, should be based on treatment of the identified psychiatric comorbidities. Clinical judgment should be used as to when it is appropriate to initiate medications to treat psychiatric comorbidities.

Cognitive behavioral therapy (CBT) is effective in FND. CBT includes education about FND and the stress response cycle, trains patients on stress management techniques and new behavioral responses, and helps patients identify and change unhelpful thought patterns that reinforce symptoms. Randomized pilot studies have shown efficacy of CBT in the treatment of PNES [51, 52]. The use of a self-guided CBT booklet showed reduction in functional neurologic symptom burden at 3 and 6 months, and the benefit was significantly different from standard medical care [53]. CBT treatment workbooks that have been validated in randomized clinical trials can be recommended to patients and mental health providers [54, 55].

Hypnosis has proven effective in a randomized trial against a waitlist control [56]. A time-controlled trial of immediate versus delayed short-term psychodynamic psychotherapy showed similar improvement in psychogenic movements in both arms, over time and irrespective of intervention [57]. Other uncontrolled interventions with promising results include other types of psychotherapy such as long-term interpersonal psychodynamic psychotherapy [58], group psychotherapy [59], prolonged exposure (for those with comorbid PTSD) [60], mindfulness-based psychotherapy [61], inpatient programs [62], psychoeducational interventions [63] and transcranial magnetic stimulation over the motor cortex [64].

There is no evidence to suggest that the effectiveness of any treatment modality is affected by sex.

Dissociative Disorders

Dissociation is defined as a "disruption of and/or discontinuity of the normal integration of consciousness, memory, identity, emotion, perception, body representation, motor control, and behavior", according to the DSM 5. The manual lists specific dissociative disorders: dissociative identity disorder (DID); dissociative amnesia (DA); depersonalization/derealization disorder; other specified dissociative disorder (dissociative disorders that do not meet full criteria for DID, DA, or depersonalization/derealization disorder, such as identity disturbance due to the prolonged and coercive persuasion of sects, cults, terror organizations, torture, etc.); and unspecified dissociative disorder (previously referred to as dissociative disorder not otherwise specified, or, DDNOS). PTSD is also distinguished as having a dissociative subtype, characterized by meeting full criteria for PTSD as well as symptoms of derealization or depersonalization [1]. Psychiatric and neurological disorders, such as panic disorder, borderline personality disorder (BPD) [65], or epileptic seizures, may present with dissociative phenomenology, and physicians caring for patients with such complaints should consider a broad differential diagnosis (see Table 3). Due to the broad array of diagnoses that may present with dissociative phenomenology and the significant comorbidity of dissociative disorders with established psychiatric illnesses, debate exists as to whether dissociative disorders should be conceptualized as independent disorders [66]. The ubiquity across multiple pathologies, however, has also been cited as an argument to define it as its own separate disorder [67]. Regardless of the specific classification, patients with pathological dissociative symptoms bear significant impairment in functioning and personal suffering [68].

Epidemiology

Although characteristically DID has been associated with female sex [69], a study of 82 inner-city, psychiatric outpatients showed no significant difference on any demographic measures, including sex, of the 29% of patients who received a diagnosis of a dissociative disorder [70]. A study of a small community in the US over 12 months revealed prevalence of

DID in 1.6% of men and 1.4% of women. Dissociative amnesia was present in 1.0% of men and 2.6% of women [71]. Depersonalization syndrome had a prevalence of 0.95% based on longitudinal data amongst a UK population based birth cohort, with a higher prevalence of women (64%) [72], though other studies showed a depersonalization and derealization disorder sex ratio of 1:1 [73].

A survey of patients with PTSD across 16 countries found 14.4% of subjects to meet criteria for dissociative subtype, and was found to be significantly higher in male demographic [74]. PTSD was the most common psychiatric comorbidity in a study of female patients with DID (97.7%) and DDNOS (90.5%). Panic disorder, somatization, FND, agoraphobia, and social phobia were also among the most common comorbidities in DID and DDNOS after PTSD [75].

Clinical Phenomenology

Dissociative experiences range broadly in severity on a continuum across general absent-mindedness, excessive daydreaming, memory impairment, and loss of sense of one's own identity [76]. Dissociation may occur in the general population and in sleep-deprived individuals [66]. DSM-5 generally characterizes symptoms into positive and negative categories. Positive symptoms are described as disruptive, unbidden intrusions into one's subjective experience, for example, experiences of detachment from one's body, mind, or self. Negative symptoms, comparatively, are associated with an inability to access information or other mental functions that are normally accessible, such as an amnestic state [1]. Several measures of dissociation have been developed, including the Multiscale Dissociation Inventory and the Multidimensional Inventory of Dissociation, though the most commonly used psychometric assessment for dissociative experiences is the self-rating Dissociative Experiences Scale (DES) [68, 77]. Whereas these questionnaires may provide screening for dissociative symptoms, they are not diagnostic, prompting further investigation and clinical assessment in subjects with high scores. In a meta-analysis of dissociation scores measured by the DES compiling more than 15,000 subjects with psychiatric disorders, dissociative identity disordered patients had the highest overall mean scores, followed by PTSD, BPD, and then depersonalization/derealization disorder. Somatic symptom disorder, substance-related and addictive disorders, eating disorders, schizophrenia, anxiety disorders, obsessive compulsive disorder, and most affective disorders also yielded scores on the DES above previously reported population norms, thus highlighting the ubiquitous and nonspecific nature of dissociative symptomatology [77].

Table 3 Differential diagnostic considerations in dissociative disorders

Disorder	Diagnostic differentiation
Bipolar disorder	Changes in mood within bipolar disorders are slower than in DID (dissociative identity disorder), which may present mood shifts within minutes
	In DID mood changes are often displayed in conjunction with overt identity change
PTSD (post-traumatic stress disorder)	Often comorbid with dissociative disorders
	PTSD may have dissociative symptoms related to the traumatic event (e.g., dissociative flashbacks, amnesia for the event)
	In dissociative disorders, however, dissociation extends beyond the traumatic event to include amnesia for everyday occurrences, disruptive occurrences of nontraumatic intrusions, or complete change in identity
Psychotic disorders	Personified, internally communicated inner voices of DID as well as hallucinatory experiences in reference to partial flashbacks may be incorrectly assumed to be secondary to a psychotic disorder
	Distinct identity change would suggest DID
	Dissociative disorders should not harbor negative symptoms seen in chronic psychoses
	Mutism in catatonia may be confused with a dissociative amnesia, though other catatonic symptoms (e.g. posturing, negativism, rigidity) would be present in catatonia
Substance induced disorders	Repeated substance misuse leading to blackouts may be confused for a dissociative amnesia
	Careful substance screening and temporal correlation to symptoms may help differentiate the two
Personality disorder	Although DID may present with identities that have characteristics of severe personality disorders, the dysfunction is not as persistently pervasive due to inconsistency amongst identities
Functional neurological disorder	Conversion disorders lack disruption in identity seen in DID
	There may be limited amnestic quality to a FND, such as during a psychogenic nonepileptic seizure, though these are more circumscribed than a dissociative amnesia
Seizures	Experiences of déjà vu, jamais vu, depersonalization, derealization, loss of consciousness, and out of body experiences may be indicative of focal seizures with impaired awareness (formerly complex partial seizures)
	Long-term monitoring on electroencephalogram (EEG) will be normal in individuals during a dissociative experience
	Patients with dissociative disorders have high scores on dissociation scores in comparison to patients with epileptic seizures
Malingering	Clear secondary gain (although this is difficult to ascertain)
	Malingering individuals will often present with encapsulated symptoms of a dissociative amnesia or identity without the comorbid mood disorders that often accompany dissociative disorders, and otherwise present psychiatrically undisturbed
	Psychologic metrics and validity assessments may be helpful to assess effort, although these measures are unable to infer motivation
Neurocognitive disorders	Intellectual and cognitive domains other than memory are preserved in dissociative amnesia, whereas neurocognitive disorders due to neurodegenerative illness will impact additional cognitive domains, especially as the illness progresses
	During early stages of neurodegenerative illnesses with amnestic presentations, amnesia is anterograde, with relative preservation of retrograde autobiographical information
TBI (traumatic brain injury)	Neurocognitive impairment due to TBI is temporally correlated to the injury and symptoms present immediately after the injury
	Additional affected cognitive and behavioral domains may include slowed processing speed, impairment in executive functioning, impulsivity
Panic disorder	Derealization/depersonalization may accompany symptoms of panic attacks
Transient global amnesia (TGA)	TGA presents with sudden onset anterograde amnesia, often presenting as the patient repeating questions related to their current situation, and generally resolves within a few hours
	TGA includes no clouding of consciousness or loss of personal identity
	TGA is rarely recurrent

Depersonalization/Derealization

Depersonalization and derealization refer to a feeling of disconnection between either oneself or their environment, respectively. Depersonalization is described as "experiences of unreality, detachment, or being an outside observer with respect to one's thoughts, feelings, sensations, body, or actions (e.g., perceptual alterations, distorted sense of time, unreal or absent self, emotional and/or physical numbing)"

[1]. Derealization is described as "experiences of unreality or detachment with respect to surroundings (e.g. individuals or objects are experienced as unreal, dream-like, foggy, lifeless, or visually distorted)." Diagnosis of depersonalization/derealization disorder requires symptomatic episodes to be recurrent and with preserved reality testing [1]. Symptoms of derealization and depersonalization may occur in anxiety disorders (including panic attacks), psychosis, chronic mood

disorders, substance use, epileptic seizures, migraines, and cerebral tumors or vascular disease [66]. A paper reviewing manifestations of depersonalization and derealization amongst organic illness suggested epilepsy and migraines as the medical illnesses most commonly associated with depersonalization, though also included traumatic brain injury (TBI), vertigo, cerebral tumors, and cerebrovascular disease. Brain pathology via imaging and electroencephalography, indicated a predominance of non-lateralizing pathology affecting the temporal lobe [78].

Dissociative Amnesia

DSM-5 defines dissociative amnesia as "an inability to recall important autobiographical information, usually of a traumatic or stressful nature, that is inconsistent with ordinary forgetting" [1]. At times, this amnesia may be accompanied by a dissociative fugue, in which the individual will wander or travel in the absence of important autobiographical information. The amnesia may be localized, with inability to recall a specific timeframe, or more rarely, a generalized amnesia with complete loss of autobiographical memory. The amnesia is generally abrupt in its development and resolution [79].

Dissociative Identity Disorder (DID)

DID is defined by DSM-5 as a disruption in one's identity and sense of self, characterized by two or more distinct personality states, disrupting one's identity as well as sense of agency. In some cultures, this experience may be linked to the concept of possession. The episode is accompanied by alterations in behavior, emotion, memory, perception, cognition, and motor functioning [1]. Signs of a transition to an altered state include a trance-like state, change in posture, eye rolling, frequently in the setting of severe stressors, depression, anger, or sexual stimulation [80]. This may lead to recurrent missing information related to day to day events, personal information, and/or traumatic events, inconsistent with ordinary forgetting [1]. Arguments criticizing the diagnosis of DID point out methodologically weak studies of its dynamic construct, vague and overinclusive diagnostic criteria, and other established illnesses that better explain such phenomenology [66] (refer to Table 3).

In all dissociative disorders, the symptoms must cause significant distress and impairment and are not to be associated with normal cultural practices nor attributable to effects of a substance or other medical condition [1].

Psychological Theories and Pathophysiology

Dissociative symptoms are frequently associated with overwhelming or traumatic experiences, especially those experienced earlier in development [67, 81–83]. Dissociation has been characterized as an extreme defense to prevent overwhelming flooding of the consciousness during times of trauma. Once learned, however, it can be generalized in response to other stressors, and while it once may have served an adaptive function, dissociation in nontraumatic situations becomes disordered [80]. Compared to other psychiatric patients, patients diagnosed with dissociative disorders were significantly more likely to report childhood physical abuse (71% vs 27%) and childhood sexual abuse (74% vs 29%) [70]. The link between trauma and dissociation has also been disputed, favoring a socio-cognitive model citing fantasy proneness, suggestibility, and cognitive failures as fostering dissociation [84].

Dissociation has been linked to increased prefrontal activity, amygdalar hypoactivity, and altered somatosensory and visual processing. Compared to controls, patients with DID have been shown to have decreased volume within amygdala, hippocampus, and parahippocampal regions on structural imaging. DID patients with comorbid PTSD also had decreased insular volumes. In functional neuroimaging studies, DID patients have shown altered amygdalar-hippocampal and fronto-parietal connectivity. Patients with depersonalization disorder have shown increased medial prefrontal and decreased striato-thalamic volumes. Depersonalization disordered patients have shown cortico-limbic disconnection, with hyperactivation of "top-down" regulatory prefrontal function and parieto-occipital regions with reduction in limbic activity [85, 86]. Patients with PTSD demonstrate increased heart rate, decreased prefrontal region activation, and increased amygdalar activity, whereas patients with the dissociative subtype show a reversed pattern, as above. This inhibition of the limbic system is theorized to be a regulatory mechanism to restrain the extreme hyperarousal in PTSD [87].

Alterations in sleep wake cycle have been implicated in dissociation. Self-reported dissociative symptoms were linked to lowered alpha power and raised delta and theta power on electroencephalogram, similar to the hypnogogic transition from alert wakefulness to sleep onset [88]. Further, patients suffering from insomnia have raised levels of dissociative symptoms [76].

Clinical Evaluation

Because dissociative symptoms have a broad differential diagnosis, clinicians must carefully consider both psychiatric and neurological etiologies. Further complicating the clinical picture, dissociative symptoms may be present in other psychiatric disorders and dissociative disorders have frequent rates of comorbidity with mood and personality disorders. Table 3 demonstrates important differentiations amongst various diagnoses. Careful discrimination of a dissociative disorder from other psychiatric, substance-induced, or other medically related symptoms is paramount to quality care. Once dissociative symptoms have been identified, further history should be gathered of current stressors in relationship to dissociative episodes, detailed description of episodes and their general course, past traumas, and past dissociative symptoms in childhood.

Treatment

Treatment may consist of psychotherapy, pharmacological intervention, and/or neuromodulation, and is dependent on appropriate diagnosis. General principles of psychotherapy are encouraged, emphasizing psychoeducation, providing a stable and secure therapeutic relationship, recognizing stressors, generating adaptive coping skills, and addressing psychiatric comorbidities. The therapist should be cautious not to promote or elaborate any further dissociative identities, but rather understand them as a potential representation of past trauma [89]. An expert consensus describes three stages of treatment of dissociative disorders. The first stage involves ego strengthening, training in affect management and impulse control techniques, grounding, interpersonal effectiveness, and an understanding that self-injurious behavior may serve as reenactments of past trauma or disruptions in forming attachments. Once stabilized, patients move to the second stage wherein they begin to gradually understand the narrative of their traumatic and nontraumatic past, acknowledging distorted self-images related to past traumas, and developing a mastery over memories. The third stage involves reconnecting with the patient's sense of self, relationship with others, and with daily life in general. The treatment may not necessarily progress in a linear fashion and depending on the patient's severity of symptoms, different therapeutic techniques are implemented (supportive therapy and coping skills in times of crisis versus psychodynamic self-reflection and examination during periods of relatively milder symptoms) [90]. Treatment of anxiety and/or PTSD symptoms with interoceptive exposure therapy has shown a reduction in associated depersonalization and derealization symptoms [91].

A non-randomized, uncontrolled study of long term (30 months), phasic, trauma-focused model treatment of patients with dissociative disorders by community therapists trained in treating DID/DDNOS led to improvement across several domains, including a reduction in self-harm, suicide attempts, dissociative, depressive, and PTSD symptoms, decreased rates of hospitalization and drug use, as well as improvement in overall global function [92]. Patients still enrolled in therapy showed continued improvement at a 6-year follow-up [93].

DID has also been considered in some cases to be worsened by therapies that encourage expression of alters [94]. Such encouragement may uncover traumatic memories too early in therapy, prior to the stabilization and ego strengthening needed to sufficiently progress to deeper stages, therefore resulting in potentially harmful effects.

Most pharmacologic interventions in DID are used for treatment of comorbid depressive and anxiety symptoms rather than specific dissociative symptoms [95]. Despite anecdotal reports of selective serotonin reuptake inhibitors use in dissociative disorders, fluoxetine therapy was inefficacious in treating depersonalization disorder in a randomized controlled trial [96]. Benzodiazepines are cautioned against as they may exacerbate dissociation [97]. A small, open label trial of lamotrigine was useful in some patients with depersonalization disorder, though showed no superiority to placebo in a placebo-controlled cross-over trial [98]. Trials of opioid antagonists have yielded some improvements in dissociative symptoms of BPD, but more rigorous studies yielded no significant improvements when compared to placebo, though overall sample size remained small [99, 100].

Repetitive 1 Hz transcranial magnetic stimulation (rTMS) to the right ventrolateral prefrontal cortex in depersonalization disorder has shown significant improvements in depersonalization symptoms, as well as depressive and anxiety symptoms. Improvement of depersonalization symptoms via low frequency rTMS, leading to inhibition of prefrontal cortex, is consistent with neurobiologic models of dissociative symptoms with reduced limbic and increased prefrontal activation [101].

Overlap Between Functional Neurological Disorder and Dissociative Disorders

FND and dissociative disorders are classified as different categories of psychiatric disorders in DSM 5. Some authors offer a broader conceptualization of dissociation [102, 103], where symptoms are categorized as "psychoform dissociation" (which includes a disruption of the normal integrative functions of consciousness, memory, identity and perception of the environment – consistent with DSM 5's dissociative disorders) and "somatoform dissociation" (which includes motor and sensory functions not well integrated into other dimensions of normal functioning – consistent with DSM 5's conversion disorder or FND). This proposed lack of integration of a motor or sensory function gives rise to a decrease in function (such as in functional weakness) or presence of a symptom that should not be present (such as in functional tremor). The same dichotomy is observed in psychoform dissociative symptoms, where access to memories can be impacted (such as in dissociative amnesia) or identities intrude into a patient's experience (such as in DID). In the

Tenth Revision of the International Statistical Classification of Diseases and Related Health Problems (ICD-10), dissociative and conversion disorders use a similar root code [104].

Measures of somatoform and psychoform dissociation have shown strong and consistent correlation with each other [105–107]. The rate of dissociative disorders or dissociation scores in FND patients is higher than the rate seen in general or psychiatric populations [108–110]. Levels of psychoform and somatoform dissociation are similar between FND and dissociative disorders and higher in FND and dissociative disorders when compared to somatization disorder and healthy controls [111].

The co-occurrence and similar behavioral profiles in FND and dissociative disorders argue for overlapping and common underlying mechanisms. From a clinical perspective, it is imperative to screen for the presence of each of these disorders (and their subtypes) when the presence of one of these syndromes is suspected.

Take Home Points
- Functional neurological disorder (FND) is frequently encountered in neurology clinics and dissociative disorders are more common than usually recognized in psychiatric practice.
- Women outnumber men in FND. Evidence of female predominance in dissociative disorders is mixed.
- Trauma and other psychiatric disorders are known risk factors for FND and dissociative disorders, and the higher frequency of trauma in women compared to men may partially explain the higher prevalence of these disorders in women. Genetically-determined sex and hormonal fluctuations may play a role in brain connectivity alterations seen in FND, however, this is highly speculative at this point.
- Evidence-based treatment for FND and dissociative disorders is emerging. There is no indication at this point that intervention effectiveness differs based on sex.
- There is a significant overlap between FND and dissociative disorders. Both disorders share a lack of integration of specific neurological functions.

References

1. American Psychiatric Association. Diagnostic and statistical manual of mental disorders. 5th ed. Arlington: American Psychiatric Association; 2013.
2. Trimble M, Reynolds EH. A brief history of hysteria: from the ancient to the modern. Hand Clin Neurol. 2016;139(Functional Neurological Disorders):3–10.
3. Stone J, Sharpe M, Rothwell PM, Warlow CP. The12-year prognosis of unilateral functional weakness and sensory disturbance. J Neurol Neurosurg Psychiatry. 2003;74(5):591–6.
4. Duncan R, Graham CD, Oto M. Outcome at 5-10 years in psychogenic nonepileptic seizures: what patients report vs. what family doctors report. Epilepsy Behav. 2014;37:71–4.
5. Carson A, Lehn A. Epidemiology. Hand Clin Neurol. 2016;139(Functional Neurological Disorders):47–60.
6. Stone J, Carson A, Duncan R, Roberts R, Warlow C, Coleman R, et al. Who is referred to neurology clinics? – the diagnoses made in 3781 new patients. Clin Neurol Neurosurg. 2010;112(9):747–51.
7. Stone J, Carson A. An integrated approach to other functional neurological symptoms and related disorders. In: Dworetzky B, Baslet G, editors. Psychogenic nonepileptic seizures: towards the integration of care. New York: Oxford; 2017. p. 290–307.
8. Ladwig KH, Marten-Mittag B, Formanek B, Dammann G. Gender differences of symptom reporting and medical health care utilization in the German population. Eur J Epidemiol. 2000;16(6):511–8.
9. Barsky AJ, Orav EJ, Bates DW. Somatization increases medical utilization and costs independent of psychiatric and medical comorbidity. Arch Gen Psychiatry. 2005;62(8):903–10.
10. Stone J, Smyth R, Carson A, Lewis S, Prescott R, Warlow C, et al. Systematic review of misdiagnosis of conversion symptoms and "hysteria". BMJ. 2005;331(7523):989.
11. Kotagal P, Costa M, Wyllie E, Wolgamuth B. Paroxysmal nonepileptic events in children and adolescents. Pediatrics. 2002;110(4):e46.
12. Duncan R, Oto M, Martin E, Pelosi A. Late onset psychogenic nonepileptic attacks. Neurology. 2006;66(11):1644–7.
13. Stone J. Functional neurological disorders: the neurological assessment as treatment. Neurophysiol Clin. 2014;44(4):363–73.
14. Morgante F, Edwards MJ, Espay AJ. Psychogenic movement disorders. Continuum (Minneap Minn). 2013;19(5 Movement Disorders):1383–96.
15. LaFrance WC, Baker GA, Duncan R, Goldstein LH, Reuber M. Minimum requirements for the diagnosis of psychogenic nonepileptic seizures: a staged approach, a report from the international league against epilepsy nonepileptic seizures task force. Epilepsia. 2013;54(11):2005–18.
16. Alving J. Serum prolactin levels are elevated also after pseudo-epileptic seizures. Seizure. 1998;7(2):85–9.
17. Chen DK, So YT, Fisher RS. Therapeutics and technology assessment subcommittee of the American Academy of Neurology. Use of serum prolactin in diagnosing epileptic seizures: report of the therapeutics and technology assessment subcommittee of the American Academy of Neurology. Neurology. 2005;65(5):668–75.
18. Matin N, Young SS, Williams B, LaFrance WC Jr, King JN, Caplan D, Chemali Z, Weilburg JB, Dickerson BC, Perez DL. Neuropsychiatric associations with gender, illness duration, work disability, and motor subtype in a U.S. functional neurological disorders clinic population. J Neuropsychiatry Clin Neurosci. 2017;29(4):375–82.
19. Hopp JL, Anderson KE, Krumholz A, Gruber-Baldini AL, Shulman LM. Psychogenic seizures and psychogenic movement disorders: are they the same patients? Epilepsy Behav. 2012;25(4):666–9.
20. Driver-Dunckley E, Stonnington CM, Locke DE, Noe K. Comparison of psychogenic movement disorders and psychogenic nonepileptic seizures: is phenotype clinically important? Psychosomatics. 2011;52(4):337–45.
21. van Merode T, de Krom MC, Knottnerus JA. Gender-related differences in non-epileptic attacks: a study of patients' cases in the literature. Seizure. 1997;6(4):311–6.
22. Gale SD, Hill SW, Pearson C. Seizure semiology in males with psychogenic nonepileptic seizures is associated with somatic complaints. Epilepsy Res. 2015;115:153–7.

23. Say GN, Tasdemir HA, Ince H. Semiological and psychiatric characteristics of children with psychogenic nonepileptic seizures: gender-related differences. Seizure. 2015;31:144–8.

24. Asadi-Pooya AA, Emami M, Emami Y. Gender differences in manifestations of psychogenic non-epileptic seizures in Iran. J Neurol Sci. 2013;332(1–2):66–8.

25. Roelofs K, Pasman J. Stress, childhood trauma, and cognitive functions in functional neurologic disorders. Hand Clin Neurol. 2016;139(Functional Neurological Disorders):139–55.

26. Oto M, Conway P, McGonigal A, Russell AJ, Duncan R. Gender differences in psychogenic non-epileptic seizures. Seizure. 2005;14(1):33–9.

27. Thomas AA, Preston J, Scott RC, Bujarski KA. Diagnosis of probable psychogenic nonepileptic seizures in the outpatient clinic: does gender matter? Epilepsy Behav. 2013;29(2):295–7.

28. Wang V, Salinsky M. Neurologic and medical factors. In: Dworetzky B, Baslet G, editors. Psychogenic nonepileptic seizures: towards the integration of care. New York: Oxford; 2017. p. 67–85.

29. Baslet G, Seshadri A, Bermeo-Ovalle A, Willment K, Myers L. Psychogenic non-epileptic seizures: an updated primer. Psychosomatics. 2016;57(1):1–17.

30. Reuber M, Brown RJ. Understanding psychogenic nonepileptic seizures-phenomenology, semiology and the integrative cognitive model. Seizure. 2017;44:199–205.

31. Edwards MJ. Neurobiologic theories of functional neurologic disorders. Hand Clin Neurol. 2016;139(Functional Neurological Disorders):131–7.

32. Liepert J, Hassa T, Tuscher O. Electrophysiological correlates of motor conversion disorder. Mov Disord. 2008;23(15):2172–6.

33. Bakvis P, Roelofs K, Kuyk J, Edelbroek PM, Swinkels WA, Spinhoven P. Trauma, stress, and preconscious threat processing in patients with psychogenic nonepileptic seizures. Epilepsia. 2009;50(5):1001–11.

34. Reinsberger C, Sarkis R, Papadelis C, Doshi C, Perez DL, Baslet G, et al. Autonomic changes in psychogenic nonepileptic seizures: toward a potential diagnostic biomarker? Clin EEG Neurosci. 2015;46(1):16–25.

35. Atmaca M, Aydin A, Tezcan E, Poyraz AK, Kara B. Volumetric investigation of brain regions in patients with conversion disorder. Prog Neuro-Psychopharmacol Biol Psychiatry. 2006;30(4):708–13.

36. Nicholson TR, Aybek S, Kempton MJ, Daly EM, Murphy DG, David AS, et al. A structural MRI study of motor conversion disorder: evidence of reduction in thalamic volume. J Neurol Neurosurg Psychiatry. 2014;85(2):227–9.

37. Aybek S, Nicholson TR, Draganski B, Daly E, Murphy DG, David AS, et al. Grey matter changes in motor conversion disorder. J Neurol Neurosurg Psychiatry. 2014;85(2):236–8.

38. Labate A, Cerasa A, Mula M, Mumoli L, Gioia MC, Aguglia U, et al. Neuroanatomic correlates of psychogenic nonepileptic seizures: a cortical thickness and VBM study. Epilepsia. 2012;53(2):377–85.

39. Aybek S, Vuilleumier P. Imaging studies of functional neurologic disorders. Hand Clin Neurol. 2016;139(Functional Neurological Disorders):73–84.

40. Voon V, Cavanna AE, Coburn K, Sampson S, Reeve A, LaFrance WC, et al. Functional neuroanatomy and neurophysiology of functional neurological disorders (conversion disorder). J Neuropsychiatry Clin Neurosci. 2016;28(3):168–90.

41. Asadi-Pooya AA. Psychogenic nonepileptic seizures and sex differences in stress responses. Epilepsia. 2016;57(5):853.

42. Hall-Patch L, Brown R, House A, Howlett S, Kemp S, Lawton G, et al. Acceptability and effectiveness of a strategy for the communication of the diagnosis of psychogenic nonepileptic seizures. Epilepsia. 2010;51(1):70–8.

43. Razvi S, Mulhern S, Duncan R. Newly diagnosed psychogenic nonepileptic seizures: health care demand prior to and following diagnosis at a first seizure clinic. Epilepsy Behav. 2012;23(1):7–9.

44. Jirsch JD, Ahmed SN, Maximova K, Gross DW. Recognition of psychogenic nonepileptic seizures diminishes acute care utilization. Epilepsy Behav. 2011;22(2):304–7.

45. Ness D. Physical therapy management for conversion disorder: case series. J Neurol Phys Ther. 2007;31(1):30–9.

46. Nielsen G, Ricciardi L, Demartini B, Hunter R, Joyce E, Edwards MJ. Outcomes of a 5-day physiotherapy programme for functional (psychogenic) motor disorder. J Neurol. 2015;262(3):674–81.

47. Jordbru AA, Smedstad LM, Klungsoyr O, Martinsen EW. Psychogenic gait disorder: a randomized controlled trial of physical rehabilitation with one-year follow-up. J Rehabil Med. 2014;46(2):181–7.

48. Voon V, Lang AE. Antidepressant treatment outcomes of psychogenic movement disorder. J Clin Psychiatry. 2005;66(12):1529–34.

49. Pintor L, Baillus E, Matrai S, Carreno M, Donaire A, Boget T, et al. Efficiency of venlafaxine in patients with psychogenic nonepileptic seizures and anxiety and/or depressive disorders. J Neuropsychiatry Clin Neurosci. 2010;22(4):401–8.

50. Kleinstäuber M, Witthöft M, Steffanowski A, van Marwijk H, Hiller W, Lambert MJ. Pharmacological interventions for somatoform disorders in adults. Cochrane Database Syst Rev. 2014;11:CD010628.

51. LaFrance WC Jr, Baird GL, Barry JJ, Blum AS, Frank Webb A, Keitner GI, Machan JT, Miller I, Szaflarski JP. NES treatment trial (NEST-T) consortium. Multicenter pilot treatment trial for psychogenic nonepileptic seizures: a randomized clinical trial. JAMA Psychiatry. 2014;71(9):997–1005.

52. Goldstein LH, Chalder T, Chigwedere C, Khondoker MR, Moriarty J, Toone BK, et al. Cognitive-behavioral therapy for psychogenic nonepileptic seizures A pilot RCT. Neurology. 2010;74(24):1986–94.

53. Sharpe M, Walker J, Williams C, Stone J, Cavanagh J, Murray G, et al. Guided self-help for functional (psychogenic) symptoms: a randomized controlled efficacy trial. Neurology. 2011;77(6):564–72.

54. Williams C, Kent C, Smith S, Carson A, Sharpe M, Cavanagh J. Overcoming functional neurological symptoms: a five areas approach. London: Hodder Arnold; 2011.

55. Reiter JM, Andrews D, Reiter C, LaFrance WC. Taking control of your seizures workbook. New York: Oxford University Press; 2015.

56. Moene FC, Spinhoven P, Hoogduin KA, van Dyck R. A randomised controlled clinical trial on the additional effect of hypnosis in a comprehensive treatment programme for in-patients with conversion disorder of the motor type. Psychother Psychosom. 2002;71(2):66–76.

57. Kompoliti K, Wilson B, Stebbins G, Bernard B, Hinson V. Immediate vs. delayed treatment of psychogenic movement disorders with short term psychodynamic psychotherapy: randomized clinical trial. Parkinsonism Relat Disord. 2014;20(1):60–3.

58. Mayor R, Howlett S, Grünewald R, Reuber M. Long-term outcome of brief augmented psychodynamic interpersonal therapy for psycho- genic nonepileptic seizures: seizure control and health care utilization. Epilepsia. 2010;51(7):1169–76.

59. Barry JJ, Wittenberg D, Bullock KD, Michaels JB, Classen CC, Fisher RS. Group therapy for patients with psychogenic nonepileptic seizures: a pilot study. Epilepsy Behav. 2008;13(4):624–9.

60. Myers L, Vaidya-Mathur U, Lancman M. Prolonged exposure therapy for the treatment of patients diagnosed with psychogenic non-epileptic seizures (PNES) and post-traumatic stress disorder (PTSD). Epilepsy Behav. 2017;66:86–92.

61. Baslet G, Dworetzky B, Perez DL, Oser M. Treatment of psychogenic nonepileptic seizures: updated review and findings from a

mindfulness-based intervention case series. Clin EEG Neurosci. 2015;46(1):54–64.

62. Kuyk J, Siffels MC, Bakvis P, Swinkels WA. Psychological treatment of patients with psychogenic non-epileptic seizures: an outcome study. Seizure. 2008;17(7):595–603.

63. Zaroff CM, Myers L, Barr WB, Luciano D, Devinsky O. Group psycho-education as treatment for psychological nonepileptic seizures. Epilepsy Behav. 2004;5(4):587–92.

64. Chastan N, Parain D. Psychogenic paralysis and recovery after motor cortex transcranial magnetic stimulation. Mov Disord. 2010;25(10):1501–4.

65. Jaeger S, Steinert T, Uhlmann C, Flammer E, Bichescu-Burian D, Tschoke S. Dissociation in patients with borderline personality disorder in acute inpatient care – a latent profile analysis. Compr Psychiatry. 2017;78:67–75.

66. Taylor MA, Viadya NA. Descriptive psychopathology; signs and symptoms of behavioral disorders. Cambridge, UK: Cambridge University Press; 2009.

67. Steinberg M. The spectrum of depersonalization: assessment and treatment. In: Tasman A, Goldfinger SM, editors. American psychiatric press review of psychiatry, vol. 10. Washington, DC: American Psychiatric Press; 1991. p. 223–47.

68. Brand BL, Lanius R, Vermetten E, et al. Where are we going? An update an assessment, treatment, and neurobiological research in dissociative disorders as we move toward the DSM-5. J Trauma Dissociation. 2012;13(1):9–31.

69. Kluft RP, editor. Childhood antecedents of multiple personality. Washington, DC: American Psychiatric Press; 1985.

70. Foote B, Smolin Y, Kaplan M, Legatt ME, Lipschitz D. Prevalence of dissociative disorders in psychiatric outpatients. Am J Psychiatr. 2006;163(4):623–9.

71. Johnson JG, Cohen P, Kasen S, Brook JS. Dissociative disorders among adults in the community, impaired functioning, and axis I and II comorbidity. J Psychiatr Res. 2006;40(2):131–40.

72. Lee WE, Kwok CHT, Hunter ECM, Richards M, David AS. Prevalence and childhood antecedents of depersonalization syndrome in a UK birth cohort. Soc Psychiatry Psychiatr Epidemiol. 2012;47(2):253–61.

73. Hunter EC, Sierra M, David AS. The epidemiology of depersonalisation and derealisation: a systematic review. Soc Psychiatry Psychiatr Epidemiol. 2004;39(1):9–18.

74. Stein DJ, Koenen KC, Friedman MJ, Hill E, McLaughlin KA, Petukhova M, et al. Dissociation in posttraumatic stress disorder: evidence from the world mental health surveys. Biol Psychiatry. 2013;73(4):302–12.

75. Rodewald F, Wilhelm-Goling C, Emrich HM, Reddemann L, Gast U. Axis-I comorbidity in female patients with dissociative identity disorder and dissociative identity disorder not otherwise specified. J Nerv Ment Dis. 2011;199(2):122–31.

76. Van Der Kloat D, Giesbrecht T, Franck E, Van Gastel A, De Volder I, Van Den Eede F, et al. Dissociative symptoms and sleep parameters – an all-night polysomnography study in patients with insomnia. Compr Psychiatry. 2013;54(6):658–64.

77. Lyssenko L, Schmahl C, Bockhacker L, Vonderlin R, Bohus M, Kleindienst N. Dissociation in psychiatric sisorders: a meta-analysis of studies using the dissociative experiences scale. Am J Psychiatry. 2017;175:37–46.

78. Lambert MV, Sierra M, Phillips ML, David AS. The organic spectrum of depersonalization. A review plus four new cases. J Neuropsychiat Clin Neurosci. 2002;14:141–54.

79. Allen JG, Smith WH. Diagnosing dissociative disorders. Bull Menn Clin. 1993;57(3):328–43.

80. Coons PM. The dissociative disorders: rarely considered and underdiagnosed. Psychiatr Clin N Am. 1998;21(3):637–64.

81. Putnam FW. Dissociation in children and adolescents: a developmental perspective. New York: The Guilford Press; 1997.

82. Dalenberg CJ, Brand BL, Gleaves DH, et al. Evaluation of the evidence for the trauma and fantasy models of dissociation. Psychol Bull. 2012;138(3):550–88.

83. Silberg J. The dissociative child. Lutherville: Sidran Press; 1996.

84. Giesbrecht T, Lynn SJ, Lilienfeld SO, Merckelbach H. Cognitive processes in dissociation: an analysis of core theoretical assumptions. Psychol Bull. 2008;134(5):617–47.

85. Krause-Utz A, Frost R, Winter D, Elzinga BM. Dissociation and alterations in brain function and structure: implications for borderline personality disorder. Curr Psychiatry Rep. 2017;19(1):6.

86. Perez DL, Matin N, Williams B, Tanev K, Makris N, LaFrance WC, et al. Cortical thickness alterations linked to somatoform and psychological dissociation in functional neurological disorders. Hum Brain Mapp. 2018;39(1):428–39.

87. Van Huijsteen J, Vermetten E. The dissociative subtype of posttraumatic stress disorder: research update on clinical and neurobiological features. Curr Top Behav Neurosci. 2017;38:229–48.

88. Giesbrecht T, Jongen EM, Smulders FTY, Merckelbach H. Dissociation, resting EEG, and subjective sleep experiences in undergraduates. J Nerv Ment Dis. 2006;194(5):362–8.

89. Okano K. Clinical handling of patients with dissociative disorders. Seishin Shinkeigaku Zasshi. 2015;117(6):399–412.

90. Myrick AC, Chasson GS, Lanius RA, Leventhal B, Brand BL. Treatment of complex dissociative disorders: a comparison of interventions reported by community therapists versus those recommended by experts. J Trauma Dissociation. 2015;16(1):51–67.

91. Weiner E, McKay D. A preliminary evaluation of repeated exposure for depersonalization and derealization. Behav Modif. 2012;37(2):226–42.

92. Brand BL, McNary SW, Myrick AC, Classen CC, Lanius R, Lowenstein RJ, et al. A longitudinal naturalistic study of patients with dissociative disorders treated by community clinicians. Psychol Trauma: Theory Res Pract Policy. 2012;5:301–8.

93. Myrick AC, Webermann AR, Loewenstein RJ, Lanius R, Putnam FW, Brand BL. Six-year follow-up of the treatment of patients with dissociative disorders study. Eur J Psychotraumatol. 2017;8(1):1344080.

94. Lilienfeld SO. Psychological treatments that cause harm. Perspect Psychol Sci. 2007;2(1):53–70.

95. Gentile JP, Dillon KS, Gillig PM. Psychotherapy and pharmacotherapy for patients with dissociative identity disorder. Innov Clin Neurosci. 2013;10(2):22–9.

96. Simeon D, Guralnik O, Schmeidler J, Knutelska M. Fluoxetine therapy in depersonalisation disorder: randomised controlled trial. Br J Psychiatry. 2004;185:31–6.

97. Stern TA, Rosenbaum JF, Fava M, et al. Massachusetts general hospital comprehensive clinical psychiatry. Waltham: Elsevier Health Sciences; 2008.

98. Sierra M, Phillips ML, Ivin G, Krystal J, David AS. A placebo-controlled, cross-over trial of lamotrigine in depersonlization disorder. J Psychopharmacol. 2003;17(1):103–5.

99. Bohus MJ, Landwehrmeyer GB, Stiglmayr CE, Limberger MF, Böhme R, Schmahl CG. Naltrexone in the treatment of dissociative symptoms in patients with borderline personality disorder: an open-label trial. J Clin Psychiatry. 1999;60:598–60.

100. Schmahl C, Kleindienst N, Limberger M, Ludascher P, Mauchnik J, Deibler P, et al. Evaluation of naltrexone for dissociative symptoms in borderline personality disorder. Int Clin Psychopharmacol. 2012;27(1):61–8.

101. Jay EL, Nestler S, Sierra M, McLelland J, Kekic M, David AS. Ventrolateral prefrontal cortex repetitive transcranial magnetic stimulation in the treatment of depersonalization disorder: a consecutive case series. Psychiatry Res. 2016;240:118–22.

102. Brown RJ, Cardena E, Nijenhuis E, Sar V, van der Hart O. Should conversion disorder be reclassified as a dissociative disorder in DSM V? Psychosomatics. 2007;48(5):369–78.

103. Nijenhuis ER. Somatoform dissociation and somatoform dissociative disorders. In: Dell P, O'Neil J, editors. Dissociation and the dissociative disorders: DSM-V and beyond. New York: Routledge; 2009. p. 259–76.

104. World Health Organization. The ICD-10 classification of mental and behavioural disorders: clinical descriptions and diagnostic guidelines. Geneva: World Health Organization; 1992.

105. Nijenhuis ER, Van Dyck R, Spinhoven P, van der Hart O, Chatrou M, Vanderlinden J, et al. Somatoform dissociation discriminates among diagnostic categories over and above general psychopathology. Aust N Z J Psychiatry. 1999;33(4):512–20.

106. Nijenhuis ER, Van Dyck R, Ter Kuile MM, Moutitis MJE, Soinhoven P, van der Hart O. Evidence for associations among somatoform dissociation, psychological dissociation and reported trauma in patients with chronic pelvic pain. J Psychosom Obstet Gynecol. 2003;24(2):87–98.

107. Sar V, Kundakci T, Kiziltan E, Bakim B, Bozkurt O. Differentiating dissociative disorders from other diagnostic groups through somatoform dissociation in Turkey. J Trauma Dissociation. 2000;1(4):67–80.

108. Sar V, Akyüz G, Kundakçi T, Kiziltan E, Dogan O. Childhood trauma, dissociation, and psychiatric comorbidity in patients with conversion disorder. Am J Psychiatry. 2004;161(12):2271–6.

109. Tezcan E, Atmaca M, Kuloglu M, Gecici O, Buyukbayram A, Tutkun H. Dissociative disorders in Turkish inpatients with conversion disorder. Compr Psychiatry. 2003;44(4):324–30.

110. Spitzer C, Spelsberg B, Grabe HJ, Mundt B, Freyberger HJ. Dissociative experiences and psychopathology in conversion disorders. J Psychosom Res. 1999;46(3):291–4.

111. Espirito-Santo H, Pio-Abreu JL. Psychiatric symptoms and dissociation in conversion, somatization and dissociative disorders. Aust N Z J Psychiatry. 2009;43(3):270–6.

Contraception in Neurologic and Psychiatric Disorders

Caryn Dutton, Andrea Hsu Roe, and Deborah Bartz

Introduction

For all reproductive-age women with neurologic or psychiatric disorders, it is essential to address contraceptive need and method selection as part of their care plan. Use of inappropriate methods, or non-use, may result in unintended pregnancy and the sequelae of unplanned pregnancy can be significant, including high-risk pregnancy in the setting of poorly controlled disease or potential exposure to teratogenic medications. Because of these risks, it is crucial to optimize timing and planning of pregnancy for women with complex medical conditions. Prevention of unplanned pregnancy should be emphasized, and paired with counseling on highly effective contraceptive methods that are compatible with the woman's medical conditions. This chapter reviews the known relationships between contraceptive method selection and both the impact on disease, and potential drug-drug interactions, for women with neurologic or psychiatric conditions.

Modern contraceptives include hormonal and non-hormonal options; for women with neurologic or psychiatric disorders there should be no reason to avoid use of non-hormonal methods such as sterilization, the copper IUD, or barrier methods. Both the copper and levonorgestrel IUDs and the contraceptive implant are the most effective reversible methods available with 1-year typical use failure rates of 0.05–0.8% [1]. Collectively, these long-acting reversible contraceptives (LARC) are safe for almost all women, including young and nulliparous patients, and have high continuation rates [2]. The next most effective methods of hormonal contraception are the progestin injectable (depot medroxyprogesterone acetate, known as DMPA or Depo-Provera™) and combined hormonal contraceptives (CHC) that contain both estrogen and progestin administered as a pill, or via a patch or ring (1 year typical use failure rates: 6–9%). Progestin-only pills (POPs) may be slightly less effective than combined pills, but are still appropriate for many women with contraindications to estrogen [1]. Counseling women regarding choice of method may include discussion of method preference, potential for adherence, and education regarding potential or expected side effects such as changes in bleeding pattern.

Throughout this chapter, we will reference evidence-based guidelines initially published by the World Health Organization and adapted for use in the United States by the Centers for Disease Control (CDC). The 2016 CDC United States Medical Eligibility Criteria (USMEC) provides a relative ranking of safety or risk for the use of various contraceptive methods compared to risks associated with unintended pregnancy in the context of chronic medical conditions, concomitant medications, or other factors [3]. The ranking system is detailed in Table 1, and provides expert consensus opinion based on proven or theoretical risks. This document is readily available on the CDC website and as a mobile application, and is a practical comprehensive resource to guide clinical practice.

C. Dutton (✉) · D. Bartz
Department of Obstetrics and Gynecology, Brigham and Women's Hospital, Boston, MA, USA

Harvard Medical School, Boston, MA, USA
e-mail: crdutton@bwh.harvard.edu; dbartz@bwh.harvard.edu

A. H. Roe
Department of Obstetrics and Gynecology, Hospital of the University of Pennsylvania, Philadelphia, PA, USA

Perelman School of Medicine, University of Pennsylvania, Philadelphia, PA, USA
e-mail: Andrea.Roe@uphs.upenn.edu

Table 1 CDC USMEC categories of medical eligibility for contraceptive use [3]

Category 1	A condition for which there is no restriction for the use of the contraceptive method
Category 2	A condition for which the advantages of using the method generally outweigh the risks
Category 3	A condition for which the theoretical or proven risks usually outweigh the advantages of using the method
Category 4	A condition that represents an unacceptable health risk if the contraceptive method is used

© Springer Nature Switzerland AG 2019
M. A. O'Neal (ed.), *Neurology and Psychiatry of Women*, https://doi.org/10.1007/978-3-030-04245-5_4

Migraine Disease

Women are disproportionately affected by migraine with a lifetime prevalence of 17–18.2%, and with peak morbidity coinciding with the reproductive years of peak fertility [4, 5]. The hormonally active events of menstruation, hormonal contraception use, pregnancy, and menopause influence the onset and severity of migraine symptoms [6]. Non-hormonal contraceptive methods (e.g. barrier methods, sterilization, copper IUD) are all safe and appropriate options in otherwise healthy migraineurs (USMEC Category 1). Because about 28% of women 15–44 years old in the US use hormonal methods of birth control, understanding the impact of contraceptive choice on migraine disease is relevant [7].

A Patient with Migraines

An otherwise healthy, non-smoking 32 year-old woman reports recent onset of migraine headaches, occurring at onset of her menses, and requests a refill of her combined oral contraceptive pills (COCs). Should you continue her pills cyclically, change to continuous use to potentially treat her headaches, or recommend switching to an alternate contraceptive method?

Migraine Disease and the Safety of Hormonal Contraception

Age, smoking status and exogenous estrogen use all independently increase women's ischemic stroke risk, a risk that is compounded when hormones are used in the setting of existing migraine disease [8, 9]. Estrogen induces the synthesis of several clotting factors resulting in increased coagulability, with changes in lipid levels and blood pressure that may further contribute to stroke risk [10]. The absolute risk of stroke in a healthy young woman is low at 5–10 per 100,000 women-years [11]. The risk of stroke in women using CHC rises with increasing age, from 3.4 per 100,000 women-years in adolescents to 64.4 events per 100,000 women-years among women 45–49 years [12].

A systematic review demonstrated two to four times increased risk of stroke associated with modern CHC doses in the setting of migraine disease [9]. Table 2 summarizes the results of a national health care claims nested case-control study of 25,887 ischemic strokes among reproductive-aged females, in which the overall incidence of stroke in the larger population was 11/100,000 [13]. The odds ratio of ischemic stroke was highest among those with migraine with aura using CHC after adjusting for hypertension, diabetes, obesity, smoking, ischemic heart disease, and valvular heart disease, compared to women with neither migraine nor CHC

Table 2 Risk of stroke in healthy women, compared to women using combined hormonal contraception (CHC), +/− migraine, with or without aura [13]

	Odds ratio (95% CI)
No migraine, no CHC	*reference*
No migraine + CHC	1.4 (1.2–1.7)
Migraine (no aura, no CHC)	1.8 (1.1–2.9)
Migraine (no aura) + CHC	2.2 (1.9–2.7)
Migraine + aura (no CHC)	2.7 (1.9–3.7)
Migraine + aura + CHC	6.1 (3.1–12.1)

use. Odds ratios were also elevated in women with migraine with aura without CHC use however the risk of stroke was similar between those women with migraine without aura who used CHC and women with migraine without aura without CHC use as compared to age-matched controls. The authors concluded that use of CHC by women with migraine but without aura did not increase stroke risk over baseline risk from their migraine disease.

Because one third of female migraineurs experience aura as part of their headache disease and others have additional risk factors for stroke, such as smoking or hypertension [14, 15]. CHC is prohibitive for many women with headache. Use of progestin-only pills, the subdermal implant or a levonorgestrel IUD (LNG-IUD) does not pose increased stroke risk, supported by a large systematic review and therefore can be used in women with migraine [16]. The USMEC also allows for the use of DMPA in women with migraine disease of all subtypes without other risk factors for stroke. Table 3 provides a summary of the USMEC guidance for use of hormonal methods in the setting of headache or migraine.

Effect of Contraceptives on the Development or Worsening of Headache Disease

New or worsening headache is among the top three reasons cited for discontinuation of a hormonal birth control method [17]. Evidence in the literature implicating hormonal contraception in the contribution to new or worsening headache disease is poor; a systematic review of this topic concluded that prior studies on exogenous hormone-induced headache are generally of low quality, have studied older contraceptive formulations with higher estrogen doses that do not reflect those in current use, have failed to distinguish migraine from other headaches, and have failed to control for baseline estimates of migraine incidence or prevalence, both of which are high and increase with age in women [18]. If new or worsening headaches are experienced after initiation of hormonal contraception, women should be counseled that these symptoms usually are transient and improve quickly. One randomized controlled trial of side effects after initiation of hormonal side effect suggests that when headache or migraine occurs

Table 3 CDC USMEC recommendations for hormonal contraceptive use in women with headaches and migraine [3]

Condition	Combined Hormonal Contraception[a] (pills, patch, ring)	Progestin-only contraception (pills, implant)	DMPA	LNG IUD
Non-migrainous headache	1	1	1	1
Migraine without aura (including menstrual migraine)	2	1	1	1
Migraines with aura, any age	4	1	1	1

[a]Classification is for women without other risk factors for stroke

in the first cycle of combination hormonal contraceptive use, there is only a one in three risk of recurrence in the second cycle, and a one in ten chance of headache in the third cycle [19]. Currently, recommendations support re-evaluation or discontinuation of a hormonal contraceptive method in women who develop escalating severity/frequency of headaches, new onset migraine with aura symptoms, or non-migraine headaches that persist beyond the first 3 months of use [11].

Hormonal Contraception as Treatment of Migraine Disease

Fluctuations in endogenous ovarian hormones modulate the nociceptive and anti-nociceptive etiologies of migraine pathogenesis, resulting in waxing and waning symptoms during hormonally active life events [20, 21]. For more than 50% of women with migraines, the withdrawal of endogenous estrogen associated with menses acts as a trigger for cyclic headache symptoms resulting in the headache subtype of menstrual migraine [22]. The mechanism of action of systemic hormonal contraceptives (COCs, POPs, the vaginal ring, the patch, DMPA and the implant) is to provide a steady state of circulating hormones that inhibit endogenous hormones and prevent ovulation [23]. Therefore, hormonal interventions have a potential biologic mechanism as a treatment strategy for migraine [6, 24]. Indeed, many women report an improvement in headache severity and frequency when they initiate hormonal contraceptives [18, 25].

Newer formulations of COCs, which provide extended (84 active/7 inactive pills) or continuous (365 active pills) hormonal dosing, may benefit women with headache. Multiple systematic reviews evaluating the COCs and vaginal ring found significantly lower rates of headache in women using continuous regimens that skip the monthly hormone-free placebo week as compared to those women who use their hormonal contraception in a cyclic fashion [24, 26, 27]. Further study is needed, but in reproductive-aged migraine patients, a trial of a systemic hormonal contraceptive used as an extended regimen may incur an improvement in headache disease.

A Patient with Migraines: Case Summary

If this patient does not report aura, and is without other risk factors that would preclude use of estrogen-containing contraception, it would be reasonable to offer continuous use of a low-dose COC. If her headaches persist or worsen, she could be advised to try a progesterone-only method to suppress menses (DMPA, implant, or possibly LNG IUD) as potential treatment for her menstrual migraine disease.

Epilepsy

There is a complex interaction between epilepsy and endogenous or exogenous hormones. While there is no known consistent impact of reproductive hormones on seizure frequency or severity, some women with epilepsy (WWE) may be more susceptible to cyclic changes. In general, estrogen is considered pro-convulsant while progestins may promote neuroinhibition [28]. In addition, metabolism of hormonal contraception can interact in a bi-directional fashion with some anti-epileptic drugs (AEDs) impacting contraceptive efficacy, or in contrast, hormonal contraceptives impacting AED levels or side effects [29]. A careful assessment of current medication use and potential interactions can help guide strategies for selecting an appropriate contraceptive method.

A Patient with Epilepsy

A 19 year-old woman with well-controlled seizures on carbamazepine (CBZ) and lamotrigine (LTG) presents with questions about her options for contraception. What can you tell her about the potential impact of hormonal contraception on her epilepsy, and what are her most appropriate contraceptive options?

Epilepsy and Safety of Hormonal Contraception

A 2002 report of large cohort study performed in the UK demonstrated that use of COCs was not associated with development of epilepsy in healthy women [30]. There are no similar analyses for WWE, and most experts agree that there is no evidence hormonal contraception negatively impacts seizure activity [3, 31]. However, any patient on AEDs should be carefully monitored with initiation of a new hormonal medication. In a recent online survey, 70% of WWE self-reported no change in seizure frequency, with the remainder reporting hormonal contraception either increased (20%) or decreased (10%) seizure frequency [32]. LARC methods (the progestin implant and IUDs) are also safe for use in WWE. A trial of levonorgestrel (LNG) IUD initiation in 20 WWE demonstrated no clinically meaningful changes in AED trough level or seizure control [33]. The USMEC guidelines assign a category 1 rating (no restriction) for all contraceptive methods, with the caveat of evaluating for potential medication interactions.

Medication Interactions: Anti-epileptic Drugs and Hormonal Contraception

Some AEDs induce the hepatic cytochrome 3A4 isoenzyme system (enzyme-inducing AEDs or EIAEDs) resulting in increased metabolism of contraceptive hormones (Table 4). This drug interaction may result in decreased efficacy for combined hormonal contraceptive methods, POPs and the implant, and therefore limits a patient's options for effective birth control [34]. One EIAED, carbamazepine (CBZ), has been studied with concurrent use of COCs or with the progestin-only implant. In both cases, serum levels of the contraceptive hormones were reduced by co-administration of CBZ [35, 36]. In the study of concurrent CBZ and COC use, there was also evidence of increased rates of ovulation in women on CBZ compared to control subjects, though the exact impact on method efficacy and risk for pregnancy is unknown. Multiple case reports have documented contraceptive failure in the setting of COC and EIAED use, even with higher dose formulations of COCs (50 mcg or more of ethinyl estradiol) [34]. Importantly, lamotrigine (LTG) has a

Table 4 Antiepileptic Drugs (AEDs) listed by CYP3A4 enzyme inducing status

Strong inducers	Weak inducers	Non-inducers
Carbamazepine	Clobazam	Clonazepam
Oxcarbazepine	Eslicarbazepine	Divalproex
Perampenel	Felbamate	Ethosuxamide
Phenobarbital	Lamotrigine	Ezogabine
Phenytoin	Rufinamide	Gabapentin
Primidone	Topiramate	Lacosamide
		Levetiracetam
		Pregabalin
		Tiagabine
		Valproate
		Vigabatrin
		Zonisamide

Table adapted from [29]

unique interaction with estrogen-containing contraceptives in that LTG clearance is increased over twofold with concomitant use [29]. Women on LTG must be carefully monitored with initiation of any estrogen-containing contraceptive to maintain therapeutic levels; likewise, if the CHC is discontinued, women may be at risk for LTG toxicity.

The efficacy of a hormonal IUD is not impacted by concomitant use of EIAEDs since the mechanism of action does not rely on systemic hormone levels. The copper IUD, barrier methods and female sterilization are all similarly appropriate contraceptive options for WWE, with no known interactions. Finally, the USMEC supports use of DMPA as an effective method of birth control for women taking EIAEDs. The guidelines state that "its effectiveness is not decreased by use of certain anticonvulsants" [37]. Figure 1 displays one strategy for approaching prescription of contraception in WWE.

A Patient with Epilepsy: Case Summary

This patient is on an enzyme-inducing anti-epileptic medication (CBZ) therefore most methods of hormonal contraception may be less effective for this patient, except for the LNG IUD and DMPA. (see Fig. 1). Non-hormonal methods should not impact her disease or interact with her medications. If she chooses to start a CHC with a barrier method, then her LTG levels should be monitored closely.

Stroke

As discussed above, use of CHC doubles the risk of stroke in healthy women to 3–9 per 10,000 women-years. However, pregnancy, and particularly the postpartum period, is also a high-risk time frame for development of stroke; the likelihood of venous thromboembolism (VTE) ranges from 7 to 27 per 10,000 women-years during pregnancy and for postpartum women, 40–65 per 10,000 women-years [38]. A woman at risk for stroke, or with a prior stroke, should therefore be strongly encouraged to use highly effective contraceptive methods to prevent pregnancy until her health status can be optimized. Non-hormonal contraceptive methods (e.g. barrier methods and the copper IUD) can be used without restriction (USMEC Category 1). The copper IUD is a well-tolerated, safe, highly effective method that may be encouraged for women with a history of stroke. However, these methods do not diminish ovulation or menstrual blood flow, and in some patients the copper IUD may result in heavier bleeding. For women on anti-coagulation therapy, use of a progestin-containing hormonal contraceptive could diminish both the risk of heavier menstrual bleeding and of potential hemorrhagic ovarian cysts.

Fig. 1 Recommending a contraceptive method for women with epilepsy [89]

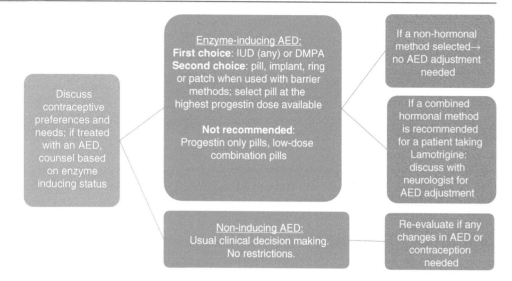

Estrogen-containing methods should be avoided in women with prior stroke (USMEC Category 4). The LNG-IUD offers highly effective, well-tolerated contraception with the lowest circulating systemic levels of hormones and thus, may be a preferred hormonal option for women with stroke. The circulating progestin level is higher in POPs and the implant, compared to the LNG-IUD. All three of these methods are USMEC Category 2 for initiation in a patient with a prior stroke due to small studies suggesting some level of increased risk for women using progestins with CV risk factors [39–41]. While there is no evidence that POPs or the subdermal implant increase the risk for VTE or stroke, the USMEC does classify *continuation* of these methods as a USMEC Category 3 if they are being used at the time of a new stroke without an otherwise obvious etiology. DMPA may cause hypoestrogenic changes in lipid profiles, and because the absolute risk of stroke in the setting of DMPA use is still under debate the theoretical risks outweigh benefits of use (USMEC Category 3) [42, 43].

Multiple Sclerosis

Sex hormones influence immunity, as evidenced by sex-based susceptibility to autoimmune diseases and fluctuations in autoimmune diseases symptoms in life events, such as pregnancy and menses. The peak prevalence of onset of multiple sclerosis (MS) occurs during childbearing years [44]. Many women with MS use novel disease modifying therapies, none of which are specifically approved for use in pregnancy, and some of which may increase risk for fetal malformations (e.g. Fingolimod, Teriflunomide) [45–48]. Women with MS should therefore have highly effective contraception as part of their treatment care plan.

There are no known interactions between the MS disease modifying therapies and hormonal or non-hormonal contraceptive methods that would affect birth control choice, though studies are limited [49]. In contrast, some of the medications used to alleviate MS symptoms have known interactions with systemic hormonal contraception (CHC, DMPA, implant). These include modafinil, commonly used to treat MS fatigue, and enzyme-inducing AEDs. Long-term users of these medications may be encouraged to use the locally acting copper- and levonorgestrel-containing IUDs for effective contraception, or barrier methods (USMEC Category 1).

Use of hormonal contraception does not appear to put women at risk for development of MS [50, 51]. A recent systematic review concluded that the use of CHC did not worsen the clinical course of MS, defined as disability level, disease severity or progression, relapse, or number of new brain lesions on magnetic resonance imaging after 96 weeks of follow-up [52]. In one prospective study, women with MS reported more pronounced symptoms during the pill-free withdrawal week in each cycle of COCs, potentially supporting extended-use dosing regimens of CHC [53].

The primary safety concern of use of hormonal contraception in women with MS surrounds disease resulting immobility and resulting increased baseline VTE risk; in this setting the risk of estrogen-containing hormonal contraception may theoretically outweigh benefits (USMEC Category 3), Patients with MS who do not have paraparesis or parathesias that affect mobility can use combined hormonal contraceptives (USMEC Category 1). It is for this same concern of VTE that DMPA is a USMEC Category 2 in MS patients with decreased mobility, though it is Category 1 for all other MS patients. Progestin-only pills, subdermal implant and the LNG-IUD are USMEC Category 1 for MS patients regardless of mobility status. Depending on disease presentation, for women with MS there may be additional issues that affect contraceptive method choice, such as difficulty swallowing pills, or manual dexterity concerns that make placing vaginal rings or barrier methods difficult.

Psychiatric Disease

Concerns about the mood effects of hormonal contraception may limit patients' interest in and providers' willingness to prescribe these methods. Among healthy women initiating oral contraceptives, one-quarter will report moodiness after 3 months of use, and this side effect leads some to discontinue the method [54]. Despite concern that hormonal contraception might worsen psychiatric disease, it is safe for women with mood disorders and even therapeutic for women with premenstrual dysphoric disorder. As with AEDs, psychiatric medications must be assessed given the possibility of drug interactions.

A Patient with Depression

A 25 year-old woman with a history of major depression on citalopram currently uses condoms for contraception. Many of her friends use the oral contraceptive pill, but she is worried that hormones may worsen her mood symptoms. Is it safe for her to start hormonal contraception?

Depression and Hormonal Contraception

A relationship between hormonal contraception and depression is biologically plausible: neurotransmitters such as serotonin and norepinephrine are insufficient in women with depression and anxiety, and steroid hormones can affect the metabolism of these same neurotransmitters [55]. Older studies did link initiation of COCs with the onset of depressive symptoms however they utilized pills with higher doses of exogenous steroids than those used today [56]. The current literature investigating modern, lower-dose hormonal contraception indicates minimal effect on mood symptoms [57].

Large population-based studies do not definitively support a clinically significant relationship between hormonal contraception and mood disorders. In the United States National Longitudinal Study of Adolescent Health, sexually active women using hormonal contraception had lower mean depressive symptom scores and lower likelihood of suicide compared to women using non-hormonal or no contraception [58]. In contrast, a Danish registry study showed that women who started hormonal contraception were more likely than non-users to subsequently start an antidepressant or be diagnosed with a psychiatric disorder for the first time [59]. The absolute risk, however, was low: the rate of first antidepressant use was 2.2 per 100 woman-years in hormonal contraception users, compared to 1.7 per 100 woman-years in non-users. The same investigators analyzed the impact of hormonal contraception on incidence of suicide

attempt or suicide. The increase in absolute risk for each of these events was small (3/10,000 person-years, and 14/100,000 person-years, respectively) [60]. Despite these findings, there is not a clear causal relationship between hormonal contraception and a diagnosis of depression, a suicide attempt or suicide. Notably, these studies excluded pregnant women, and the comparison groups were never-users of hormonal contraception, rather than users of non-hormonal contraception.

These data also do not parse out the effects of hormonal contraception in sub-populations of women with pre-existing mental illness. Smaller, prospective studies of women with depression support the safety of hormonal contraception, showing that the initiation and continuation of COCs did not adversely impact on depression scores among adolescents and women who were at risk for or screened positive for depression [61–63]. While some case-control studies suggest that women with underlying mood disorders may be at greater risk for worsening mood symptoms on COCs, the majority (75%) of women with a psychiatric history experienced no deterioration in mood [64, 65].

Based on this evidence, all hormonal contraceptive methods are USMEC category 1 for women with depressive disorders. Therefore, women with mood disorders may initiate any method, though as for all patients, follow-up is recommended to assess side effects and interest in continuation.

Antidepressant Use and Hormonal Contraception

Hormonal contraceptives are metabolized by the hepatic cytochrome P450 system which can lead to drug interactions with some AEDs, which may be used in treatment of psychiatric disease. While selective serotonin reuptake inhibitors (SSRIs) do inhibit certain hepatic enzymes, pharmacokinetic studies show that they do not affect the pathway of contraceptive metabolism, CYP3A4 [66, 67]. In clinical studies, COCs did not worsen depression scores in women taking fluoxetine [68]. Similarly, hormonal contraception did not worsen depression scores, and in fact was associated with greater remission, in women with major depression who were treated with citalopram [69]. In the absence of any documented interaction, the USMEC considers all contraceptive methods to be category 1 for women taking SSRIs.

In contrast, tricyclic antidepressants and bupropion may interact with hormonal contraception. Clinically, depression response to clomipramine did not differ among users and non-users of COCs [70, 71]. However, compared to women not using contraception, women taking COCs had significantly higher serum levels of imipramine and amitriptyline [72, 73]. Given the narrow therapeutic range of tricyclic antidepressants, these pharmacokinetic data suggest an increased risk of toxicity when taken with hormonal contraception [74]. Bupropion exhibits a decrease in its serum concentration among women using oral contraceptive pills [75]. For other antidepressants, such as serotonin-norepinephrine reuptake inhibitors and monoamine oxidase inhibitors, there is no published research to guide clinical decision-making.

Premenstrual Dysphoric Disorder and Non-contraceptive Benefits of Hormonal Contraception

Premenstrual dysphoric disorder (PMDD) is a cyclic depressive disorder with symptoms that present in the late luteal phase of the menstrual cycle. Treatment of PMDD includes antidepressants and/or hormonal contraception. Monophasic oral contraceptive formulations, especially extended or continuous regimens, provide a stable dose of steroid hormones and thereby reduce cyclic mood symptoms in women who have them [76]. Drospirenone-containing oral contraception has received FDA approval for PMDD treatment. Both drospirenone and levonorgestrel-based COCs reduce premenstrual depressive symptoms in women with PMDD, although the placebo effects have been notable in these trials [77, 78]. Other forms of hormonal contraception that suppress endogenous hormone variation, such as the contraceptive implant and the injection, may also improve premenstrual mood changes but have not been investigated for this indication.

Other Psychiatric Disorders and Hormonal Contraception

Hormonal contraception for women with less common psychiatric illnesses has not been well studied. In women with bipolar disorder, psychiatric hospitalizations did not differ among those using the progestin injection, progestin IUD, copper IUD, or sterilization for contraception [79]. COCs may act as a mood stabilizer for bipolar women, reducing mood variations across the menstrual cycle [80]. Contraception has not been explicitly studied at all in women with schizophrenia and other psychotic disorders. However, pharmacokinetic data demonstrate the safety of co-administering atypical antipsychotics and hormonal contraception [81–83].

Selecting the Best Method for a Woman with a Psychiatric Disorder

Psychiatric disease appears to impact patients' choice of contraception: compared to other women, those with depressive symptoms are more likely to not use any form of contraception, or to select a less effective method [84]. Mental illness is also associated with lower contraceptive adherence and continuation [85, 86]. Unfortunately, there are few studies that investigate the use of contraception in women with psychiatric disease. What limited data exist support the safety of hormonal contraception in women with mood disorders and those using antidepressants and atypical antipsychotics. Though COCs are the most studied form of contraception in women with psychiatric disease, other methods may be equally, if not more appropriate, options to consider based on a patient's priorities and preferences. Long-acting reversible contraception methods (the implant, LNG IUD, and copper IUD) have the highest efficacy compared to other reversible methods, and the American College of Obstetricians and Gynecologists and the American Academy of Pediatrics recommend these methods as first-line contraception for adults and adolescents alike [87, 88]. Figure 2 provides guidance on selection of an appropriate contraceptive method for women with psychiatric disease.

A Patient with Depression: Case Summary

Neither the patient's depression diagnosis nor her treatment with an SSRI limits her contraceptive options. She would be eligible to try the oral contraceptive pill should she choose. Thorough contraceptive counseling would include a review of all available contraceptive methods, including long-acting reversible options such as the implant and IUD, which have the highest effectiveness.

Summary

- Addressing appropriate contraceptive need and method choice for patients with neurologic or psychiatric disease prevents sequelae of unplanned pregnancy, including high-risk pregnancy in the setting of poorly controlled disease or potential exposure to teratogenic medications.
- There are no contraindications for use of any progestin-only method or IUD in women with any type of migraine. However, combined hormonal contraception is contraindicated in women with aura as part of their migraine disease due to increased risk of stroke.
- Continuous use of hormonal contraception may be used to treat migraine disease in women who have cyclic headache symptoms.
- For women with epilepsy there are known complex interactions between hormones, seizures, and medicines used to treat epilepsy. Despite these potential interactions hormonal methods are generally regarded as safe, and selection of method(s) based on AED type will provide reliable efficacy.

Fig. 2 Recommending a contraceptive method for women with psychiatric disease

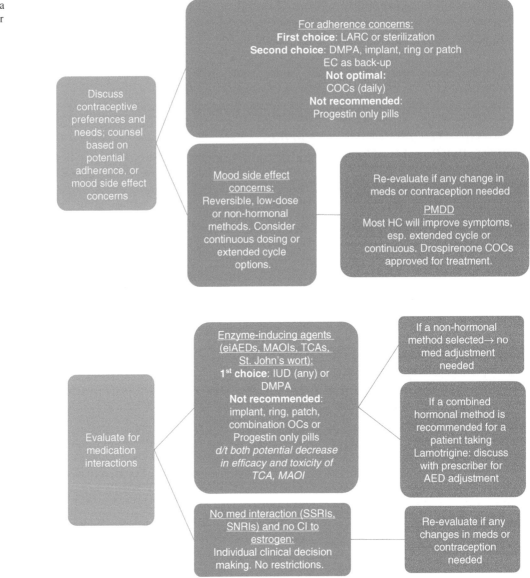

For adherence concerns:
First choice: LARC or sterilization
Second choice: DMPA, implant, ring or patch
EC as back-up
Not optimal:
COCs (daily)
Not recommended:
Progestin only pills

Discuss contraceptive preferences and needs; counsel based on potential adherence, or mood side effect concerns

Mood side effect concerns:
Reversible, low-dose or non-hormonal methods. Consider continuous dosing or extended cycle options.

Re-evaluate if any change in meds or contraception needed
PMDD
Most HC will improve symptoms, esp. extended cycle or continuous. Drospirenone COCs approved for treatment.

Evaluate for medication interactions

Enzyme-inducing agents (eiAEDs, MAOIs, TCAs, St. John's wort):
1st choice: IUD (any) or DMPA
Not recommended: implant, ring, patch, combination OCs or Progestin only pills
d/t both potential decrease in efficacy and toxicity of TCA, MAOI

If a non-hormonal method selected→ no med adjustment needed

If a combined hormonal method is recommended for a patient taking Lamotrigine: discuss with prescriber for AED adjustment

No med interaction (SSRIs, SNRIs) and no CI to estrogen:
Individual clinical decision making. No restrictions.

Re-evaluate if any changes in meds or contraception needed

- For women with depression and bipolar disorder, hormonal contraception is safe to use; for women with PMDD, it can be therapeutic. SSRIs and atypical antipsychotics may be used concurrently with hormonal contraception.

References

1. Trussell J. Contraceptive failure in the United States. Contraception. 2011;83:397–404.
2. Curtis K, Peipert J. Long-acting reversible contraception. N Engl J Med. 2017;376:461–8.
3. Curtis K, Tepper N, Jatlaoui T, Berry-Bibee E, Horton L, Zapata L, et al. U.S. medical eligibility criteria for contraceptive use, 2016. MMWR Recomm Rep. 2016;65:1–104.
4. Lipton R, Bigal M. Migraine: epidemiology, impact, and risk factors for progression. Headache. 2005;45:S3–S13.
5. Buse D, Manack A, Fanning K, et al. Chronic migraine prevalence, disability, and sociodemographic factors: results from the American Migraine Prevalence and Prevention Study. Headache. 2012;52:1456–70.
6. Faubion S, Casey P, Shuster L. Hormonal contraception and migraine: clinical considerations. Curr Pain Headache Rep. 2012;16:461–6.
7. Daniels K, Daugherty J, Jones J, Mosher W. Current contraceptive use and variation by selected characteristics among women aged 15–44: United States, 2011–2013. Natl Health Stat Rep. 2015;86:1–14.
8. Etminan M, Takkouche B, Isorna F, Samii A. Risks of ischaemic stroke in people with migraine: systematic review and meta-analysis of observational studies. BMJ. 2005;330:63.
9. Tepper N, Whiteman M, Zapata L, Marchbanks P, Curtis K. Safety of hormonal contraceptives among women with migraine: a systematic review. Contraception. 2016;94:630–40.

10. Fazio G, Ferrara F, Barbaro G, Alessandro G, Ferrro G, Novo G, et al. Prothrombotic effects of contraceptives. Curr Pharm Des. 2010;16:3490–6.

11. Bousser M, Conard J, Kittner S, de Lignieres B, MacGregor E, Massiou H, et al. Recommendations of the risk of ischaemic stroke associated with use of combined oral contraceptives and hormone replacement therapy in women with migraine. The International Headache Society Task Force on Combined Oral Contraceptives & Hormone Replacement Therapy. Cephalalgia. 2000;20:155–6.

12. Lidegaard O, Lokkegaard E, Jensen A, Skovlund C, Keiding N. Thrombotic stroke and myocardial infarction with hormonal contraception. N Engl J Med. 2012;366:2257–66.

13. Champaloux S, Tepper N, Monsour M, Curtis K, Whiteman M, Marchbanks P, et al. Use of combined hormonal contraceptives among women with migraines and risk of ischemic stroke. Am J Obstet Gynecol. 2017;216:489.e1–7.

14. Russell M, Rasmussen B, Fenger K, Olesen J. Migraine without aura and migraine with aura are distinct clinical entities: a study of four hundred and eight-four male and female migraineurs from the general population. Cephalalgia. 1996;16:239–45.

15. Kurth T, Chabriat H, Bousser M. Migraine and stroke: a complex association with clinical implications. Lancet Neurol. 2012;11:92–100.

16. Tepper N, Whiteman M, Marchbanks P, James A, Curtis K. Progestin-only contraception and thromboembolism: a systematic review. Contraception. 2016;94:678–700.

17. Rosenberg M, Waugh M. Oral contraceptive discontinuation: a prospective evaluation of frequency and reasons. Am J Obstet Gynecol. 1998;179:577–82.

18. Loder E, Buse D, Golub J. Headache and combination estrogen-progestin oral contraceptives: integrating evidence, guidelines, and clinical practice. Headache. 2005;45:224–31.

19. Berger G, Edelman D, Talwar P. The probability of side effects with ovral, norinyl 1/50 and norlestrin. Contraception. 1979;20:447–53.

20. Martin V, Behbehani M. Ovarian hormones and migraine headache: understanding mechanisms and pathogenesis—part 1. Headache. 2006;46:3–23.

21. Loder E, Rizzoli P, Golub J. Hormonal management of migraine associated with menses and the menopause: a clinical review. Headache. 2007;47:329–40.

22. MacGregor A. Migraine associated with menstruation. Funct Neurol. 2000;15:143–5.

23. Hatcher R, Trussell J, Nelson A, Cates W, Kowal D, Policar M. Contraceptive technology. 20th ed. Atlanta: Bridging the Gap Communications; 2011.

24. Calhoun A, Ford S, Pruitt A. The impact of extended-cycle vaginal ring contraception on migraine aura: a retrospective case series. Headache. 2012;52:1246–53.

25. Larsson-Cohn U, Lundberg P. Headache and treatment with oral contraceptives. Acta Neurol Scand. 1970;46:267–78.

26. De Leo V, Scolaro V, Musacchio M, Di Sabatino A, Morgante G, Cianci A. Combined oral contraceptives in women with menstrual migraine without aura. Fertil Steril. 2011;96:917–20.

27. Sulak P, Willis S, Kuehl T, Coffee A, Clark J. Headaches and oral contraceptives: impact of eliminating the standard 7-day placebo interval. Headache. 2007;47:27–37.

28. Harden C, Pennell P. Neuroendocrine considerations in the treatment of men and women with epilepsy. Lancet Neurol. 2013;12:72–83.

29. Pennell P, Davis A. Selecting contraception for women treated with antiepileptic drugs. In: Klein A, Angela O'Neal M, Scifres C, Waters JFR, Waters JH, editors. Neurological illness in pregnancy: principles and practice. 1st ed: Wiley; 2016. p. 110–21.

30. Vessey M, Painter R, Yeates D. Oral contraception and epilepsy: findings in a large cohort study. Contraception. 2002;66:77–9.

31. Harden C, Leppik I. Optimizing therapy of seizures in women who use oral contraceptives. Neurology. 2006;67:s56–8.

32. Herzog A, Mandle H, Cahill K, Fowler K, Houser W. Differential impact of contraceptive methods on seizures varies by anti-epileptic drug category: findings of the epilepsy birth control registry. Epilepsy Behav. 2016;60:112–7.

33. Davis A, Saadatmand H, Pack A. Women with epilepsy initiating a progestin IUD: a prospective pilot study of safety and acceptability. Epilepsia. 2016;57:1143–8.

34. Dutton C, Foldvary-Shafer N. Contraception in women with epilepsy: pharmacokinetic interactions, contraceptive options and management. Int Rev Neurobiol. 2008;83:113–34.

35. Davis A, Westhoff C, Stanczyk F. Carbamazepine co-administration with an oral contraceptive: effects on steroid pharmacokinetics, ovulation and bleeding. Epilepsia. 2011;52:243–7.

36. Lazorwitz A, Swartz M, Davis A, Guihai M. The effect of carbamazepine on etonogestrel concentrations among contraceptive implant users. Contraception. 2016;94:571–7.

37. Curtis K, Tepper N, Jatlaoui T, Berry-Bibee E, Horton L, Zapata L, et al. U.S. medical eligibility criteria for contraceptive use, 2016. MMWR Recomm Rep. 2016;65:48.

38. U.S. Food and Drug Administration. FDA Drug Safety Communication: updated information about the risk of blood clots in women taking brith control pills containing drospirenone. 2011. Available from: http://www.fda.gov/drugs/drugsafety/ucm299305. htm.

39. World Health Organization Collaborative Study of Cardiovascular Disease and Steroid Hormone Contraception. Cardiovascular disease and use of oral and injectable progestogen-only contraceptives and combined injectable contraceptives: Results of an international, multicenter, case-control study. Contraception. 1998;57:315–24.

40. Heinemann L, Assmann A, DoMinh T, Garb E. Oral progestogen only contraceptives and cardiovascular risk: results from the transnational study on oral contraceptives and the health of young women. Eur J Contracept Reprod Health Care. 1999;4:67–73.

41. Vasilakis C, Jick H, del Mar Melero-Montes M. Risk of idiopathic venous thromboembolism in users of progestagens alone. Lancet. 1999;354:1610–1.

42. Bergendal A, Persson I, Odeberg J, Sundstrom A, Holmstrom M, Schulman S, et al. Obstet Gynecol. 2014;124:600–9.

43. Mantha S, Karp R, Raghavan V, Terrin N, Bauer K, Zwicker J. Assessing the risk of venous thromboembolic events in women taking progestin-only contraception: a meta-analysis. BMJ. 2012;345:e4944.

44. Bove R, Alwan S, Friedman J, Hellwig K, Houtchens M, Koren G, et al. Management of multiple sclerosis during pregnancy and the reproductive years: a systematic review. Obstet Gynecol. 2014;124:1157–68.

45. Houtchens M, Kolb C. Multiple sclerosis and pregnancy: therapeutic considerations. J Neurol. 2013;260:1202–4.

46. Fragoso Y, Adoni T, Alves-Leon S, Azambuja NJ, Barreira A, Brooks J, et al. Long-term effects of exposure to disease-modifying drugs in the offspring of mothers with multiple sclerosis: a retrospective chart review. CNS Drugs. 2013;27:955–61.

47. Sahin L, Nallani S, Tassinari M. Medication use in pregnancy and the pregnancy and lactation labeling rule. Clin Pharmacol Ther. 2016;100:23–5.

48. Vukusic S, Marignier R. Multiple sclerosis and pregnancy in the 'treatment era. Nat Rev Neurol. 2015;11:280–9.

49. David O, Ocwieja M, Meise K, Emotte C, Jakab A, Wemer J, et al. Pharmacokinetics of fingolimod (FTY720) and a combined oral contraceptive coadministered in healthy women: drug-drug interaction study results. Int J Clin Pharmacol Ther. 2012;50:540–4.

50. Villard-Mackintosh L, Vessey M. Oral contraceptives and reproductive factors in multiple sclerosis incidence. Contraception. 1993;47:161–8.

51. Thorogood M, Hannaford P. The influence of oral contraceptives on the risk of multiple sclerosis. Br J Obstet Gynecol. 1998;105:1296–9.

52. Zapata L, Oduyebo T, Whiteman M, Houtchens M, Marchbanks P, Curtis K. Contraceptive use among women with multiple sclerosis: a systematic review. Contraception. 2016;94:612–20.

53. Kempe P, Hammar M, Brynhildsen J. Symptoms of multiple sclerosis during use of combined hormonal contraception. Eur J Obstet Gynecol Reprod Biol. 2015;19:1–4.

54. Westhoff C, Heartwell S, Edwards S, Zieman M, Stuart G, Cwiak C, et al. Oral contraceptive discontinuation: do side effects matter? Am J Obstet Gynecol. 2007;196:412.e1–7.

55. Parry B, Rush A. Oral contraceptives and depressive symptomatology: biologic mechanisms. Compr Psychiatry. 1979;20:347–58.

56. Herzberg B, Johnson A, Brown S. Depressive symptoms and oral contraceptives. Br Med J. 1970;4:142–5.

57. Pagano H, Zapata L, Berry-Bibee E, Nanda K, Curtis K. Safety of hormonal contraception and intrauterine devices among women with depressive and bipolar disorders: a systematic review. Contraception. 2016;94(6):641–9.

58. Keyes K, Cheslack-Postava K, Westhoff C, Heim C, Haloossim M, Walsh K, et al. Association of hormonal contraceptive use with reduced levels of depressive symptoms: a national study of sexually active women in the United States. Am J Epidemiol. 2013;178:1378–88.

59. Skovlund C, Morch L, Kessing L, Lidegaard O. Association of hormonal contraception with depression. JAMA Psychiat. 2016;73:1154–62.

60. Skovlund C, Morch L, Kessing L, Lange T, Lidegaard O. Association of hormonal contraception with suicide attempts and suicides. AJP Adv. 2017. https://doi.org/10.1176/appiajp201717060616.

61. O'Connell K, Davis A, Kerns J. Oral contraceptives: side effects and depression in adolescent girls. Contraception. 2007;75:299–304.

62. Duke J, Sibbritt D, Young A. Is there an association between the use of oral contraception and depressive symptoms in young Australian women? Contraception. 2007;75:27–31.

63. Herzberg B, Draper K, Johnson A, Nicol G. Oral contraceptives, depression, and libido. Br Med J. 1971;3:495–500.

64. Joffe H, Cohen L, Harlow B. Impact of oral contraceptive pill use on premenstrual mood: predictors of improvement and deterioration. Am J Obstet Gynecol. 2003;189:1523–30.

65. Segebladh B, Borgstrom A, Odlind V, Bixo M, Sundstrom-Poromaa I. Prevalence of psychiatric disorders and premenstrual dysphoric symptoms in patients with experience of adverse mood during treatment with combined oral contraceptives. Contraception. 2009;79:50–5.

66. Bergstrom R, Goldberg M, Cerimele B, Hatcher B. Assessment of the potential for a pharmacokinetic interaction between fluoxetine and terfenadine. Clin Pharmacol Ther. 1997;62:643–51.

67. Chen G, Lee R, Hojer A, Buchbjerg J, Serenko M, Zhao Z. Pharmacokinetic drug interactions involving vortioxetine (Lu AA21004), a multimodal antidepressant. Clin Drug Investig. 2013;33:727–36.

68. Koke S, Brown E, Miner C. Safety and efficacy of fluoxetine in patients who receive oral contraceptive therapy. Obstet Gynecol. 2002;187:551–5.

69. Kornstein S, Toups M, Rush A, Wisniewski S, Thase M, Luther J, et al. Do menopausal status and use of hormone therapy affect antidepressant treatment response? Findings from the sequenced treatment alternatives to relieve depression (STAR*D) study. J Women's Health. 2013;22:121–31.

70. Beaumont G. Drug interactions with clomipramine (Anafranil). J Int Med Res. 1973;1:480–4.

71. Gringras M, Beaumont G, Grieve A. Clomipramine and oral contraceptives: an interaction study–clinical findings. J Int Med Res. 1980;8:76–80.

72. Abernethy D, Greenblatt D, Shader R. Imipramine disposition in users of oral contraceptive steroids. Clin Pharmacol Ther. 1984;35:792–7.

73. Edelbroek P, Zitman F, Knoppert-van der Klein E, van Putten P, de Wolff F. Therapeutic drug monitoring of amitriptyline: impact of age, smoking and contraceptives on drug and metabolite levels in bulimic women. Clin Chim Acta. 1987;165:177–87.

74. Berry-Bibee E, Kim M, Simmons K, Tepper N, Riley H, Pagano H, et al. Drug interactions between hormonal contraceptives and psychotropic drugs: a systematic review. Contraception. 2016;94:650–67.

75. Palovaara S, Pelkonen O, Uusitalo J, Lundgren S, Laine K. Inhibition of cytochrome P450 2B6 activity by hormone replacement therapy and oral contraceptive as measured by bupropion hydroxylation. Clin Pharmacol Ther. 2003;74:326–33.

76. Edelman A, Micks E, Gallo M, Jensen J, Grimes D. Continuous or extended cycle vs. cyclic use of combined hormonal contraceptives for contraception. Cochrane Database Syst Rev. 2014;7:CD004695.

77. Lopez L, Kaptein A, Helmerhorst F. Oral contraceptives containing drospirenone for premenstrual syndrome. Cochrane Database Syst Rev. 2012;2:CD006586.

78. Freeman E, Halbreich U, Grubb G, Rapkin A, Skouby S, Smith L, et al. An overview of four studies of a continuous oral contraceptive (levonorgestrel 90 mcg/ethinyl estradiol 20 mcg) on premenstrual dysphoric disorder and premenstrual syndrome. Contraception. 2012;85(5):437–45.

79. Berenson A, Asem H, Tan A, Wilkinson G. Continuation rates and complications of intrauterine contraception in women diagnosed with bipolar disorder. Obstet Gynecol. 2011;118:1331–6.

80. Rasgon N, Bauer M, Glenn T, Elman S, Whybrow P. Menstrual cycle related mood changes in women with bipolar disorder. Bipolar Disord. 2003;5:48–52.

81. Chiu Y, Ereshefsky L, Preskorn S, Poola N, Loebel A. Lurasidone drug–drug interaction studies: a comprehensive review. Drug Metabol Drug Interact. 2014;29:191–202.

82. Muirhead G, Harness J, Holt P, Oliver S, Anziano R. Ziprasidone and the pharmacokinetics of a combined oral contraceptive. Clin Pharmacol. 2000;49:49S–56S.

83. Haslemo T, Refsum H, Molden E. The effect of ethinylestradiol-containing contraceptives on the serum concentration of olanzapine and N-desmethyl olanzapine. Clin Pharmacol. 2011;71:611–6155.

84. Garbers S, Correa N, Tobier N, Blust S, Chiasson M. Association between symptoms of depression and contraceptive method choices among low-income women at urban reproductive health centers. Matern Child Health J. 2010;14:102–9.

85. Hall K, White K, Rickert V, Reame N, Westhoff C. Influence of depressed mood and psychological stress symptoms on perceived oral contraceptive side effects and discontinuation in young minority women. Contraception. 2012;86:518–25.

86. Callegari L, Zhao X, Nelson K, Borerro S. Contraceptive adherence among women veterans with mental illness and substance use disorder. Contraception. 2015;91:386–92.

87. American College of Obstetricians and Gynecologists. Increasing use of contraceptive implants and intrauterine devices to reduce unintended pregnancy. ACOG Committee Opinion No. 450. Obstet Gynecol. 2009;14:1434–8.

88. Ott M, Sucato G. Contraception for adolescents. Pediatrics. 2014;134:e1244–5.

89. Davis A, Pack A, Dennis A. Contraception for women with epilepsy. In: Allen RH, Cwiak C, editors. Contraception for the medically challenging patient. New York: Springer Science+Business Media; 2014.

Neuroendocrine Disorders in Women

Alexandra J. Lovett and Whitney W. Woodmansee

Introduction

Neuroendocrine disorders can cause hormonally-mediated symptoms in patients and are most commonly due to structural lesions of the pituitary or hypothalamic region. Pituitary adenomas are the most common of these lesions and are thought to account for approximately 15% of all intracranial tumors [1, 2]. Epidemiologic studies have shown variable numbers based on the population examined, with higher prevalence rates reported in radiologic and autopsy studies due to the fact that these tumors may be clinically silent and thus under diagnosed [1, 2]. These tumors can cause symptoms due to hormonal hypersecretion, hormonal deficiency or mass effects on surrounding brain structures. Patients can present with a wide variety of hormonal, neurologic and psychiatric manifestations depending on the size and location of the lesion, as well as the type of hormonal system disrupted. Due to the location of the pituitary gland and its close proximity to the optic chiasm, patients can develop visual disturbances including diplopia and visual field deficits. Other mass effect symptoms can include headache, facial numbness, and stroke if the integrity of the internal carotid artery is compromised. Hormonal imbalance in these patients can lead to a number of clinical symptoms depending on whether they have hormonal hypersecretion or deficiency. These hormonal alterations can also lead to psychiatric (i.e. depression, anxiety, psychosis) and neurocognitive (impaired memory and executive function) symptoms. Very large sellar masses can cause mass effect on the frontal lobes, which can lead to abulia, personality change, weakness, or seizures. When sellar pathology is suspected, the evaluation should include a detailed history and physical exam, appropriate imaging of the cavernous sinus and pituitary gland as well as laboratory testing to evaluate for hormonal excess and deficiency [3].

Pituitary Adenomas and Sellar Tumors

The sellar space, located between both cavernous sinuses and behind the sphenoid sinus, contains the pituitary gland (Fig. 1). The pituitary can be the source of primary tumors and additionally is susceptible to compression by other tumors that invade the sella. There are a multitude of sellar and parasellar lesions that can arise, with the most common being pituitary adenomas but with other possibilities including but not limited to meningiomas, craniopharyngiomas, chordomas, germ cell tumors, neuronal tumors, infiltrative lesions such as sarcoidosis, and vascular lesions such as internal carotid artery (ICA) aneurysms [4].

When pituitary tumors or other sellar lesions grow, they can produce damaging mass effects by applying pressure on surrounding structures. For example, invasion of the tumor into the suprasellar region may cause compression of the optic chiasm leading to visual loss. Mass effect on the optic chiasm classically causes a bitemporal hemianopia but can cause a quadrantopia depending on the path of tumor expansion. Depending on the growth trajectory, pituitary tumors can cause headaches secondary to either to stretching of pain-sensitive structures or increased intracranial pressure, cranial neuropathies (specifically of cranial nerves III, IV, V1, V2, and VI which travel within the cavernous sinus), stenosis of the internal carotid arteries, or impingement of the infundibulum and optic chiasm.

Without a mass lesion, pituitary enlargement can also occur in the physiologic setting. In pituitary hyperplasia, a known stimulus causes proliferation of a certain pituitary cell type, which typically resolves when the stimulus is removed [4, 5]. This can be physiologically driven, such as during pregnancy when prolactin-secreting cells, called lactotrophs, proliferate leading to increased prolactin produc-

A. J. Lovett
Massachusetts General Hospital, Boston, MA, USA
e-mail: ajlovett@partners.org

W. W. Woodmansee (✉)
Division of Endocrinology, Diabetes and Metabolism, University of Florida, Gainesville, FL, USA
e-mail: whitney.woodmansee@medicine.ufl.edu

© Springer Nature Switzerland AG 2019
M. A. O'Neal (ed.), *Neurology and Psychiatry of Women*, https://doi.org/10.1007/978-3-030-04245-5_5

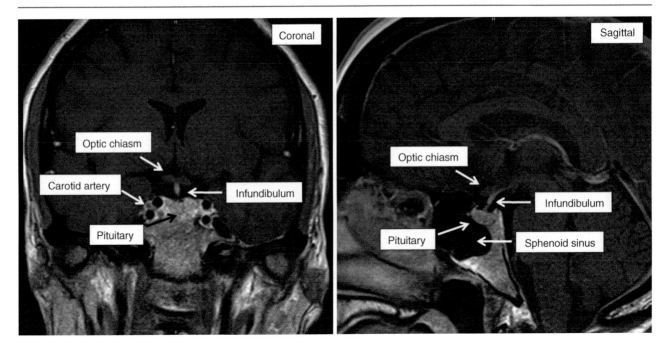

Fig. 1 Pituitary MRI images, T1 with gadolinium contrast showing normal pituitary

tion [5]. Secondary pituitary hyperplasia is uncommon but can occur when negative feedback is lacking, which occurs in end-organ dysfunction such as with primary hypothyroidism [6].

Pituitary adenomas are classified based on size, pituitary cell lineage and whether they are secretory (functional) [7]. Microadenomas are defined as less than 1 centimeter (cm) in size, whereas macroadenomas are greater than 1 cm in size. Additionally, pituitary adenomas are characterized as nonfunctioning or functioning based on whether they secrete an active hormone. They most often arise from the adenohypophysis where thyrotrophic, lactotrophic, gonadotrophic, corticotrophic, and somatotrophic hormones are secreted, with these hormones being thyroid stimulating hormone (TSH), prolactin, follicule-stimulating hormone (FSH), luteinizing hormone (LH), adrenocorticotropic hormone (ACTH), and growth hormone (GH) respectively. Lactotrope tumors secreting prolactin (prolactinomas) are thought to be the most common secretory adenoma at about 40% and occur more frequently in women compared to men [1, 8, 9].

Pituitary adenomas are relatively common and are an incidental finding in an estimated 10–15% of patients based on combined autopsy data and imaging [1, 4, 8]. They are found incidentally on imaging quite often (4–20% of computed tomography (CT) and 10–38% of magnetic resonance imaging (MRI) [8]. If not found incidentally and there are no contraindications, the ideal imaging modality for clinically suspected pituitary adenomas is a contrast-enhanced coronal and sagittal MRI to visualize the pituitary gland. All patients with newly discovered sellar/pituitary masses should undergo full clinical and laboratory evaluation assessing for mass

effects, hormonal hyperfunction and hormonal deficiencies [3, 8]. Laboratory testing should include TSH, free thyroxine (free T4), morning cortisol, prolactin, insulin-like growth factor I (IGF-I), LH, FSH, estradiol in women (E2), and testosterone (T) in men [3, 8]. Asymptomatic and non-functional pituitary incidentalomas may be monitored with serial MRIs, with more frequent imaging in macroadenomas, given that surgery may be required if there is any evidence on history, physical exam, or imaging of impending mass effect on the optic chiasm [8, 10]. In addition, macroadenomas should be serially monitored clinically and biochemically for signs of hypopituitarism [3, 8, 10]. All patients require long term management and assessment of hormonal status and tumor progression.

Prolactinomas and Hyperprolactinemia

Prolactinomas are the most common pituitary adenoma subtype and account for approximately 40% of pituitary adenomas [9, 11–13]. They are more common in women and often diagnosed in women presenting with amenorrhea/oligomenorrhea or galactorrhea, or in the setting of infertility in young women trying to conceive [9, 11–13]. Because of these symptoms prompting earlier presentation, most of the prolactinomas in premenopausal women are microadenomas. Men and postmenopausal women often present later in the course of the disease with macroadenomas. A prolactin level is often obtained in women with abnormal menses and infertility, and elevated levels of at least 100–150 mcg/L are suggestive of an underlying prolactinoma, with levels greater than 250 mcg/L suggestive of a macroprolactinoma [9, 11–13]. Hyperprolactinemia not in excess of 150 mcg/L should prompt a search for other possible etiologies, including but not limited to medication effect from dopamine antagonists, stalk effect from inflammatory or compressive lesions, or elevated levels of estrogen [9, 11–13]. Multiple medications have been associated with hyperprolactinemia, with antidepressants and antipsychotics, used for depression and other psychiatric illnesses such as schizophrenia, being the most common culprits for medication-induced hyperprolactinemia [12, 14]. Metoclopramide, commonly used as an abortive therapy for migraines as well as for gastrointestinal dysmotility, can also cause hyperprolactinemia. Although less common with the newer prolactin assays, the presence of "hook effect" should be evaluated in select cases particularly when the prolactin level is lower than expected in a large tumor [12, 14]. The hook effect occurs when high levels of prolactin cause antibody saturation in the assay causing artificially low results. Testing for hook effect, by repeating the prolactin level with sample dilution, should be considered in every patient presenting with a large pituitary macroadenoma with a normal or minimally elevated prolactin levels.

Treatment of prolactinomas is done to prevent mass effect and restore gonadal and sexual function [9, 11, 12, 15]. However, if found incidentally and there are no symptoms, close surveillance with serial imaging, visual fields, and prolactin levels may be appropriate [9, 11, 12, 15]. Medical therapy with a dopamine agonist (most commonly bromocriptine or cabergoline) is the treatment of choice for prolactinomas as these agents are highly effective at normalizing prolactin levels and decreasing tumor size. Cabergoline is the preferred agent due to higher efficacy and tolerability of the medication [12]. Medical therapy alone is often sufficient to reduce the serum level of prolactin and decrease the tumor burden. However, prolactinomas refractory to dopamine agonist therapy, patients with intolerability of medical therapy, or tumors with significant mass effect at time of diagnosis may require surgical resection or much less commonly radiation therapy, with potential side effects including hypopituitarism [16, 17].

Patients with prolactinomas who are trying to conceive or become pregnant should be closely followed given that these tumors can increase in size during pregnancy. Most women do not have symptomatic tumor growth during pregnancy (>95%), but certainly if a macroadenoma enlarges during pregnancy it can cause considerable mass effects depending on its proximity to surrounding structures. Less than 3% of microadenomas show clinically apparent enlargement with pregnancy, whereas approximately 20–30% of macroadenomas may demonstrate enlargement with pregnancy [9, 12]. Trending serum prolactin levels during pregnancy is unreliable and gadolinium should be avoiding during pregnancy making it difficult to follow these tumors with imaging.

However, progressive headaches or new visual field deficits in these patients during pregnancy should prompt a noncontrast MRI. Bromocriptine and cabergoline have been deemed safe in prior studies during pregnancy, though more safety data is available for bromocriptine [15, 18]. Despite these findings, limiting the fetal exposure to these medications is optimal, and thus it is usually recommended that medical therapy be stopped once pregnancy is achieved [12].

Patients who wish to breast-feed in the post-partum period should not be given dopamine agonists. In addition, breastfeeding usually does not appear to increase the size of these tumors. A study of prolactinomas in the setting of pregnancy and lactation demonstrated that, on MRI at 3 months postpartum, the majority of women had either decrease or stability in the size of their tumor with 9% having an increase in tumor burden [19]. Some patients may be in prolonged remission from their prolactinoma after pregnancy, with both a smaller adenoma size at diagnosis and normalization of the pituitary on post-partum MRI serving as independent predictors of remission [19].

In the setting of medication-induced hyperprolactinemia without an underlying adenoma, treatment involves stopping the offending agent if possible. Dopamine agonists are not generally recommended for drug induced hyperprolactinemia, particularly in patients on antidepressants or antipsychotic agents, as this can exacerbate psychiatric symptoms [12]. Restoration of the menstrual cycle or treatment of hypogonadism can be achieved by hormonal replacement (example, oral contraceptives in women or testosterone in men).

Cushing's Syndrome

Cushing's syndrome occurs in the setting of elevated cortisol levels from either exogenous or endogenous sources. Endogenous etiologies are divided into ACTH dependent or ACTH independent causes. Cushing's disease refers specifically to the syndrome of cortisol excess caused by an ACTH-secreting pituitary adenoma [20, 21]. Cushing's disease is at least three times more prevalent in women than in men [21]. Hypercortisolemia can be present in many other settings, including but not limited to pregnancy, depression, alcohol dependence, obesity, diabetes, physical stress, and malnutrition [20]. Signs and symptoms of Cushing's syndrome include fatigue, memory difficulties, poor concentration, menstrual irregularities, acne, pedal edema, easy bruising, poor wound healing, infertility, proximal muscle weakness, weight gain with fat deposition in the trunk and abdomen as well as the face, hirsutism, purple striae, and acanthosis nigricans. Cushing's syndrome can cause additional medical comorbidities including hypertension, hyperlipidemia, diabetes, polycystic ovary syndrome, hypercoagulability with venous thromboembolism, and osteoporosis [20–23]. Cushing's disease is associated with increased risk of cardiovascular and cerebrovascular disease as well as increased mortality [21, 24–26].

Mood disorders, such as depression and anxiety, and cognitive impairment are common in patients with Cushing's syndrome [27]. Patients can develop mental fatigue, which is often seen after performing strenuous tasks, even in the setting of disease remission, as well as deficits in memory and executive function [27]. Cognitive impairments may be subtle, but can have significant effects on quality of life and mood. Multiple studies have shown impaired quality of life in these patients which often persists even after biochemical remission [28]. Although the reason for the persistent deficits despite treatment is not entirely clear, newer studies have shown chronic changes in brain MRI's of Cushing's disease patients that do not reverse with remission and are correlated with adverse behavioral outcomes [29, 30]. Structural correlates with cognitive dysfunction have not been fully elucidated, but do correlate with cardiovascular risk [31].

The evaluation and ultimately diagnosis of Cushing's syndrome/disease is often quite laborious and can require extensive biochemical testing to confirm the diagnosis. Diagnosis involves first reviewing the patient's medication list to look for exogenous sources of steroids [20, 32]. If this is excluded, the next step in the evaluation is to confirm hypercortisolism. This can be done by performing a combination of screening tests including: at least two 24 h urine cortisol measures, an overnight 1 milligram (mg) dexamethasone suppression test, and/or at least two late night salivary cortisol measurements [20, 32]. Patients with normal test results in whom there is a high pretest probability should undergo further evaluation with an endocrinologist. They should also undergo a thorough review of their medication list, as drugs that induce or inhibit the cytochrome P450 3A4 enzyme (CYP3A4), with anti-epileptic medications being a known culprit, and drugs that increase cortisol-binding globulin (CBG) can alter results of cortisol testing. One abnormal test result should be confirmed with a subsequent evaluation.

Once hypercortisolism is confirmed, then it is important to determine whether the cause is ACTH dependent or independent by measuring ACTH levels. The direction of additional testing and imaging is based on the ACTH level. Normal or elevated ACTH levels suggest a pituitary or ectopic ACTH producing tumor and the next step would be brain imaging with a pituitary MRI. Low ACTH levels indicate a potential adrenal source for the hypercortisolism and adrenal imaging would be the initial imaging modality of choice. Additional studies are sometime indicated depending initial imaging and laboratory results and may include inferior petrosal sinus sampling (to differentiate pituitary vs ectopic source of ACTH excess production) or chest imaging (for an ectopic source) which can be expanded to full-body imaging if the chest is unrevealing [20, 32]. The treatment of choice is typically surgical resection of the ACTH-secreting tumor, followed by medical therapy or radiation as second line options [33]. Post-operatively, laboratory testing should be performed to confirm biochemical remission and then periodically or as clinically indicated to follow for long term remission, as late recurrences are not uncommon.

There are several medication options for patients who do not have biochemical remission with surgery alone. These options include medical therapy with steroidogenesis inhibitors (i.e. ketoconazole), glucocorticoid antagonists (mifepristone) or pituitary directed medications, cabergoline or pasireotide [33, 34]. Mifeprisone antagonizes the action of cortisol as well as progesterone, and can be an effective therapy. It is somewhat challenging to manage as response to therapy cannot be monitored by measuring cortisol levels. ACTH-secreting tumors may express dopamine 2 (D2) receptors, making some tumors responsive to medical therapy with cabergoline. Finally, corticotrophic tumors can express somatostatin receptors and the somatostatin receptor agonist, pasireotide, has been shown to reduce cortisol production [35] and is FDA approved for medical therapy. For persistent Cushing's disease refractory to surgical and medical therapy, pituitary radiation therapy or bilateral adrenalectomy may be considered.

Hypopituitarism

Hypopituitarism occurs when there is partial or total loss of pituitary function of the anterior and/or posterior pituitary gland (reviews see [36, 37]). Depending on the cause, hypopituitarism can present chronically after years of hormone deficiency or acutely which can require emergent management. Causes of hypopituitarism include compressive lesions such as sellar tumors (either primary or metastatic), vascular lesions such as ICA aneurysms and cavernous sinus thrombosis; ischemic necrosis of the pituitary and pituitary apoplexy; infectious disease such as tuberculosis and HIV; infiltrative/inflammatory disease such as sarcoidosis and lymphocytic hypophysitis; primary empty sella syndrome; iatrogenic via surgical destruction or radiation-induced; secondary to traumatic brain injury; hormone induced; genetic; or idiopathic. Surgical resection of a pituitary adenoma can cause hypopituitarism. Much of this is related to the size and nature of the adenoma, as well as the surgical technique and experience of the surgeon, with endoscopic surgery in a series of 80 patients documenting only a 6.3% incidence of worsened pituitary function from pre-operative baseline [38]. Somatotrophs are the most susceptible to pressure-related insults, followed by gonaotrophs with the lactotrophs being the most resilient. GH deficiency is clinically most obvious in children where it is associated with impaired linear growth and can be treated with GH therapy to optimize the final adult height [39, 40]. GH deficiency in adults is also associated with multiple comorbidities including central obesity, impaired exercise capacity, bone loss, poor quality of life, unfavorable lipid profile and increased risk of cardiovascular disease and mortality [41, 42].

Women with gonadotropin deficiency may report amenorrhea and infertility, as well as loss of libido, osteoporosis, and premature atherosclerotic disease. ACTH deficiency can be dangerous if the hypopituitarism occurs acutely and will be further discussed below. Hypotension is less problematic in chronic ACTH deficiency, given that the supply of mineralocorticoids from the renin-angiotensin-aldosterone system is intact. TSH deficiency will cause typical symptoms of hypothyroidism, which can include fatigue, weight gain, constipation, cold intolerance, and cognitive slowing. Given that TSH cannot be reliably interpreted in central hypothyroidism, the free thyroxine (T4) level must be used to guide therapy. Deficiency in prolactin in women will only be manifest in the patient who is lactating, as the symptom would be difficulty with breast feeding. In hypopituitarism, the functions of the posterior pituitary can also be affected, leading to diabetes insipidus which is caused by deficiency of anti-diuretic hormone (ADH). This will manifest with polydipsia, polyuria, and nocturia due to inability to concentrate the urine. In the acute setting if patients do not have access to free water, patients can develop life threatening hypernatremia.

Hypopituitarism is diagnosed by testing each axis with measurement of basal anterior pituitary and target organ hormone levels, specifically prolactin, FSH, LH, estradiol (women), testosterone (men), TSH, free T4, cortisol and IGF-1. The ACTH, and GH axes usually require stimulation testing to confirm the diagnosis [3, 36, 37]. Diabetes insipidus is diagnosed in the appropriate clinical setting by demonstrating inability of the patient to concentrate urine in response to the appropriate stimuli and can be confirmed by performing a water deprivation test [43].

Hypopituitarism treatment involves replacing the deficient target organ hormones. Fortunately, all of the target endocrine hormones can be replaced with the exception of prolactin. The Endocrine Society has recently published guidelines outlining strategies for optimal hormonal replacement in hypopituitarism [37]. Adrenal insufficiency should be treated with replacement glucocorticoids, and can include hydrocortisone, prednisone, cortisone or dexamethasone. Hydrocortisone is often preferred due to its shorter half life that allows more physiologic dosing throughout the day. Daily doses are variable between patients and depend on weight and how the patient feels clinically, though stress doses are needed when patients become ill or undergo surgical procedures. It is important to use the lowest possible dose of glucocorticoid replacement that controls symptoms of

adrenal insufficiency to avoid complications of over-replacement. Stress dose steroids are usually two to threefold increased for mild stress, such as an upper respiratory tract illness that is managed at home, with higher doses for severe stress such as peri-operatively or severe critical illness [37]. Steroids should be replaced prior to thyroid hormone replacement to prevent precipitation of an adrenal crisis. Patients with very mild diabetes insipidus can often drink to thirst to maintain adequate hydration but many require a synthetic analogue of vasopressin called desmopression or DDAVP.

Post-menopausal women with FSH or LH insufficiency do not require hormone replacement. Pre-menopausal women without contraindications should consider replacement therapy, often with a conjugated estrogen and progesterone, at least until at least menopause for cardiovascular benefit and prevention of osteoporosis [36, 37].

Fertility can be difficult to manage in these patients. One study done in 2006 of 19 women with hypopituitarism with gonadotropin deficiency presenting to a fertility clinic documented a 47% rate of pregnancy, with a live birth rate of 42% [44]. Patients were receiving estrogen and progesterone replacement and underwent anywhere between 1 and 11 ovulatory induction cycles [44]. All women were deficient in at least one additional axis including gonadotropin deficiency in this study, and the study suggested that deficiency in TSH, ACTH, or GH could also have negative fertility outcomes [44].

Finally, GH replacement therapy is approved for use in children and adults. GH therapy in GH deficient children improves final height [39, 40] and many studies in GH deficient adults have shown that comorbidities improve with replacement therapy [41, 42]. A discussion of risks, benefits and expectations of therapy would be indicated prior to initiation of GH replacement in adults and it is contraindicated in patients with an active malignancy or those with a growing residual pituitary adenoma.

Pituitary Apoplexy and Sheehan's Syndrome

Pituitary apoplexy is caused by ischemic or hemorrhagic necrosis of the pituitary gland, often within a pre-existing tumor, which is most commonly a macroadenoma [45]. An MRI example is shown in Fig. 2. The pre-existing adenomas are most commonly non-functioning, followed by prolactinomas and GH-secreting adenomas [45]. Other risk factors for pituitary apoplexy include cardiac or vascular surgery, iatrogenic in the setting of gonadotropin-releasing hormone (GnRH) and somatostatin analogues and dopamine agonists, hypertension, use of anticoagulant medications, diabetes mellitus, head trauma, radiation therapy, and use of oral contraceptives [45]. The mechanism is felt to be secondary to blood pressure fluctuations, hormonal stimulation of the pituitary, vascular compromise, or impaired coagulation

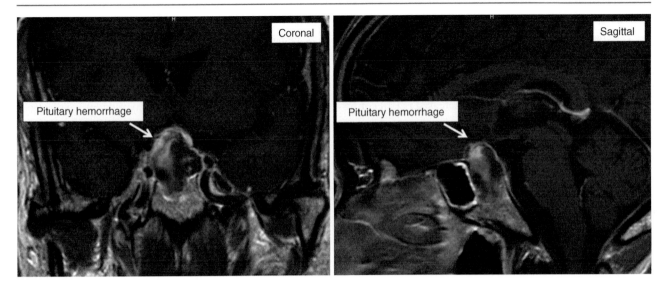

Fig. 2 Pituitary MRI images, T1 with gadolinium contrast showing pituitary apoplexy. Acute hemorrhage noted in the center of the lesion

[45]. Patients will often clinically present with severe sudden-onset headache which is often retro-orbital, nausea, emesis, ophthalmoplegia, and visual field deficit often accompanied by hormonal dysfunction in several axes, with the most clinically relevant being ACTH and ADH deficiency (often preceded by increased ADH secretion). Acute adrenal insufficiency leading to hypotension and vascular collapse can be fatal if unrecognized. Pituitary apoplexy may additionally lead to altered mental status and subsequently coma in the most clinically severe cases. Hyperprolactinemia is often present secondary to stalk compression or an underlying prolactinoma. The third cranial nerve controlling most of the extraocular muscles as well as the levator palpebrae is most commonly affected given that it is the most medial of the cranial nerves within the cavernous sinus, placing it in close proximity to the pituitary gland [45]. Urgent MRI with thin cuts through the pituitary is recommended, though computed tomography (CT) can be obtained if there is contraindication to MRI, or if the patient is experiencing rapid clinical deterioration to avoid delay in diagnosis.

Sheehan syndrome is ischemic necrosis of the adenohypophysis, which occurs postpartum following peripartum hemorrhagic shock [45, 46]. Pituitary hyperplasia is a normal occurrence during pregnancy, and in the setting of hypotension the impaired blood supply to the pituitary causes necrosis with subsequent hypopituitarism [46], though in the setting of hypercoagulability in pregnancy the etiology could also be due to thrombosis or vasospasm of the arterial supply to the pituitary [47]. Symptoms can be nonspecific and include fatigue, weakness, and anorexia, which can lead to a missed or delayed diagnosis in many cases. One study of 114 patients with Sheehan syndrome documented an average delay of 19.7 years after pregnancy to attain the diagnosis [47]. The frequency of complications at the last deliveries

included stillbirth in 17.5%, miscarriage in 1.8%, and massive uterine bleeding leading to hysterectomy in 4.4% of patients [47]. Eighty-five percent of these patients with Sheehan syndrome had amenorrhea immediately after delivery, and 42% of patients had agalactia after delivery which can be symptoms to clue the provider in to a possible diagnosis of Sheehan syndrome [47]. 55.3% of these patients had panhypopituitarism with deficiency of all hormones of the adenohypophysis, with all of the remainder of women being deficient in at least gonadotropins and GH [47].

Patients with suspected pituitary apoplexy should undergo a full set of basic laboratory studies including a complete metabolic panel, complete blood count, coagulation studies, and pituitary axis labs in addition to urgent imaging. Stress-dose steroids should be administered promptly assuming the patient has adrenal insufficiency until further confirmatory testing can be performed. Once patients are clinically stable, formal visual fields should be obtained. Management can be supportive or surgical, and early involvement of a neurosurgeon is crucial while the patient is monitored in the acute setting, with surgical management being most strongly considered in patients who are clinically unstable or have visual field deficits or neurologic symptoms [45]. Untreated pituitary apoplexy, whether peri-partum or spontaneous, can lead to significant morbidity and mortality if unrecognized.

Lymphocytic Hypophysitis

Lymphocytic hypophysitis, or autoimmune hypophysitis, is a presumed autoimmune disorder characterized by inflammation of the pituitary gland via lymphocytic infiltration, with subsequent fibrosis [48–50]. Other subtypes of primary hypophysitis include granulomatous, xanthomatous and plasmacytic [48, 50]. The type of hypophysitis is based on the histopathology as well as certain characteristics of the diseases processes. Granulomatous hypophysitis can occur together with lymphocytic hypophysitis and has been hypothesized to represent a later form of the disease, though it does not have the same epidemiology as lymphocytic hypophysitis. Granulomatous hypophysitis is characterized by pituitary infiltration of multinucleated giant cells and histiocytes as well as lymphocytes and plasma cells [48]. Lymphocytic, granulomatous and xanthomatous hypophysitis all show a higher prevalence in women compared to men [50]. Unlike other forms of hypophysitis, lymphocytic hypophysitis can involve infiltration of the infundibulum and neurohypophysis, or posterior pituitary [48, 50]. Xanthomatous hypophysitis on histopathology demonstrates cystic areas with infiltration by lipid-rich foamy histiocytes and lymphocytes, and has been theorized to be an inflammatory response to ruptured cysts [48]. Secondary hypophysitis is pituitary inflammation from a neighboring lesion or a systemic disease process, as can be seen in sarcoidosis and Langerhans cell histiocytosis, among other disorders. Medication induced hypophysitis is secondary cause of hypophysitis that has been observed more frequently in recent years as a consequence of immunomodulatory therapy for certain malignancies. Specifically, immunotherapy with immune check point inhibitors, anti-CTLA-4 and anti-PD-1, used for malignancies such as malignant melanoma have been associated with the development of hypophysitis as well as other endocrinopathies [51].

Lymphocytic hypophysitis has a higher incidence in women, as well as an association with pregnancy/postpartum and other autoimmune diseases [48, 50]. Most patients affected during pregnancy manifest with symptoms in the last month of pregnancy or the first 2 months post-partum [48]. The reason for the association with pregnancy is unknown, but has been postulated to be related to pituitary hyperplasia leading to release of pituitary antigens, as well as changes in pituitary blood flow with more blood being derived from the systemic circulation as opposed to the hypothalamic-pituitary portal circulation [48]. Patients typically present with symptoms from sellar compression (headaches, visual disturbances), hypopituitarism (corticotroph deficiency is common), diabetes insipidus (secondary to direct immune destruction or compression of the neurohypophysis or infundibulum), and hyperprolactinemia (felt to be secondary to compression of the infundibulum, destruction of lactotrophs causing prolactin release into the vasculature, compromise of dopamine production in the hypothalamus or expression of dopamine receptors, or production of stimulatory antibodies) [48–50]. The symptoms will depend on the extent of inflammation of the pituitary and the infundibulum and hormonal deficiencies.

Diagnosis involves, as previously described, laboratory evaluation of pituitary function and pituitary imaging. Because of the temporal relationship with pregnancy, it can be difficult to distinguish clinically between lymphocytic hypophysitis and Sheehan syndrome. Although infrequently utilized given poor sensitivity and poor specificity, laboratory assessment for pituitary antibodies can be performed [48, 49]. On MRI, the pituitary affected by lymphocytic hypophysitis is often symmetrically enlarged, stalk can be thickened, and the gland is often homogenously enhancing with gadolinium, which are all characteristics that can aid in differentiating between hypophysitis and an adenoma [48, 50]. When the neurohypophysis is affected, there can be loss in intrinsic T1 hyperintensity [48, 50].

Current treatment for lymphocytic hypophysitis is symptomatic, and can include surgery or radiation to minimize mass effect, immunosuppressive medications such as glucocorticoids, and always includes hormone replacement therapy for the affected pituitary axis.

Conclusion

Neuroendocrine disorders, with more specific reference to pituitary dysfunction, can lead to a complex clinical picture of hormonal dysregulation as well as neurologic sequelae from mass effect or infiltration of structures close in proximity to the pituitary gland. Recognizing pituitary pathology requires a high index of suspicion, specifically with the female patient, given that symptoms can be non-specific and thought to be from cyclical hormonal changes. Treating neuroendocrine disease in women is also more complex given consideration of fertility and the partum and post-partum period. Imaging with MRI and a laboratory evaluation to ensure integrity of the pituitary gland can aid the clinician in diagnosing the pathology in such patients, which will guide the treatment required.

References

1. Ezzat S, Asa SL, Couldwell WT, Barr CE, Dodge WE, Vance ML, McCutcheon IE. The prevalence of pituitary adenomas: a systematic review. Cancer. 2004;101(3):613–9.
2. Aflorei ED, Korbonits M. Epidemiology and etiopathogenesis of pituitary adenomas. J Neuro-Oncol. 2014;117:379–94.
3. Woodmansee WW, Carmichael J, Kelly D, Katznelson L. American Association of Clinical Endocrinologists and American College of endocrinology disease state clinical review: postoperative management following pituitary surgery. Endocr Pract. 2015;21(7):832–8.
4. Bresson D, Herman P, Polivka M, Froelich S. Sellar lesions/pathology. Otolaryngol Clin N Am. 2016;29(1):63–93.
5. Horvath E, Kovacs K, Scheithauer BW. Pituitary hyperplasia. Pituitary. 1999;1(3–4):169–79.

6. Joshi AS, Woolf PD. Pituitary hyperplasia secondary to primary hypothyroidism: a case report and review of the literature. Pituitary. 2005;8(2):99–103.

7. Lopes MBS. The 2017 World Health Organization classification of tumors of the pituitary gland: a summary. Acta Neuropathol. 2017;134(4):521–35.

8. Freda PU, Beckers AM, Katznelson L, Molitch ME, Montori VM, Post KD, et al. Pituitary incidentaloma: an endocrine society clinical practice guideline. J Clin Endocrinol Metab. 2011;96(4):894–904.

9. Casaneuva FF, Molitch ME, Schlechte JA, Abs R, Bonert V, Bronstein MD, et al. Guidelines of the Pituitary Society for the diagnosis and management of prolactinomas. Clin Endocrinol. 2006;65(2):265–73.

10. Orija IB, Weil RJ, Hamrahian AH. Pituitary incidentaloma. Best Pract Res Clin Endocrinol Metab. 2012;26(1):47–68.

11. Klibanski A. Prolactinomas. New Engl J Med. 2010;362:1219–26.

12. Melmed S, Casanueva FF, Hoffman AR, Kleinberg DL, Montori VM, Schlechte JA, Wass JAH. Diagnosis and treatment of hyper-prolactinemia: an Endocrine Society clinical practice guideline. J Clin Endocrinol Metab. 2011;96(2):273–88.

13. Wong A, Eloy JA, Couldwell WT, Liu JK. Update on prolactino-mas. Part 1: clinical manifestations and diagnostic challenges. J Clin Neurosci. 2015;22:1562–7.

14. Vilar L, Abucham J, Albuquerque JL, Araujo LA, Azevedo MF, Boguszewski CL, Casulari LA, Cunha Neto MBC, Czepielewski MA, Duarte FHG, Faria MDS, Gadelha MR, Garmes HM, Glezer A, Gurgel MH, Jallad RS, Martins M, Miranda PAC, Montenegro RM, Musolino NRC, Naves LA, Ribeiro-Oliveira Júnior A, Silva CMS, Vieceeli C, Bronstein MD. Controversial issues in the management of hyperprolactinemia and prolactinomas – an overview by the Neuroendocrinology Department of the Brazilian Society of Endocrinology and Metabolism. Arch Endocrinol Metab. 2018;62(2):236–63.

15. Wong A, Eloy JA, Couldwell WT, Liu JK. Update on prolactino-mas. Part 2: treatment and management strategies. J Clin Neurosci. 2015;22:1568–74.

16. Molitch ME. Pharmacologic resistance in prolactinoma patients. Pituitary. 2005;8:43–52.

17. Smith TR, Hulou MM, Huang KT, Gokoglu A, Cote DJ, Woodmansee WW, Laws ER. Current indications for the surgical treatment of prolactinomas. J Clin Neurosci. 2015;22:1785–91.

18. Maiter D. Prolactinoma and pregnancy: from the wish of concep-tion to lactation. Ann Endocrinol (Paris). 2016;77(2):128–34.

19. Domingue ME, Devuyst F, Alexopoulou O, Corvilain B, Maiter D. Outcome of prolactinoma after pregnancy and lactation: a study on 73 patients. Clin Endocrinol. 2014;80(5):642–8.

20. Nieman LK, Biller BM, Findling JW, Newell-Price J, Savage MO, Stewart PM, Montori VM. The diagnosis of Cushing's syndrome: an endocrine society clinical practice guideline. J Clin Endocrinol Metab. 2008;93(5):1526–40.

21. Pivonello R, De Leo M, Cozzolino A, Colao A. The treatment of Cushing's disease. Endocr Rev. 2015;36(4):385–486.

22. Van der Pas R, Leebeek FW, Hofland LJ, de Herder WW, Feelders RA. Hypercoagulability in Cushing's syndrome: prevalence, patho-genesis, and treatment. Clin Endocrinol. 2013;78(4):481–8.

23. Sharma ST, Nieman LK, Feelders RA. Comorbidities in Cushing's disease. Pituitary. 2015;18:188–94.

24. Webb SM, Mo D, Lamberts SW, Melmed S, Cavagnini F, Pecori Giraldi F, Strasburger CJ, Zimmermann AG, Woodmansee WW, International HypoCCS Advisory Board. Metabolic, cardiovas-cular, and cerebrovascular outcomes in growth hormone-deficient subjects with previous Cushing's disease or non-functioning pitu-itary adenoma. J Clin Endocrinol Metab. 2010;95(2):630–8.

25. Dekkers OM, Biermasz NR, Pereira AM, Roelfsema F, van Aken MO, Voormolen JH, Romijn JA. Mortality in patients treated for Cushing's disease is increased, compared with patients treated for

26. Van Haalen FM, Broersen LH, Jorgensen JO, Pereira AM, Dekkers OM. Management of endocrine disease: mortality remains increased in Cushing's disease despite biochemical remission: a systematic review and meta-analysis. Eur J Endocrinol. 2015;172(4):R143–9.

27. Papakokkinou E, Johansson B, Berglund P, Ragnarsson O. Mental fatigue and executive dysfunction in patients with Cushing's syn-drome in remission. Behav Neurol. 2015;2015:173653.

28. Santos A, Crespo I, Aulinas A, Resmini E, Valassi E, Webb SM. Quality of life in Cushing's syndrome. Pituitary. 2015;18(2):195–200.

29. Pires P, Santos A, Vives-Gilabert Y, Webb SM, Sainz-Ruiz A, Resmini E, Crespo I, de Juan-Delago M, Gómez-Anson B. White matter alterations in the brains of patients with active, remitted, and cured Cushing syndrome: a DTI study. AJNR Am J Neuroradiol. 2015;36(6):1043–8.

30. Andela CD, van Haalen FM, Ragnarsson O, Papakokkinou E, Johannsson G, Santos A, Webb SM, Biermasz NR, van der Wee NJ, Pereira AM. Mechanisms in endocrinology: Cushing's syndrome causes irreversible effects on the human brain: a systematic review of structural and functional magnetic resonance imaging studies. Eur J Endocrinol. 2015;173(1):R1–14.

31. Santos A, Resmini E, Gómez-Ansón B, Crespo I, Granell E, Valassi E, Pires P, Vives-Gilabert Y, Martínez-Momblán MA, de Juan M, Mataró M, Webb SM. Cardiovascular risk and white matter lesions after endocrine control of Cushing's syndrome. Eur J Endocrinol. 2015;173(6):765–75.

32. Loriaux DL. Diagnosis and differential diagnosis of Cushing's syn-drome. N Engl J Med. 2017;376(15):1451–9.

33. Nieman LK, Biller BM, Findling JW, Murad MH, Newell-Price J, Savage MO, Tabarin A. Treatment of Cushing's syndrome: an endocrine society clinical practice guideline. J Clin Endocrinol Metab. 2015;100(8):2807–31.

34. Nieman LK. Update in the medical therapy of Cushing's disease. Curr Opin Endocrinol Diabetes Obes. 2013;20(4):330–4.

35. Colao AM, Petersenn S, Newell-Price J, Findling JW, Gu F, Maldonado M, Schoenherr U, Mills D, Salgado LR. Biller BKM for the Pasireotide B2305 Study Group. A 12 month phase 3 study of pasireotide in Cushing's disease. N Engl J Med. 2012;366:914–24.

36. Kim SY. Diagnosis and treatment of hypopituitarism. Endocrinol Metab (Seoul). 2015;30(4):443–55.

37. Fleseriu M, Hashim IA, Karavitaki N, Melmed S, Murad MH, Salvatori R, et al. Hormonal replacement in hypopituitarism in adults: an endocrine society clinical practice guideline. J Clin Endocrinol Metab. 2016;101(11):3888–921.

38. Laws ER, Iuliano SL, Cote DJ, Woodmansee W, Hsu L, Cho CH. A Benchmark for preservation of normal pituitary function after endoscopic transsphenoidal surgery for pituitary macroadenomas. World Neurosurg. 2016;91:371–5.

39. Richmond E, Rogol AD. Treatment of growth hormone deficiency in children, adolescents and at the transitional age. Best Pract Res Clin Endocrinol Metab. 2016;30(6):749–55.

40. Pfäffle R. Hormone replacement therapy in children: the use of growth hormone and IGF-I. Best Pract Res Clin Endocrinol Metab. 2015;29(3):339–52.

41. Molitch ME, Clemmons DR, Malozowski S, Merriam GR, Vance ML, Endocrine Society. Evaluation and treatment of adult growth hormone deficiency: an Endocrine Society clinical practice guide-line. J Clin Endocrinol Metab. 2011;96(6):1587–609.

42. Jorgensen JOL, Juul A. Therapy of endocrine disease: growth hor-mone replacement therapy in adults: 30 years of personal clinical experience. Eur J Endocrinol. 2018;179(1):R47–56.

43. Leroy C, Karrouz W, Douillard C, Cao CD, Cortet C, Wemeau JL, Vantyghem MC. Diabetes insipidus. Ann Endocrinol. 2013;74:496–507.

44. Hall R, Manski-Nankervis J, Goni N, Davies MC, Conway GS. Fertility outcomes in women with hypopituitarism. Clin Endocrinol. 2006;65(1):71–4.

45. Capatina C, Inder W, Karavitaki N, Wass JA. Management of endocrine disease: pituitary tumour apoplexy. Eur J Endocrinol. 2015;172(5):R179–90.

46. Karaca Z, Laway BA, Dokmetas HS, Atmaca H, Kelestimur F. Sheehan syndrome. Nat Rev Dis Prim. 2016;2:16092.

47. Diri H, Tanriverdi F, Karaca Z, Senol S, Unluhizarci K, Durak AC, et al. Extensive investigation of 114 patients with Sheehan's syndrome: a continuing disorder. Eur J Endocrinol. 2014;171(3):311–8.

48. Caturegli P, Newschaffer C, Olivi A, Pomper MG, Burger PC, Rose NR. Autoimmune hypophysitis. Endocr Rev. 2005;26(5):599–614.

49. Kyriacou A, Gnanalingham K, Kearney T. Lymphocytic hypophysitisis: modern day management with limited role for surgery. Pituitary. 2017;20(2):241–50.

50. Faje A. Hypophysitis: evaluation and management. Clin Diabetes Endocrinol. 2016;2:15.

51. Joshi MN, Whitelaw BC, Palomar MT, Wu Y, Carroll PV. Immune checkpoint inhibitor-related hypophysitis and endocrine dysfunction: clinical review. Clin Endocrinol. 2016;85(3):331–9.

Somatoform Disorders

Timothy M. Scarella

Patients who present to medical settings with health concerns and associated for which no diagnosable medical causes for their distress can be found are described as having somatoform disorders. The fifth edition of the Diagnostic and Statistical Manual of Mental Disorders (DSM5) includes four primary somatoform disorders- Illness Anxiety Disorder (IAD), Somatic Symptom Disorder (SSD), Conversion Disorder (CD), and Factitious Disorder (FD).

A Clinically Useful Framework for "Unexplained" Symptoms

Saying a symptom "no known medical cause" is problematic in discussions of patient suffering. It may covertly suggest that symptoms are feigned, exaggerated, not real, or "in the patient's head". Though some patients intentionally fake or exaggerate symptoms, it is more important to note that subjective symptoms are real *as experienced by the patient*. As objective observers, clinicians have no ability to deny that a certain symptom is experienced; the presence of symptom does not depend on the existence of a definitive explanation.

The utility of calling a symptom unexplained is limited, as saying that a symptom has no known medical cause is not equivalent to saying that there is no cause. One can imagine that many illnesses readily and reliably diagnosed today were once unknown and confidently described as medically unexplainable.

Defining a clear etiology for a symptom is certainly useful for treatment planning, but deciding that symptoms is "functional" in nature- that is, a problem with organ function rather than a definable structural or metabolic deficit-does not make the symptom less important for a patient's well-being and quality of life. Most patients present with a combination of explainable and unexplainable symptoms, and the majority of symptoms reported to general practitioners turn out to be unexplained [1, 2]. The presence and burden of symptoms predicts functional limitations and health outcomes, whether or not the symptoms are explainable [3, 4]. Such a framework helps reduce pejorative attitudes towards patient with these syndromes and helps the clinician align with the patients suffering rather than focus on the presence or absence of definable pathology.

In this chapter, the phrases "medically unexplained", "no known medical cause", and similar ones should not be understood as saying that no pathology exists, but rather that the cause of symptoms is not known.

Somatic Symptom Disorder

The hallmark of SSD is the presence of one or more symptoms that cause significant distress or disruption to a person's life. There are significantly distressing thoughts about symptoms, elevated anxiety regarding health or the symptoms, and/or maladaptive behaviors related to the symptoms or associated health concerns [5]. Importantly, DSM-5 does not include a requirement that the symptom be medically unexplained.

This distinction is important, as traditionally, diagnostic criteria for somatoform disorders emphasized that symptoms were medically unexplainable and of a presumed psychologic origin [6]. This created diagnostic confusion with functional syndromes defined by positive criteria. For example, irritable bowel syndrome (IBS) involves difficulty with recurrent abdominal pain and diarrhea or constipation, and is diagnosed with validated positive criteria despite no clear "medical cause" for this "functional illness" [7].

The DSM-5 criteria refocus assessment from the origin and number of symptoms to the associated psychologic distress, leading to increased identification of more psychologically impaired and functionally limited patients [8, 9].

Therefore, though many symptoms involved in SSD are medically unexplained or "functional" in nature, an

T. M. Scarella (✉)
Department of Psychiatry, Beth Israel Deaconess Medical Center/Harvard Medical School, Boston, MA, USA
e-mail: tscarell@bidmc.harvard.edu

© Springer Nature Switzerland AG 2019
M. A. O'Neal (ed.), *Neurology and Psychiatry of Women*, https://doi.org/10.1007/978-3-030-04245-5_6

unexplained symptom is neither necessary nor sufficient for a diagnosis of SSD. A patient with acute leukemia may have excessive and maladaptive thoughts, affects, and behaviors related to medically explained symptoms and thus meet the definition of SSD, whereas a person with unexplained and persistent lower back pain may not. Specific functional syndromes may or may not be associated with SSD. For example, a significant association with somatization in IBS [10], interstitial cystitis [11], and chronic pelvic pain [12] has been demonstrated, but not between somatization and functional dyspepsia [13] or chronic lower back pain [14].

The descriptors "somatoform disorder", "somatization disorder", and "somatic symptom disorder" should be distinguished from the concept of "somatization". Somatization is a tendency to experience psychological distress as bodily sensations; it is a potential mechanism for a somatoform disorder, but it cannot be assumed that all "medically unexplained" symptoms are a result of displaced experience of psychologic distress.

Neuropsychologic Characteristics

Patients with SSD catastrophize bodily sensations and are prone to awareness of physiologic sensations. They are more intolerant of body sensations and more anxious about their health than others, though in both cases to lesser degrees than those with IAD [15]. While patients with somatic symptom disorders are more likely to attribute bodily sensations to disease, they are also more likely than patients with non-somatoform medical illnesses to acknowledge and emotional component to their illness [16].

The construct of Somatosensory Amplification has been proposed as a neuropsychologic framework within which to understand the marked emotional distress of SSD [17, 18]. There is attentional bias towards bodily sensations with increased focus on relatively insignificant or physiologic sensations. A disposition towards reacting to bodily sensation with fear, negative anticipatory cognitions, and catastrophization subsequently increases attentional bias towards bodily sensations in a vicious cycle that serves to amplify the sensations and their related affects. This process is mediated by connections between visceral and somatic sensory systems, prefrontal regions associated with attentional regulation and outcome expectation, and the limbic system [18].

Alexithymia (a deficiency in recognizing internal emotional experience) is associated with somatosensory amplification [18, 19], and increased alexithymia may adversely affect treatment [20]. This suggests that increased affective responses to bodily sensations may result from poor differentiation between internal affects and external sensations and/or difficulty connecting emotional states to changes in symptoms [18, 19].

Epidemiology

Rates of somatic symptom disorders in general medical settings are significant; estimates range from 9% to 38% in general practice settings [2, 21, 22], 12% in general medical settings [23] and up to 30% among referrals to neurology clinics [24]. Somatization has been associated with older age, lower socio-economic class, living in urban settings, lower educational level, and separated/divorced/widowed marital status [25, 26]. Most studies have found a significantly higher rate in women than men, though as is described below, the influence of sex on somatization is complex [27].

Somatic symptom disorders may be chronic, with around 20% of patients continuing to show symptoms at 5 years of follow-up [28]. Presence of a greater number of symptoms is associated with worsening of self-rated health through time [29].

Somatization increases utilization of medical services and associated costs independent of any other medical or psychiatric illnesses that are present, placing significant burden on the healthcare system [20, 30]. Somatoform disorders involving unexplained symptoms are a significant contributor to functional disability and lost productivity; in one study, about 20% of subjects with somatoform disorder were receiving disability benefits, a number which was sustained over 10 years [21, 31–33].

There is a well-established association between somatoform disorders and disorders of mood and anxiety [12, 21, 34, 35]. In addition to clinical studies showing high rates of co-morbidity, studies have shown that depressed mood and trait anxiety are associated with significantly increased sensation of and affective response to somatic and visceral pain [36–39]. This relationship between somatization and mood and anxiety disorders is reciprocal, as increased somatization is associated with future development of depressive and anxiety disorders [40].

Treatment

There is significant uncertainty regarding the effective treatment of somatic symptom disorders and medically unexplained symptoms [41].

Medication trials for reducing burden of medically unexplained symptoms show potential benefit for SSRIs and SNRIs [42–44], with some interval benefit over SSRIs when they are augmented with antipsychotics [45, 46]. However, the data are from relatively small studies with significant heterogeneity in the data and high rates of dropout [47]. Small studies have shown benefit with St. John's Wort, with lower rates of drop-out than antidepressants [48, 49].

The hallmark of treatment for somatic symptoms disorders are cognitive and behavioral interventions, though effect sizes are modest [50]. Individual CBT [51–58], group CBT [59–62], and behavioral therapy [63] have shown benefit for reducing burden of somatic symptoms that is sustained long-term [64]. More recent iterations of CBT incorporating mindfulness have shown mixed results [65, 66], though relatively few randomized studies have been published. Short-term psychodynamic psychotherapies have been shown to be effective in the group and individual settings [67–69].

A major barrier to the treatment of somatic symptom disorders is the reluctance of patients to engage in psychiatric treatment and high rates of drop-out, owing to patients' beliefs in the bodily nature of their symptoms. Interventions meant to be delivered in primary care settings have been developed. Studies have not demonstrated that training general practitioners in basic cognitive and behavioral interventions is beneficial, and any positive effects on symptoms are not necessarily functionally relevant [70–75]. Training general practitioners in communicating with patients with unexplained symptoms has shown mixed results in terms of improving physician and patient satisfaction with clinical encounters around unexplained symptoms [72, 76, 77].

Adding psychiatric specialist consultation to treatment centered in the primary care setting improves its efficacy, as consultation may help diagnose and manage co-morbid psychiatric illnesses and provide specific recommendations for management [78–83]. Consulting psychiatrists can confirm the diagnosis of a somatic symptom disorder and explain that the course is often chronic and relapsing. Recommendations typically include regularly scheduled brief appointments with the general practitioner that include brief physical examination with focus on any particular systems of concern to the patient, minimization of unplanned "as-needed" visits, a focus on use of objective signs to drive diagnostic testing and treatment, minimization of any diagnostic or therapeutic interventions that are not clearly indicated, and avoidance of invalidation of the patient's symptoms or suffering [81].

Illness Anxiety Disorder

The hallmark of IAD, a diagnostic entity derived from Hypochondriasis (HC) in previous editions of the DSM, is intense fear about the possibility of having or developing a serious illness. Transdiagnostically, the syndrome is often referred to as "health anxiety", a term which will be used here to incorporate the spectrum of individuals with clinically significant health-related worry. Diagnosis of IAD in DSM-5 requires preoccupation with having or acquiring a serious illness, absence of somatic symptoms (or, if present, symptoms that are only mild in severity), a high level of anxiety about health, proneness to alarm regarding health status, and either excessive health-related behaviors or maladaptive avoidance of medical settings [5].

Neuropsychologic Characteristics

There are three core components of health anxiety. The first is *disease conviction*: belief that one has a serious illness from which one cannot be dissuaded despite negative diagnostic evaluation. Often, there is one specific disease that is feared [84]. Second, there is *disease fear*: worry about developing serious illness. Finally, there is *bodily preoccupation*: heightened salience of physiologic functions, benign bodily sensations and sources of discomfort, and physical limitations. These are subjected to intense scrutiny with the goal of identifying warning signs of illness [85–88].

With health anxiety, there is overestimation of probability of catastrophic and severe illnesses, as opposed to minor conditions [89–92]. They rate their global health as poorer than others with similar burdens of known medical illness [93]. Individuals with health anxiety perceive their overall health as being poor, catastrophize somatic symptoms, and believe most somatic sensations are indicative of illness [91, 93].

These characteristics are likely mediated by aberrant neural connectivity among frontal, subcortical, and limbic regions related to planning, outcome anticipation, and attention. While these are similar in some ways to other anxiety disorders, there may be a specific sensitivity to stimuli relating to bodily sensations. This leads to negative attentional bias towards and catastrophization of bodily sensations, with subsequent behavioral modifications [18, 94–96].

Maladaptive behaviors include self-examination, reassurance seeking, and research into illness and signs/symptoms of disease. Some patients may present to clinicians for reassurance frequently, but many avoid medical settings due to fear of confirming the presence of a serious illness [97]. Reassurance behaviors may not be limited to the patient's own health; for example, mothers with health anxiety report a higher burden of symptoms in their children and bring their children to the practitioners more often in comparison with mothers without health anxiety. This difference is despite only small and mostly non-significant differences in the health anxiety of their children and the children's' report of symptom burden [98].

Rates of co-morbid mood and anxiety disorders are high in HC/IAD, though a wide range of prevalence of mood and anxiety disorders has been reported [12, 99–103]. Up to 65% of individuals have at least one co-morbid psychiatric condition [12].

Epidemiology

The epidemiology of IAD as defined in DSM-5 is unclear. The point prevalence of DSM-IV HC has been reported to be 0.04–4.5% in population based studies, 0.3–8.5 of patients in general practice settings [104–109], and 12–20% of patients in specialty clinics [110, 111]. In the general population, the prevalence of clinically significant health anxiety is 2.1–13.1% [109]. Screening in psychiatric populations found 1.6–3.5% of individuals meeting criteria for HC and 19–31% with clinically significant health anxiety [109, 112–115].

Studies of the socio-demographic characteristics of patients with health anxiety have had inconsistent findings. Many, but not all, studies have found a relatively even distribution between men and women [12, 116, 117]. There have not been consistent findings of differences between HC/IAD patients and the general population in terms of age, socio-economic status, race, ethnicity, or level of education [12, 85, 89, 104, 116, 118, 119].

Health anxiety incurs significant cost for health-care systems. It is associated with higher outpatient costs, higher laboratory and procedure costs, more office visits to primary care and specialist physicians, greater number of specialists seen, increased inpatient medical hospitalizations, and increased presentations to emergency departments [93, 103, 108, 120–122]. Health anxiety also carries substantial risk of functional limitation. Populations with clinically significant health anxiety demonstrate more days of work lost, increased functional impairment, and higher rates of use of disability benefits as compared to both the general population and medical populations without health anxiety [118, 123–127].

In up to 70% of patients with DSM-IV HC, the diagnosis persists in long term follow-up [103, 118, 128–131]. Poorer outcomes are associated with more severe illness, but presence of co-morbid psychiatric illness has not been shown to be a significant factor in remission status [118, 129–133]. When the onset is in childhood, health anxiety tends to persist into adolescence [121].

Treatment

Effective psychopharmacologic and psychotherapeutic treatments exist for healthy anxiety. Fluoxetine [134–136], paroxetine [101, 137], and fluvoxamine [100] have been shown to be beneficial, though most trials are relatively small. Rates of sustained improvement among those who remit approach 60%, with even higher rates of sustained remission with prolonged use of medication [135, 138].

There is robust evidence for the use of individual [139–152] and group [153–156] CBT), including delivery in an internet-based model [157–159]. Treatment with CBT is sustained through time [104, 145, 149, 152, 153], cost-effective [149, 156], and preferred by patients over medications [160]. Acceptance and Commitment Therapy (ACT) and Mindfulness Based Cognitive Therapy (MBCT) have also shown benefit for health anxiety [161–164].

The relative benefits of medications and psychotherapy is less studied. One study found CBT to be equivalent to paroxetine [101]. Another found fluoxetine alone to be superior to CBT alone, with a small but notable incremental effect of fluoxetine plus CBT as compared to fluoxetine alone [136].

While several studies have reported positive treatment effects measured by response/remission rates and continuous measures, benefits of treatment in terms of functional status, social activities, health-related quality of life, and days of lost work have not consistently been demonstrated [118, 124, 142, 149].

Illness Anxiety Disorder and Somatic Symptom Disorder: An Important Diagnostic Distinction

The pattern of worry about being sick and seeking reassurance is the defining characteristic of IAD. In contrast, the prominence of somatic symptoms (whether or not they are explainable) and related affects, behaviors, and cognitions, defines SSD.

Distinguishing between these conditions comes down answering the questions "Why is the patient here" and "What are they looking for?". Patients with IAD are *worried* that they are sick, and seek *reassurance*; those with SSD are *distressed by symptoms*, and they seek *relief from symptoms*. These two patterns of distress may co-occur, but when one is distinctly present, reliable delineation is important for treatment planning.

Conversion Disorder

CD, also referred to as Functional Neurologic Symptom Disorder, involves symptoms of altered sensory or voluntary motor function for which no identifiable neurologic or medical cause has been found. The definition of CD in DSM-5 does not presume a psychologic origin for the symptoms, but acknowledges that the symptoms are not due to a known neurologic condition [5].

Motor manifestations include weakness [165], paralysis [166], and involuntary movements [167]. Among functional involuntary movements, tremor is most common, with dystonia, myoclonus, tics, and dyskinesia also observed [167–169]. A significant proportion have more than one movement symptom [167]. More complex motor phenomenologies of CD include Parkinsonism, gait disturbance, aphonia, and dysarthria [167, 170–172]. Paroxysmal episodes of involuntary complex motor activity resembling epileptic seizures, termed psychogenic non-epileptic seizures (PNES), are a particularly dramatic manifestation of CD [173].

Disturbances may involve somatosensory or special sensory systems, including numbness, paraesthesias, vertigo [171, 174–176], and changes to vision [177], olfaction [178], taste [179], and hearing [180]. Cognitive symptoms are an underappreciated manifestation of CD, and may include impairment of specific cognitive functions or more global impairment [181, 182].

The onset of symptoms is often sudden [183] and commonly associated with physical injury [184, 185]. While symptoms can be associated with an identifiable stress [167], a precipitating psychologic factor is not required for diagnosis of conversion disorder (nor is identification of a stressful event preclude the diagnosis of an organic disorder) [5]. Despite a high burden of psychiatric symptoms and co-morbidity, most patients with CD do not have a diagnosable co-morbid mood or anxiety disorder [1].

Distinguishing organic from functional neurologic symptoms based on exam can be challenging. Though several findings more typical of functional rather than structural/metabolic illness have been elucidated, (Table 1)

Table 1 Test characteristics for physical exam findings in CD

Exam finding		
Motor weakness [187]	PPV	NPV
Hoover sign	99%	96%
Downward pressure of contralateral LE when testing hip flexion of a paretic leg		
Collapsing/give-away weakness	96%	65%
Sudden collapse of strength during testing		
Co-contraction	100%	55%
Simultaneous contraction of agonist and antagonist muscles, resulting in no movement		
Inconsistency	67%	75%
Sensory loss [187]	PPV	NPV
Midline splitting	40%	82%
Loss of sensation occurs exactly at midline		
Vibration splitting	22%	92%
Loss of vibration splits midline when tested on sternum or frontal bone		
Non-anatomic sensory loss	100%	79%
Inconsistency	61%	85%
Gait [170]	PPV	NPV
Dragging gait	100%	32%
Paretic leg drags behind hip instead of circumducting		
Chair test	100%	90%
Able to propel self in rolling chair better than walking		
PNES [186, 189]	Sensitivity	Specificity
Fluctuating course	69%	96%
Asynchronous movements	44–96%	93–96%
Pelvic thrusting	1–31%	96–100%
Side-to-side movements	25–63%	96–100%
Eye closure	34–88%	74–100%
Ictal crying	13–14%	100%
Ictal stuttering	8.5%	100%

Abbreviations: PPV positive predictive value, *NPV* negative predictive value

[165, 186–189] no single finding definitively rules out organic illness, and many features classically associated with CD are not validated in systematic studies [175, 186]. For example, *la belle indifference*, an inappropriate lack of concern from the patient regarding the extent of symptoms, has long been taught as a common phenomenon in CD. This finding has not been validated in formal studies [165, 190]. Diagnosis therefore relies on accurate synthesis of all available information from the clinical interview, physical exam, and diagnostic testing.

Neurologic disorders with complex manifestations represent a particular challenge. For example, specific semiologies of PNES as opposed to epileptic seizures have been described, but the wide range of potential manifestations of frontal-lobe seizures makes definitive use of these signs difficult [169, 187, 191], and video-observed electroencephalography (EEG) of spells remains the gold standard for diagnosis. Multiple sclerosis (MS) is a neurologic disease with diverse potential manifestations and variable course, where diagnosis and identification of relapses is often difficult. Symptoms of CD may mimic MS [192, 193], and patients with a clear diagnosis of MS may develop functional neurologic symptoms [194, 195] and functional symptoms in other organ systems [196].

CD is a common diagnosis in neurologic clinics. One study found that 22% of patients presenting to neurology clinics had symptoms (other than headache) unexplained by neurologic disease, with 5.4% of all presenting patients having diagnosable CD [197]. Additionally, 2–7% of patients presenting to movement disorder clinics [167, 169, 189, 198] and 30% of patients admitted for video EEG monitoring [199] are diagnosed with conversion disorder.

Functional neurologic symptoms often co-exist with other somatoform processes, as other medically unexplained symptoms are present in most patients with conversion disorders [165]. Co-existence of functional and organic neurologic symptoms is also common; around one-quarter of patients with unexplainable neurologic symptoms have a co-existing neurologic or medical condition [197]. Among patients with FMDs, 16% also have an identifiable organic movement disorder, and epileptic seizures occur in up to 30% of patients with PNES [173, 200–202].

Neuropsychologic Characteristics

Initial theories on the pathogenesis of CD focused on symptoms as manifestations of unconscious conflicts, with later psychoanalysts focusing on symptoms as a coping mechanism for interpersonal problems. Societal expectations regarding the behavior of those suffering from illness and those treating them was later recognized as an important factor. Cognitive-behavioral theorists noted the complex interactions between the environment, emotions, and maladaptive thoughts, which combined with physiologic sensations and behavioral responses to induce and maintain the symptoms of CD [203]. As knowledge of functional neuroanatomy has improved, explanations of CD in terms of aberrant connectivity among executive function, limbic, sensory, and motor brain neural networks have emerged [204].

CD is associated with a high burden of co-morbid mood and anxiety symptoms [165, 167, 205]. Rates of depression are between 20% and 40% [205–207], and up to 40% have an anxiety disorder [208]. Rates of psychiatric co-morbidity are significantly higher than for those with neurologic illness and similar levels of disability [205, 206, 209].

Like SSD, CD is associated with alexithymia [205], harkening back to classic explanations of CD as being rooted in physical manifestations of unconscious affects. However, it is more likely that CD, alexithymia, and related affective disturbances are varied outcomes of a common neurodevelopmental vulnerability mediated by large-scale disturbances in somatosensory, motor, and limbic networks [204]. CD is also associated with certain personality profiles including high neuroticism and low conscientiousness [210].

Patients with CD acknowledge psychologic factors to physical symptoms less than those with known organic pathology [165], and often experience greater levels of psychologic distress related to symptoms than those with identifiable illness [211].

Epidemiology

The overall prevalence of CD in the general adult population is around 5 per 10,000, with an incidence of 4–12 per 100,000 per year in adults and up to 4 per 100,000 per year in children. Though CD is diagnosed throughout the lifespan, the most common onset is between 35 and 50 years of age [1]. Rates of CD are consistent across cultures [168, 212] and through time [213]. An association between socioeconomic status or educational level and CD has not been consistently demonstrated [165, 209, 214–218].

The relationship between gender and CD prevalence is complex. In general, studies have shown conversion disorder to be more prevalent in women than men [167, 169, 201, 202, 219]. These studies are mostly based on surveys of populations presenting to clinics; thus, as women are more likely to present to health services in general, the data may be skewed. For example, although women presenting with neurologic symptoms are more likely to be diagnosed as having a functional component to their symptoms [197], in one study, the proportion of women among patients diagnosed with functional disorders was similar to the percentage of women among patients diagnosed with organic neurologic illness [165]. In line with this, despite the traditional finding

that CD is more prevalent in women, some studies have shown no differences between sexes in CD prevalence [220].

In long term follow-up, rates of persistence of functional neurologic symptoms are high, with 40–60% of patients continuing to have significant symptoms in long-term follow-up [189, 202, 217], often with marked functional disability [32, 167]. Disability from conversion disorder can be significant and equivalent to that which is seen in those with known organic etiology of neurologic symptoms [165, 211].

Poor outcome in CD is strongly associated with patient expectations of non-recovery, lack of acceptance of the diagnosis of a functional disorder, and receiving financial benefit from illness, demonstrating the strong influence of environmental pressures and pathogenic cognitions on functional symptoms [201, 202, 221]. Number of symptoms, level of disability, and psychologic distress are not shown to influence outcome [211].

Treatment

Very few trials of psychotherapy in the treatment of CD exist. One small trial showed benefit for CBT, with or without structured physical activity, as being superior to treatment as usual for functional movement disorders [222], while small studies of individual psychodynamic psychotherapy in CD with motor symptoms have not shown clear benefit [223, 224].

In PNES specifically, treatment with CBT informed psychotherapy, either alone or in combination with sertraline, decreases the frequency of spells [225, 226]. Small studies show potential benefit for MBCT [227] and Dialectical Behavioral Therapy (DBT) emotional regulation skills training [228]. Several non-controlled studies have shown symptom reduction with individual and group psychodynamic psychotherapy and structured group psychoeducation sessions [229–232]. Studies have not shown a robust positive effect for SSRIs alone on PNES [226, 233, 234].

Newer somatic therapies, such as Transcranial Magnetic Stimulation (TMS), are beginning to be studied for treatment of CD but have not yet been proven effective [235]. Hypnosis, used as a treatment for CD beginning in the nineteenth century, lacks robust evidence for utility, though principles of suggestion are often incorporated into other psychotherapeutic techniques [236].

While traditional CBT is not well studied for CD, standardized protocols for multi-disciplinary rehabilitative interventions which draw from behavioral therapy principles and incorporate intensive physical and occupational therapy exist and have been shown to be beneficial across a spectrum of manifestations of CD [237–242]. The mix of strengthening and motor retraining exercises and psychological treatment likely serves to rework functional aberrations in the associated neural networks [237, 239]. Separate from structured rehabilitation settings, physical activity in general is a useful treatment for CD [222].

As with other somatoform disorders, a definitive diagnosis of conversion disorder and clear communication of the diagnosis to the patient and treatment team has therapeutic benefit. For example, in PNES, informing the patient of the diagnosis reduces hospitalizations, emergency department visits, and general practitioner visits [243, 244]. Communication of the diagnosis has also been shown to decrease episode frequency [245] and improves patient satisfaction with clinic visits [246]. The focus of communication should be on explaining the difference between a functional disorder and one due to identifiable pathology, and developing a plan for appropriate follow-up [173, 245–247].

Factitious Disorder

Factitious disorder involves the deliberate and conscious feigning of symptoms or production of illness with associated deceptive behaviors [5]. The term "Munchausen's Syndrome" has often been used interchangeably with FD, but will not be used here.

FD is included in the Somatoform Disorders chapter in DSM-5 based on the common presentation of the disorder to medical rather than psychiatric settings. However, it is distinct from the others in that physical symptoms associated with the above disorders are subjectively experienced without conscious production or exaggeration, and the associated affects and behaviors are reactions to these symptoms. The motivation, presumed to be unconscious, is to adopt the sick role, the result of which is a centering of one's life around being a medical patient [248]. The patient is consciously aware of his or her efforts to falsify or induce illness, though the patient may not be consciously aware of the motivation driving the behavior.

A diagnosis of FD is indicated when there is no clear external reward associated with the patient's illness behavior. FD must be differentiated from malingering, in which intentional feigning or production of illness is performed with a conscious and concrete goal (for example, faking symptoms of illness to obtain disability benefits). Malingering is not considered a mental illness.

The clinical definition of FD encompasses instances of deliberate feigning of symptoms or illness as well as deliberate induction of illness. Among reported cases, 70% involve illness induction [249].

FD may present to any medical specialty [249], including urology [250], oncology [251], cardiology [252], and gynecology [253]. A particularly high prevalence has been reported in dermatology [254, 255], and guidelines have been published for specific management of these conditions [256].

Differentiating FD from SSD, CD, and malingering is challenging. In cases where FD involves subjective symptom reports as opposed to observable findings, it can be difficult to differentiate from SSD, as an examiner has no ability to objectively measure whether the patient is reporting a genuine experience of symptoms or deliberately feigning or exaggerating them. Additionally, a patient with SSD may escalate affective responses and behaviors in response to feeling unheard by doctors and in context of ongoing somatic distress, which may mimic the consciously falsified reports of those with FD. Given these similarities, as well as observation that both conditions can be formulated as having major contributions from the unconscious benefits of being in the sick role, some have suggested that FD should be considered a subtype of SSD [257].

When the presentation is neurological, distinguishing FD from CD is especially problematic [182]; data suggest that physicians may in general be more comfortable assigning a diagnosis of CD over FD when there is ambiguity [258]. No clear clinical findings have been validated to discriminate between the two, and diagnosis relies mostly on the examiner's subjective impression [259].

Discrimination between FD and malingering relies on the clinician's knowledge of an external motivation for adopting the sick role. However, identification of such a factor relies on report from the patient or another source of collateral information, and while the presence of such a factor is helpful in diagnosis, its absence does not preclude a diagnosis of malingering. Additionally, the concept of conscious versus unconscious motivation for symptom feigning or production is likely not binary, but exists on a continuum [248, 252].

The most common observations used to support a diagnosis of FD are diagnostic and exam findings that do not explain the presenting complaints [249], though obviously this is a common experience in all somatoform disorders. Classic signs of FD include an inconsistent or unlikely history given by the patient, evidence from outside records that contradicts the patient's history, observation of illness-producing behaviors, atypical presentations, and unexplainable laboratory results; however, in case series, none of these were individually present in a majority of patients [249, 260].

Over 90% of presentations in one series involved a complaint of pain, though this is a non-specific sign [260]. Half of patients are self-referred, and one third have previously accessed healthcare services for the presenting problem [249, 260]. Other common features include atypical course of illness, a patient's eager agreement to invasive tests or procedures, patients who explicitly predict clinical decompensations, employment in the healthcare field, and patient opposition to psychiatric assessment [249, 254, 260].

Among those diagnosed with FD, 30–40% have a comorbid psychiatric condition [260], with high rates of depression, personality disorder, substance abuse, and anxiety disorders [249, 260–262]. Suicidality is common, with 14% reporting suicidal ideation or a history of suicide attempts at the time of diagnosis of FD [249].

FD may also present as the induction of illness in another person, almost always by a parent or caregiver towards a child. This is described as Factitious Disorder Imposed on Another (FD-O) DSM-5 and also referred to as "Medical Child Abuse" [5, 263]. FD-O has almost exclusively been described in cases of parents inducing or fabricating signs of illness in children [263], including a case of induced illness towards a fetus [264]. Potential mechanisms include fabrication of clinical history, administration of substances to invoke symptoms, or tampering with test samples. Depression is significantly less common in FD-O (14% of reported cases) than FD, but there are similar rates of personality disorder, substance abuse, and suicidality, and 30% of reported cases with FD-O have a history of FD towards the self [263].

Epidemiology

Given the inherent difficulty in definitively diagnosing FD and the fact that the nature of the illness makes systematic study difficult, obtaining reliable data on epidemiologic characteristics is challenging.

Estimates of 1-year prevalence of FD range from 0.5% to 2%, though rates among different specialties vary widely [53, 254]. Estimations of FD prevalence in neurology are among the highest among medical specialties, together with dermatology. Studies have generally found FD to be more prevalent (60–70%) in women, and 44–57% of identified FD cases have worked in healthcare. The majority have at least a high-school education and are employed [249, 254]. FD-O is overwhelmingly more prevalent in women, and much more commonly identified in married women as opposed to unmarried, divorced, or widowed women [263].

Data on precise cost of FD to the healthcare system have not been published, but estimating costs from individual cases indicates the financial burden is significant [265].

Treatment

Ultimately, the course of FD is often chronic, and full recovery is thought to be rare. Morbidity from illness inducing behaviors and suicide have been reported [266].

Treatment is complicated by the core psychopathology of the illness, namely, that there is unconscious motivation to be seen as medically ill. In one series, three quarters of patients were confronted with the diagnosis of FD but less than 20% were able to acknowledge having a factitious illness. While 20% of patients in this sample agreed to some type of psychiatric follow-up, the outcome of treatment was unknown. In scarce case reports of patients who have recovered from FD, contributing factors include new affiliation with religion and external pressures which make illness-inducing behaviors antithetical to conscious goals [267–269].

Goals of treatment in FD include avoiding serious injury or death due to illness-inducing behavior and avoidance of iatrogenic harm from unnecessary testing. Though guidelines for communication of diagnosis and management of FD patient exist, no strategy has been empirically validated to improve outcomes.

As in other somatoform disorders, communication of the diagnosis to members of the health care team and the patient is an important first step. A supportive, non-punitive approach that avoids blaming the patient is key. One should place emphasis on the patient being ill and in need of help. Allowing the patient to maintain this identity, such as encouraging identification with being "survivor" or "in recovery" may aid in therapeutic alliance [248].

One framework for supportive confrontation suggests the following elements: collection of evidence of illness fabrication, consultation of a psychiatrist or member of the hospital legal team, holding a meeting among team members to clarify facts and strategy, supportive delivery of diagnosis to the patient, discussion among the team of the outcome of this confrontation, and thorough documentation of the intervention [248].

Assessment of Somatoform Disorders

Clinical assessment begins with proper diagnostic testing for known medical conditions. Though some consider SSD a diagnosis of exclusion, such an attitude may lead to unnecessary testing; decisions on testing should be made based on the clinical context and the usefulness of the test rather than the level of patient affect. For example, consider a non-overweight woman in her early 20s with no family history of early heart disease and no personal history of diabetes, hyperlipidemia, or hypertension who presents with intermittent sharp pain in her right chest wall that only occurs at rest and lasting less than 1 min. She likely does not warrant a cardiac stress test regardless of her level of conviction that she has coronary artery disease, as even with a positive test, her probability of having cardiac disease is exceedingly low.

Once appropriate medical work-up is done, a standard psychiatric diagnostic interview should be performed to assess symptoms of somatoform disorders and any comorbid psychiatric symptoms. The Health Preoccupation Diagnostic Interview is a structured assessment tool to diagnoses and differentiate between SSD and IAD [270]. A specific structured interview for IAD, the Anxiety Disorder Interview Schedule (ADIS-5) has also been developed [271].

The most commonly used instrument for dimensional measurement of health anxiety symptoms is the Whitely Index, a 14-item self-report questionnaire that includes items regarding disease fear, disease conviction, and bodily preoccupation [86–88, 272]. Measurement of somatic symptom burden can be performed using the Patient Health Questionnaire 15 (PHQ15) [273], a self-report instrument encompassing several organ systems. Despite higher burden of symptoms being the hallmark of SSD, those with HC/IAD also show higher PHQ-15 scores than those without somatoform disorders, and there is a positive correlation between scores on the Whiteley Index and PHQ15 [12, 34]. Care must be taken to consider the presence of known pathology in the interpretation of scores. For CD, the Psychogenic Movement Disorders Rating Scale is available when motor symptoms predominate [273]. Additional instruments used to measure symptoms of health anxiety, somatic symptoms, and bodily awareness are listed in Table 2 [87, 273–277, 279–283].

Standardized rating scales of depression and anxiety are useful adjuncts in assessment, somatoform disorders are associated with elevated scores on these measures [8, 12, 43, 64, 85, 86].

Table 2 Standardized rating scales for somatoform disorders

Scale	Scoring	Comment
Whiteley Index [87]	Self-report	Measurement of health anxiety
Illness Attitudes Scale [87]	Self-report	Measurement of health anxiety
Health Anxiety Inventory [274]	Self-report	Measurement of health anxiety
H-YBOCS-M [275]	Clinician-rated	Modified version of Y-BOCS targets at illness related thoughts, behaviors, and avoidance
Childhood Illness Attitudes Scale [276]	Self-report	Measurement of health anxiety in children
Cyberchondria Severity Scale [277]	Self-report	Measures health anxiety-related internet use
PHQ-15 [278]	Self-report	Index of overall somatic symptom burden
Somatosensory Amplification Scale [279]	Self-report	Measures awareness of bodily sensations
Somatoform Dissociation Questionnaire [280]	Self-report	Index of somatic symptoms related to dissociative processes
Bodily Awareness Scale [281]	Self-report	Measures awareness of bodily sensations
Bodily Vigilance Scale [282]	Self-report	Measures awareness of bodily sensations
Scale of Bodily Connection [283]	Self-report	Measures awareness of bodily sensations
PMDRS [273]	Clinician-rated	Objective rating of psychogenic movements disorders

Abbreviations: Y-BOCS Yale-Brown Obsessive Compulsive Rating Scale, *H-YBOCS-M* Modified Hypochondriasis Yale-Brown Obsessive Compulsive Rating Scale, *PMDRS* Psychogenic Movement Disorders Rating Scale

Differential Diagnosis of Somatoform Disorders

In addition to somatoform disorders, other psychiatric conditions often include elements of somatic symptoms and health anxiety. Panic Disorder and Generalized Anxiety Disorder often include distressing somatic symptoms and significant health anxiety [102, 284, 285]. Obsessive-compulsive disorder may manifest as obsessions regarding health status with related compulsive checking behaviors [99, 286].

Unexplained somatic symptoms are commonly seen in depression [287, 288], and complaints of symptoms or worries about health may be manifestations of somatic delusions in psychotic disorders [285]. Despite not being among the DSM-5 criteria for PTSD, unexplained somatic symptoms and functional illness are very common in this condition, especially when individuals have experienced extensive trauma throughout childhood and adolescence [289].

Influences of Sex and Gender on Somatoform Disorders

Symptoms without known cause were first attributed to displacement of the uterus in Egypt in the second millennium BC, and since then a strong connection has remained between the diagnosis and treatment of somatoform disorders and cultural attitudes towards and expectations of women. Uterine pathology and its relation to women's sexual practices continued to be used to explain somatoform disorders in Greece and Rome through the first few centuries AD. The relative moral, spiritual, and physiologic inadequacies of women in relation to men remained prominent in theories of somatization up through the nineteenth century, despite increased consideration of biologic and societal factors. As understanding about the complex relationships between the brain and behavior has improved, a more medical model has emerged, though formulation, diagnosis, and treatment of these conditions remains largely impacted by cultural biases regarding sex and gender [290].

Through time, a higher burden of somatic symptoms [2, 27, 291–297], greater number of symptoms reported [2, 105, 291–294, 296, 298], and higher prevalence of somatic symptom disorders [27, 295, 299–306], have been observed in women. Notably, HC/IAD (with its focus on health anxiety rather than symptoms) does not show increased prevalence in women as compared to men [2, 12, 116]. Women are also more likely than men to have somatic symptoms of depression such as fatigue, appetite disturbance, and changes in sleep [33, 307, 308].

Many defined functional syndromes such as IBS [309], IC [310], PNES [173], fibromyalgia [311], temporomandibular joint syndrome [312], and chronic fatigue syndrome [313]

show female predominance, though as noted above, not all have shown an association with somatic symptom disorders. Defined functional syndromes specific to women, such as chronic pelvic pain, women's orgasmic disorder, vaginismus, and dyspareunia have been associated with somatization and somatoform disorders [314, 315].

However, the complex interactions between biologic, psychologic, and sociologic influences on sex-specific manifestations of somatic symptoms make it difficult to tease out their relative contributions.

Sex-specific biologic influences on non-neuropsychiatric organ systems are likely important contributors to discrepancies between women and men on symptom reporting and experience [27, 314, 316–321] though a true biologic influence of sex on the clinical presentation of somatoform disorders may be far less than previously thought once confounding factors are accounted for [27, 293, 322, 323]. The burden of symptoms related to female sex organs, including disruptions in the menstrual cycle, pelvic pain, and dyspareunia, may bias diagnosis, especially as many categorical diagnoses (such as Somatization Disorder in DSM-IV) rely on reaching a threshold number of distinct somatic symptoms [324]. Additionally, affects, cognitions, and bodily sensations related to fertility, pregnancy, and childbirth represent niduses of somatoform concern that do not pertain to men [325–327].

For a somatic symptom to be distressing, the intensity of the symptom must be sufficient enough to be perceived as salient. Evidence exists that women are more aware of somatic sensations than men, which is mediated by biologic and sociologic factors [27, 295, 323, 328, 329]. Women may remember pain more intensely than men (though this is not a consistent finding) [330, 331], which influences affective responses to the anticipation of pain. Somatic amplification has not been found to be greater in women than men [279], perhaps suggesting psychologic and sociologic influences may be more important than biologic factors in increased symptom perception in woman.

From a psychologic perspective, the hallmark of somatoform disorders is not the lack of medical explanation for symptoms, but the marked emotional distress related to them. It has been suggested that women may have more prominent affective response to somatic symptoms than men or that women may be more likely than men to attribute bodily sensations to illness, though little empiric evidence exists [305, 323, 324, 332, 333].

Women may be more likely than men to report health-related distress, independent of whether they are more likely to experience symptoms [27, 323, 334, 335]. For example, in one study, women were much more likely to feel anxious in response to pain and seek to disclose it to others, while men were more likely to react with embarrassment and reluctance to disclose pain. Importantly, this effect was seen despite no sex differences in appraisal of the seriousness of the pain or any related danger [334].

Women have been noted to be more likely to describe distressing symptoms in the context of functional disruption, an approach that may increase the likelihood of seeking help [336].

The tendency of societal pressures suggesting that stoicism in the face of physical and mental discomfort is expected of men may lead to decreased reporting of physical symptoms, as opposed to women in whom it is more accepted and expected [279, 305, 323, 332]. Women tend to report more hypochondriacal traits on dimensional measures of personality than men, though the observation that this gap has decreased with time may reflect changing societal attitudes regarding gender roles and acceptability of certain forms of distress reporting [323].

Though biologic differences between men and women are important, gender (which is influenced by both genetic and developmental) is a key mediating factor. Data has suggested that women do not have a lower threshold of pain experience than men but may have a lower threshold for the point at which pain becomes distressing [337]. However, this effect has been shown to be strongly mediated by self-perception of gender and one's perception of gender-normative behavior [329, 335, 338, 339]. There is evidence that somatization aggregates among women in the same family, but male relatives of women with somatic symptom disorders do not have increased rates of somatization [340], again suggesting that psychosocial influences are important.

Differences in somatoform phenomenology between men and women have been found. Somatic symptom disorders in women are more likely to involve numerous episodes of discrete illness with many different complaints, as opposed to men who were more likely to have complaints that were more limited in number but more chronically disabling (such as chronic fatigue or weakness) [341, 342].

Certain manifestations of CD including functional weakness, functional cognitive complaints, and late-onset PNES are more common in men [201, 343, 344]. Specific features of PNES have been shown to be more common in adolescent girls (atonic falls aka 'swooning', longer episode duration) or boys (tonic-clonic extremity movements) [345] though studies in adults have not found gender differences in PNES semiology [346, 347].

Clinical biases may encourage the diagnosis of one somatoform disorder from another. As noted above, differentiating FD from CD can be quite challenging. Despite findings in case series that women present with FD more often than men [260], a study of neurology patients found that men made up the majority of FD diagnoses [258]. One study also found a trend suggesting that, among patients where a somatoform disorder is suspected, men are more likely than women to receive a diagnosis of FD [258]. As above, this may suggest that the finding that FD is more common in women than men may in part be explained by the overall higher rate at which women present to medical settings in general, or by a cultural bias that makes clinicians more likely to diagnosis CD in women and FD in men when there is ambiguity [258].

Manifestations of FD are also influenced by gender. Though case series indicate 60–70% of FD cases are women, diagnoses of FD are more common in men in cardiology, HIV/sexual health clinics, and neurology, and more evenly distributed between the sexes in urology/nephrology and orthopedics [249].

Physical and sexual trauma, often found to be more prevalent in women, are strongly associated with a high burden of somatic symptoms [289, 347–351] and somatoform disorders [352–354]. Trauma may be a mediating factor in gender differences in somatoform disorders; while early-life adversity is associated with chronic pain in both men and women, it is specifically associated with chronic pain in multiple sites in men but not women [355]. Women with motor conversion disorders are more likely than men to have experienced physical or sexual trauma [201, 347]. Thus, trauma may be a specific risk factor for the development of conversion disorder in women. Supporting the connection between trauma and somatization is the observation that both CD [204, 205, 354] and somatization [355] are associated with dissociation, another common manifestation of early trauma [289].

The ambiguities in the relationships among sex, gender, functional disorders, and somatoform disorders have implications for clinical practice, and the true nature of their relationship. The practitioner should be aware of innate biases towards assuming strong emotional contributions to physical symptoms in women [356, 357], which may lead to decreased likelihood of attributing presenting symptoms to physical illness [27, 358]. This is of importance as data exists to suggest that it is more difficult to tell "organic" from "functional" pathology in women as opposed to men [330]. To quote Barsky et al.:

> One should not conclude that women are over-reporters who dramatize and exaggerate trivial sensations and benign dysfunction; it can be equally concluded that men are insensitive perceivers and poor historians who ignore, suppress, or are unaware of much bodily experience […] Men's and women's styles of symptom reporting are simply different [27].

Clinical Care of Patients with Somatoform Disorders

Listening to concerns with empathy, adopting an active and curious attitude towards the patient's experience, and asking respectful questions fosters a useful therapeutic relationship. Patients come to the medical setting with pre-existing explanatory models for their distress and the connection between mind and body, and listening empathically rather than inflexibly attempting to impose a medical explanatory model facilitates therapeutic alliance. It is important to empathize with the patient's distress without colluding with false beliefs; agreeing with distorted ideas will likely lead to disappointment.

Individuals with somatoform disorders often report feelings like they are treated with suspicion, dismissal, and contempt by the medical field. Practitioners should be mindful of their countertransference, clearly express empathy, and avoid blaming the patient for symptoms or suggesting symptoms are not real or "in the patient's head".

When a diagnostic test is ordered, it is helpful to tell the patient clearly and explicitly the reasons for the test, what results would be considered abnormal, and what next steps would be in the case of a positive, negative, or equivocal test. Clear documentation in the medical record of this plan helps other providers understand what was discussed.

Direct communication between providers caring for a patient is absolutely vital in order to avoid iatrogenic risk from testing that is repetitive or not clinically indicated. When an appropriate diagnostic work-up is conducted, an erroneous diagnosis of a somatoform disorder is rare [197, 359–363]. The diagnosis of somatoform disorder should be explicitly discussed with the patient and all members of the treatment team, as medical decision making in any specialty is best made with knowledge of all conditions, psychiatric and somatic, that are present, and a shared understanding of that which is being treated.

Conclusion

The somatoform disorders represent a broad range of psychopathology involving the connection between body and mind. Disturbances include excessive worry about being sick, intense distress over symptoms that may not be explainable, alterations in neurologic function without known cause, and the deliberate fabrication or induction of symptoms in order to be in a sick role. One must be mindful that all patients, whether suffering from diagnosable or undiagnosable illness, present because they are distressed, and that the clinicians job is to reduce this distress by utilizing whichever biologic, psychologic, and social treatments are available and indicated.

References

1. Carson A, Lehn A. Epidemiology. Handb Clin Neurol. 2016;139:47–60.
2. Steinbrecher N, Koerber S, Frieser D, Hiller W. The prevalence of medically unexplained symptoms in primary care. Psychosomatics. 2011;52:263–71.

3. Kisely S, Goldber D, Simon G. A comparison between somatic symptoms with and without clear organic cause: results of an international study. Psychol Med. 1997;27:1011–9.

4. Tomenson B, Essau C, Jacobi F, Ladwig KH, Leiknes KA, Liet R, Meinlschmidt G, McBeth J, Rosmalen J, Rief W, Sumathipala A, Creed F. Total somatic symptom score as a predictor of health outcome in somatic symptom disorders. Br J Psychiatry. 2013;203:373–80.

5. American Psychiatric Association. Diagnostic and statistical manual of mental disorders. 5th ed. Arlington: American Psychiatric Publishing; 2013.

6. American Psychiatric Association. Diagnostic and statistical manual of mental disorders. 4th ed., text rev. Washington, DC: American Psychiatric Publishing; 2000.

7. Drossman DA, Hasler WL. Rome IV-functional GI disorders: disorders of gut-brain interaction. Gastroenterology. 2016;150:1257–61.

8. Claassen-van Dessel N, van der Wouden JC, Dekker J, van der Horst HE. Clinical value of DSM IV and DSM 5 criteria for diagnosing the most prevalent somatoform disorders in patients with medically unexplained symptoms (MUPS). J Psychosom Res. 2016;82:4–10.

9. Voigt K, Wollburg E, Wienmann N, Herzog A, Beyer B. Predictive validity and clinical utility of DSM-5 somatic symptom disorder-comparison with DSM-IV somatoform disorders and additional criteria for consideration. J Psychosom Res. 2012;73:345–50.

10. Patel P, Bercik P, Morgan DF, Bolino C, Pintos-Sanchez MI, Moayyedi P, et al. Irritable bowel syndrome is significantly associated with somatisation in 840 patients, which may drive bloating. Aliment Pharmacol Ther. 2015;41:449–58.

11. Chen IC, Lee M, Lin HH, Wu S, Chang K, Lin HY. Somatoform disorder as a predictor of interstitial cystitis/bladder pain syndrome: evidence from a nested case control study and a retrospective cohort study. Medicine. 2017;96:18.

12. Scarella TM, Laferton JA, Ahern DK, Fallon BA, Barsky A. The relationship of hypochondriasis to anxiety, depressive, and somatoform disorders. Psychosomatics. 2016;57(2):200–7.

13. Gracie DJ, Bercik P, Morgan DG, Bolino C, Pintos-Sanchez MI, Moayyed P, et al. No increase in prevalence of somatization in functional vs organic dyspepsia: a cross-sectional study. Neurogastroenterol Motil. 2015;27:1024–31.

14. Ramond-Roquin A, Pecquenard F, Schers H, van Weel C, Oskam S, van Boven K. Psychosocial, musculoskeletal and somatoform comorbidity in patients with chronic low back pain: original results from the Dutch Transition Project. Fam Pract. 2015;32(3):297–304.

15. Rief W, Hiller W, Margraf J. Cognitive aspects of hypochondriasis and the somatization syndrome. J Abnorm Psychol. 1998;107(4):587–95.

16. Frostholm L, Ornbol E, Fink PK. Physical symptoms attributions: a defining characteristic of somatoform disorders? Gen Hosp Psychiatry. 2015;37:147–52.

17. Barsky AJ, Goodson JS, Lane RS, Cleary PD. The amplification of somatosensory symptoms. Psychosom Med. 1988;50:510–9.

18. Perez DL, Barsky AJ, Vago DR, Baslet G, Silbersweig DA. A neural circuit framework for somatosensory amplification in somatoform disorders. J Neuropsychiatr Clin Neurosci. 2015;27:e40–50.

19. Kleiman A, Kramer KA, Wegener I, Kock AS, Geiser F, Imbierowicz K, et al. Psychological decoupling in alexithymic pain disorder patients. Psychiatry Res. 2016;237:316–22.

20. Barksy AJ, Orav J, Bates DW. Somatization increases medical utilization and costs independent of psychiatric and medical co-morbidity. Arch Gen Psychiatry. 2005;62:903–10.

21. De Waal MWM, Arnold IA, Eekhoff JAH, van Hemert AM. Somatoform disorders in general practice: prevalence, functional impairment, and co-morbidity with anxiety and depressive disorders. Br J Psychiatry. 2004;184:470–6.

22. Haller H, Cramer H, Lauche R, Dobos G. Somatoform disorders and medically unexplained symptoms in primary care- a systematic review and meta-analysis of prevalence. Dtsh Arztebl Int. 2015;112:279–87.

23. Fink P, Hansen MS, Oxhoj ML. The prevalence of somatoform disorders among internal medicine inpatients. J Psychosom Res. 2004;56:413–8.

24. Fink P, Hansen MS, Sondergaard L. Somatoform disorders among first-time referrals to a neurology service. Psychosomatics. 2005;46(6):540–8.

25. Obimakinde AM, Ladipo MM, Irabor AE. Familial and socio-economic correlates of somatisation disorder. Afr J Prim Health Care Fam Med. 2015;7(1):746.

26. Swartz M, Landerman R, Blazer D, George L. Somatization in the community: a rural/urban comparison. Psychosomatics. 1989;30:44–53.

27. Barsky AJ, Peekna HM, Borus J. Somatic symptom reporting in women and men. J Gen Intern Med. 2001;16:266–75.

28. Jackson JL, Kroenke K. Prevalence, impact, and prognosis of multisomatoform disorder in primary care: a 5-year follow-up study. Psychosom Med. 2008;70(4):430–4.

29. Hansen HS, Rosendal M, Oernboel E, Fink P. Are medically unexplained symptoms and functional disorders predictive for the illness course? A two-year follow-up on patients' health and health care utilization. J Psychosom Res. 2011;71:38–44.

30. McAndrew LM, Phillips IA, Helmer DA, Maestro K, Engel CC, Greenberg LM, et al. High healthcare utilization near the onset of medically unexplained symptoms. J Psychosom Res. 2017;98:98–105.

31. Lee S, Creed FH, Ma Y, Leung CMC. Somatic symptom burden and health anxiety in the population and their correlates. J Psychosom Res. 2015;78:71–6.

32. Rask MT, Rosendal M, Fenger-Gron M, Bro F, Ornbol E, Fink P. Sick leave and work disability in primary care patients with recent onset multiple medically unexplained symptoms and persistent somatoform disorders: a 10-year follow-up of the FIP study. Gen Hosp Psychiatry. 2015;37:53–9.

33. Silverstein B. Gender differences in the prevalence of somatic versus pure depression: a replication. Am J Psychiatry. 2002;159:1051–2.

34. Clarke DM, Piterman L, Byrne CJ, Austin DW. Somatic symptoms, hypochondriasis and psychological distress: a study of somatisation in Australian general practice. Med J Aust. 2008;189(10):560–4.

35. Escobar JI, Burnam A, Karno M, Forsythe A, Golding JM. Somatization in the community. Arch Gen Psychiatry. 1987;44:713–8.

36. Berna C, Leknes S, Holmes EA, Edwins RR, Goodwin GM, Tracey I. Induction of depressed mood disrupts emotion regulation neurocircuitry and enhances pain unpleasantness. Biol Psychiatry. 2010;67:1083–90.

37. Coen SJ, Yaguez L, Aziz Q, Mitterschiffthaler MT, Brammer M, Williams SC, et al. Negative mood affects brain processing of visceral sensation. Gatroenterology. 2009;137:253–61.

38. Ploner M, Lee MC, Wiech K, Bingel U, Tracey I. Prestimulus functional connectivity determines pain perception in humans. Proc Natl Acad Sci U S A. 2010;107:355–60.

39. Wagner G, Koschke M, Leuf T, Schlosser R, Bar KJ. Reduced heat pain threshold after sad-mood induction are associated with changes in thalamic activity. Neuropsychologia. 2009;47:980–7.

40. Dijkstra-Kersten SMA, Sitnikova K, van Marwijk HMWJ, Gerrits MMJG, van der Wouden JC, Penninx BWJH, et al. Somatisation as a risk factor for incident depression and anxiety. J Psychosom Res. 2015;79:614–9.

41. Den Boeft M, Claasseen-van Dessel N, van der Wouden JC. How should we manage adults with persistent unexplained physical symptoms? BMJ. 2017;256:j268.

42. Kroenke K, Messina N, Benattia I, Graepel J, Musgnung J. Venlafaxine extended release in the short-term treatment of depressed and anxious primary care patients with multisomatoform disorder. J Clin Psychiatry. 2006;67(1):72–80.

43. Luo YL, Zhang MY, Wu WY, Li CB, Lu Z, Li QW. A randomized double-blind clinical trial on analgesic efficacy of fluoxetine for persistent somatoform pain disorder. Prog Neuropsychopharmacol Biol Psychiatry. 2009;33(8):1522–5.

44. Müller JE, Wentzel I, Koen L, Niehaus DJ, Seedat S, Stein DJ. Escitalopram in the treatment of multisomatoform disorder: a double-blind, placebo-controlled trial. Int Clin Psychopharmacol. 2008;23(1):43–8.

45. Huang M, Luo B, Hu J, Wei N, Chen L, Wang S, et al. Combination of citalopram plus paliperidone is better than citalopram alone in the treatment of somatoform disorder: results of a 6-week randomized study. Int Clin Psychopharmacol. 2012;27(3):151–8.

46. Li G, Jin W. Comparison study of paroxetine and paroxetine combined with quetiapine in treatment of somatoform disorder. Chin J Behav Med Sci. 2006;15(7):598–9.

47. Kleinstäuber M, Witthöft M, Steffanowski A, van Marwijk H, Hiller W, Lambert MJ. Pharmacological interventions for somatoform disorders in adults. Cochrane Database Syst Rev. 2014;(11):CD010628.

48. Müller T, Mannel M, Murck H, Rahlfs VW. Treatment of somatoform disorders with St. John's wort: a randomized, double-blind and placebo-controlled trial. Psychosom Med. 2004;66(4):538–47.

49. Volz HP, Murck H, Kasper S, Möller HJ. St John's wort extract (li 160) in somatoform disorders: results of a placebo-controlled trial [Johanniskrautextrakt (LI 160) bei somatoformen Stoerungen: Ergebnisse einer plazebokontrollierten Studie]. Psychopharmacology. 2002;164(3):294–300.

50. van Dessel N, den Boeft M, van der Wouden JC, Kleinstauber M, Leone SS, Terluin B, et al. Non-pharmacological interventions for somatoform disorders and medically unexplained physical symptoms (MUPS) in adults. Cochrane Database Syst Rev. 2014;(11):CD011142.

51. Allen LA, Woolfolk RL, Escobar JI, Gara MA, Hamer RM. Cognitive-behavioral therapy for somatization disorder: a randomized controlled trial. Arch Intern Med. 2006;166:1512–8.

52. Burton C, Weller D, Marsden W, Worth A, Sharpe M. A primary care symptoms clinic for patients with medically unexplained symptoms: pilot randomised trial. BMJ Open. 2012;2:e000513.

53. Escobar JI, Gara MA, Diaz-Martinez AM, Interian A, Warman M, Allen LA, et al. Effectiveness of a time-limited cognitive behavior therapy type intervention among primary care patients with medically unexplained symptoms. Ann Fam Med. 2007;5:328–35.

54. Kashner TM, Rost K, Cohen B, Anderson M, Smith GR Jr. Enhancing the health of somatization disorder patients. Effectiveness of short-term group therapy. Psychosomatics. 1995;36:462–70.

55. Martin A, Rauh E, Fichter M, Rief W. A one-session treatment for patients suffering from medically unexplained symptoms in primary care: a randomized clinical trial. Psychosomatics. 2007;48:294–303.

56. Moreno S, Gili M, Magallón R, Bauzá N, Roca M, Del Hoyo YL, et al. Effectiveness of group versus individual cognitive-behavioral therapy in patients with abridged somatization disorder: a randomized controlled trial. Psychosom Med. 2013;75:600–8.

57. Schweickhardt A, Larisch A, Wirsching M, Fritzsche K. Short-term psychotherapeutic interventions for somatizing patients in the general hospital: a randomized controlled study. Psychother Psychosom. 2007;76:339–46.

58. Sumathipala A, Hewege S, Hanwella R, Mann AH. Randomized controlled trial of cognitive behaviour therapy for repeated consultations for medically unexplained complaints: a feasibility study in Sri Lanka. Psychol Med. 2000;30:747–57.

59. Lidbeck J. Group therapy for somatization disorders in primary care: maintenance of treatment goals of short cognitive-behavioural treatment one-and-a-half-year follow-up. Acta Psychiatr Scand. 2003;107:449–56.

60. Magallón R, Gili M, Moreno S, Bauzá N, García-Campayo J, Roca M, et al. Cognitive-behaviour therapy for patients with abridged somatization disorder (SSI 4,6) in primary care: a randomized, controlled study. BMC Psychiatry. 2008;8:47.

61. Zonneveld LN, van Rood YR, Kooiman CG, Timman R, van't Spijker A, Busschbach JJ. Predicting the outcome of a cognitive-behavioral group training for patients with unexplained physical symptoms: a one-year follow-up study. BMC Public Health. 2012;12:848.

62. Zonneveld LN, van Rood YR, Timman R, Kooiman CG, Van't Spijker A, Busschbach JJ. Effective group training for patients with unexplained physical symptoms: a randomized controlled trial with a non-randomized one year follow-up. PLoS One. 2012;7:e42629.

63. Katsamanis M, Lehrer PM, Escobar JI, Gara MA, Kotay A, Liu R. Psychophysiologic treatment for patients with medically unexplained symptoms: a randomized controlled trial. Psychosomatics. 2011;52:218–29.

64. Chowdhury S, Burton C. Associations of treatment effects between follow-up times and between outcome domains in interventions for somatoform disorders: review of three Cochrane reviews. J Psychosom Res. 2017;98:10–8.

65. Fjorback LO, Arendt M, Ornbol E, Walach H, Rehfeld E, Schroder A, et al. Mindfulness therapy for somatization disorder and functional somatic syndromes-randomized trial with one year follow-up. J Psychosom Res. 2013;74(1):31–40.

66. Van Ravesteijn H, Lucassen P, Bor H, van Weel C, Speckens A. Mindfulness-based cognitive therapy for patients with medically unexplained symptoms: a randomized controlled trial. Psychother Psychosom. 2013;82:299–310.

67. Sattel H, Lahmann C, Gunder H, Guthrie E, Kruse J, Noll-Hussong M, et al. Brief psychodynamic interpersonal psychotherapy for patients with multisomatoform disorder: randomized controlled trial. Br J Psychiatry. 2012;200(1):60–7.

68. Chavooshi B, Mohammadkhani P, Dolatshahi B. A randomize double-blind controlled trial comparing Davanloo intensive short-term dynamic psychotherapy as internet delivered vs. treatment as usual for medically unexplained pain: a 6-month pilot study. Psychosomatics. 2016;57(3):292–300.

69. Schaefert R, Kaufmann C, Wild B, Schellberg D, Boelter R, Faber R, et al. Specific collaborative group intervention for patients with medically unexplained symptoms in general practice: a cluster randomized controlled trial. Psychother Psychosom. 2013;82:106–19.

70. Aiarzaguena JM, Grandes G, Gaminde I, Salazar A, Sanchez A, Arino J. A randomized controlled clinical trial of a psychosocial and communication intervention carried out by GPs for patients with medically unexplained symptoms. Psychol Med. 2007;37:283–94.

71. Larisch A, Schweickhardt A, Wirsching M, Fritzsche K. Psychosocial interventions for somatizing patients by the general practitioner: a randomized controlled trial. J Psychosom Res. 2004;57:507–14.

72. Morriss RK, Gask L, Ronalds C, Thompson H, Goldberg D. Clinical and patient satisfaction outcomes of a new treatment for somatized mental disorder taught to general practitioners. Br J Gen Pract. 1999;49:263–7.

73. Rosendal M, Olesen F, Fink P, Toft T, Sokolowski I, Bro F. A randomized trial of brief training in the assessment and treatment of somatization in primary care: effects on patient outcome. Gen Hosp Psychiatry. 2007;29(4):364–73.

74. Shaefert R, Kaufmann C, Wild B, Schellberg D, Boelter R, Faber R, et al. Specific collaborative group intervention for patients with medically unexplained symptoms in general practice: a cluster randomized controlled trial. Psychother Psychosom. 2013;82(2):106–19.

75. Toft T, Rosendal M, Ornbol E, Olesen F, Frostholm L, Fink P. Training general practitioners in the treatment of functional somatic symptoms: effects on patient health in a cluster-randomised controlled trial (the Functional Illness in Primary Care study). Psychother Psychosom. 2010;79(4):227–37.

76. Frostholm L, Fink P, Oernboeel E, Christensen KS, Toft T, Olesen F, et al. The uncertain consultation and patient satisfaction: the impact of patients' illness perceptions and a randomized controlled trial on the training of physicians' communication skills. Psychosom Med. 2005;67(6):897–905.

77. Rosendal M, Bro F, Sokolowski I, Fink P, Toft T, Olesen F. A randomized controlled trial of brief training in assessment and treatment of somatisation: effects on GP's attitudes. Fam Pract. 2005;22(4):419–27.

78. Dickinson WP, Dickinson LM, DeGruy FV, Main DS, Candib LM, Rost K. A randomized clinical trial of a care recommendation letter intervention for somatization in primary care. Ann Fam Med. 2003;1:228–35.

79. Rost K, Kashner TM, Smith GR. Effectiveness of psychiatric intervention with somatization disorder patients: improved outcomes at reduced costs. Gen Hosp Psychiatry. 1994;16:381–7.

80. Smith GR, Monson RA, Ray DC. Psychiatric consultation in somatization disorder. N Engl J Med. 1986;314:1407–13.

81. Smith GR, Rost K, Kashner M. A trial of the effect of a standardized psychiatric consultation on health outcomes and costs in somatizing patients. Arch Gen Psychiatry. 1995;52:238–43.

82. van der Feltz-Cornelis CM, van Oppen P, Ader HJ, van Dyck R. Randomised controlled trial of a collaborative care model with psychiatric consultation for persistent medically unexplained symptoms in general practice. Psychother Psychosom. 2006;75(5):282–9.

83. Van der Feltz-Cornelis CM, Van Os TWDP, van Marwijk HWJ, Leentjens AFG. Effect of psychiatric consultation models in primary care. A systematic review and meta-analysis of randomized controlled trials. J Psychosom Res. 2010;68:521–33.

84. Schutte K, Vocks S, Waldorf M. Fears, coping styles, and health behaviors: a comparison of patients with hypochondriasis, panic disorder, and depression. J Nerv Ment Dis. 2016;204:778–86.

85. Barsky A, Wyshak G, Klerman G. Hypochondriasis: an evaluation of the DSM-III criteria in medical outpatients. Arch Gen Psychiatry. 1986;43(5):493–500.

86. Speckens AEM, Spinhoven P, Slockers PPA, Bolk JH, van Helmert AM. A validation of the whitely index, the illness attitude scales, and the somatosensory amplification scale in general medical and general practice patients. J Psychosom Res. 1996;40:95–104.

87. Pilowsky I. Dimensions of hypochondriasis. Br J Psychiatry. 1967;113:89–93.

88. Pilowsky I. A general classification of abnormal illness behaviours. Br J Med Psychol. 1978;51:131–7.

89. Barsky AJ, Ahern DK, Bailey ED, Saintfort R, Liu EB, Peekna HM. Hypochondriacal patients' appraisal of health and physical risks. Am J Psychiatry. 2001;158:783–7.

90. Hadjistavropoulos HD, Craig KD, Hajistavropoulos T. Cognitive and behavioural responses to illness information: the role of health anxiety. Behav Res Ther. 1998;36:149–64.

91. Schwind J, Nenh JMB. Changes in free symptom attributions in hypochondriasis after cognitive therapy and behavioral therapy. Behav Cogn Psychother. 2016;44(5):601–14.

92. Wells A, Hackmann A. Imagery and core beliefs in health anxiety: contents and origins. Behav Cogn Psychother. 1993;21:265–73.

93. Barksy AJ, Coueytaux RR, Sarnie MK, Cleary PD. Hypochondriacal patients' beliefs about good health. Am J Psychiatry. 1993;150:1085–9.

94. Abramovitz J, Olantuji B, Deacon B. Health anxiety, hypochondriasis, and the anxiety disorders. Behav Ther. 2007;38:86–94.

95. van den Heuvel OA, Veltman DJ, Groenewegen HJ, Witter MP, Merkelbach J, Cath DC, et al. Disorder-specific neuroanatomincal correlates of attentional bias in obsessive-compulsive disorder, panic disorder, and hypochondriasis. Arch Gen Psychiatry. 2005;62:922–33.

96. van den Heuvel OA, Mataix-Cols D, Zwister G, Cath DC, ven der Werf YD, Groenewegen HJ, et al. Common limbic and frontal-striatal disturbances in patients with obsessive-compulsive disorder, panic disorder, and hypochondriasis. Psychol Med. 2011;41(11):2399–410.

97. Newby JM, Hobbs MJ, Mahoney AEJ, Wong S, Andrews G. DSM-5 illness anxiety disorder and somatic symptom disorder: comorbidity, correlates, and overlap with DSM-IV hypochondriasis. J Psychosom Res. 2017;101:31–7.

98. Thorgaard MV, Frostholm L, Walker LS, Stengaard-Pedersen K, Karlsson MM, Jensen JS, Fink P, Rask CU. Effects of maternal health anxiety on children's health complaints, emotional symptoms, and quality of life. Eur Child Adolesc Psychiatry. 2017;26:591–601.

99. Barsky A. Hypochondriasis and obsessive-compulsive disorder. Psychiatr Clin N Am. 1992;15(4):791–801.

100. Fallon B, Qureshi A, Schneider F, Sanchez-Lacay A, Vermes D, Reinstein R, et al. An open trial of fluvoxamine for hypochondriasis. Psychosomatics. 2003;44:298–303.

101. Greeven A, van Balkom A, Visser S, Merkelbach J, van Rood Y, van Dyck R, et al. Cognitive behavior therapy and paroxetine in the treatment of hypochondriasis: a randomized controlled trial. Am J Psychiatry. 2007;164:91–9.

102. Hiller W, Leibbrand R, Rief W, Fichter MM. Differentiating hypochondriasis from panic disorder. J Anxiety Disord. 2005;19(1):29–49.

103. Noyes R, Kathol RG, Fisher MM, Phillips BM, Suelzer MT, Woodman CL. Psychiatric co-morbidity among patient with hypochondriasis. Gen Hosp Psychiatry. 1994;16:78–87.

104. Barsky A, Wyshak G, Klerman GL, Latham S. The prevalence of hypochondriasis in medical outpatients. Soc Psychiatry Psychiatr Epidemiol. 1990;25(2):89–94.

105. Kirmayer LJ, Robbins JM. Three forms of somatization in primary care: prevalence, co-occurrence, and sociodemographic characteristics. J Nerv Ment Dis. 1991;179:647–55.

106. Noyes RJ, Kathol RG, Fisher MM, Philips BM, Suelzer MT, Holt CS. The validity of DSM III hypochondriasis. Arch Gen Psychiatry. 1993;50(12):961–70.

107. Spitzer RL, Williams JB, Kroenke K, Linzer M, deGruy FV, Hahn SR, et al. Utility of a new procedure for diagnosing mental disorders in primary care. The PRIME-MD 1000 study. JAMA. 1994;272:1749–56.

108. Sunderland M, Newby JM, Andrews G. Health anxiety in Australia: prevalence, comorbidity, disability and service use. Br J Psychiatry. 2013;202:56–61.

109. Weck F, Richtberg S, Neng J. Epidemiology of hypochondriasis and health anxiety: comparison of different diagnostic criteria. Curr Psychiatr Rev. 2014;10:14–23.

110. Seivewright H, Mulder R, Tyrer P. Prevalence of health anxiety and medically unexplained symptoms in general practice and hospital clinics. Aust N Z J Psychiatry. 2007;41(suppl2):A159.

111. Tyrer P, Cooper S, Crawford M, Dupont S, Green J, Murphy D, et al. Prevalence of health anxiety problems in medical clinics. J Psychosom Res. 2011;71:392–4.

112. Bleichhardt G, Hiller W. Krankheitsangst bei Patienten in ambulanter Verhaltenstherapie: Psychopathologie, medizinische Inanspruchnahme und Mediennutzung [Pathological features, medical consulting behaviour and media consume in outpatients with health anxiety]. Verhaltenshtherapie Verhaltensmedizin. 2006;27:29–41.

113. Garyfallos G, Adamopoulou A, Karastergiou A, Voikli M, Ikonomidis N, Donias S, et al. Somatoform disorders: comorbidity with other DSM-III-R psychiatric diagnosis in Greece. Compr Psychiatry. 1999;40:299–307.

114. Pieh C, Lahmann C, von Heymann F, Tritt K, Loew T, Busch V, et al. Prävalenz und Komorbidität der somatoformen Störung: Eine Multicenter-Studie [Prevalence and comorbidity of somatoform disorder in psychosomatic inpatients: a multicentre study]. Z Psychosom Med Psychother. 2011;57:244–50.

115. Weck F, Harms G, Neng J, Stangier U. Hypochondrische Merkmale bei Patienten einer psychotherapeutischen Ambulanz: Prävalenz und prädisponierende Faktoren [Hypochondriacal characteristics in psychotherapeutic outpatients: prevalence and predisposing factors]. Z Klin Psychol Psychother. 2011;40:124–32.

116. Creed F, Barsky A. A systematic review of the epidemiology of somatization disorder and hypochondriasis. J Psychosom Res. 2004;56(4):391–408.

117. Jacobi F, Wittchen HU, Holting C, Hofler M, Pfister H, Muller N, et al. Prevalence, co-morbidity, and correlates of mental disorders in the general population: results from the German Health Interview and Examination Survey (GHS). Psychol Med. 2004;34:597–611.

118. Barsky AJ, Fama JM, Bailey D, Ahern DKA. Prospective 4- to 5-year study of DSM-III-R hypochondriasis. Arch Gen Psychiatry. 1998;55:737–44.

119. Gropalis M, Bleichhardt G, Witthoft M, Hiller W. Hypochondriasis, somatoform disorders, and anxiety disorders: sociodemographic variables, general psychopathology, and naturalistic treatment effects. J Nerv Ment Dis. 2012;200:406–12.

120. Fink P, Ørnbøl E, Christensen KS. The outcome of health anxiety in primary care. A two-year follow-up study on health care costs and self-rated health. PLoS One. 2010;5(3):e9873.

121. Hedman E, Lekander M, Ljotsson B, Lindefors N, Ruck C, Andersson G, et al.. 2015Optimal cut-off points on the health anxiety inventory, illness attitude scales, and whitely index to identify severe health anxiety. PLoS One. 2015;10(4):e0123412.

122. Palsson N. Functional somatic symptoms and hypochondriasis among general practice patients: a pilot study. Acta Psychiatr Scand. 1998;78:191–7.

123. Bobevski I, Clarke DM, Meadows G. Health anxiety and its relationship to disability and service use: findings from a large epidemiological survey. Psychosom Med. 2015;78:13–25.

124. Eilenberg T, Frostholm L, Schroder A, Jensen JS, Fink P. Long-term consequences of severe health anxiety on sick leave in treated and untreated patients: analysis alongside a randomised controlled trial. J Anxiety Disord. 2015;32:95–102.

125. Gureje O, Ustun TB, Simon GE. The syndrome of hypochondriasis: a cross-national study in primary care. Psychol Med. 1997;27(5):1001–10.

126. Martin A, Jacobi F. Features of hypochondriasis and illness worry in the general population in Germany. Psychosom Med. 2006;68(5):770–7.

127. Mykletun A, Heradstveit O, Eriksen K, Glozier N, Overland S, Maeland JG, et al. Health anxiety and disability pension award: the HUSK Study. Psychosom Med. 2009;71(3):353–60.

128. Barsky AJ, Cleary PD, Sarnie MK, Klerman GL. The course of transient hypochondriasis. Am J Psychiatry. 1993;150:484–8.

129. Barsky AJ, Bailey ED, Fama JM, Ahern DK. Predictors of remission in DSM hypochondriasis. Compr Psychiatry. 2000;41:179–83.

130. Fernandez C, Fernandez R, Isaac Amigo D. Characteristics and one year follow-up of primary care patients with health anxiety. Prim Care Community Psychiatry. 2005;10:81–93.

131. Noyes R, Kathol RG, Fisher MM, Phillips BM, Suelzer MT, Woodman CL. One-year follow-up of medical outpatients with hypochondriasis. Psychosomatics. 1994;35(6):533–45.

132. Olde-Hartman TC, Borghuis MS, Lucassen PLBJ, van de Laar FA, Speckens AE, van Weel C. Medically unexplained symptoms, somatisation disorder, and hypochondriasis: course and prognosis. A systematic review. J Psychosom Res. 2009;66:363–77.

133. Simon GE, Gureje O, Fullerton C. Course of hypochondriasis in an international primary care study. Gen Hosp Psychiatry. 2001;23:51–5.

134. Fallon B, Liebowitz M, Salman E. Fluoxetine for patients without major depression. J Clin Psychopharmacol. 1993;13:438–41.

135. Fallon B, Petkova E, Skritskaya N. A double-masked placebo controlled study of fluoxetine for hypochondriasis. J Clin Psychopharmacol. 2008;28:638–45.

136. Fallon BA, Ahern DK, Pavlicova M, Slavov I, Skritskya N, Barsky AJ. A randomized controlled trial of medication and cognitive behavioral therapy for hypochondriasis. Am J Psychiatry. 2017;174(8):756–64.

137. Oosterbaan D, van Balkom A, van Boeijen C, de Meij T, van Dyck R. An open study of paroxetine in hypochondriasis. Prog Neuropsychopharmacol Biol Psychiatry. 2001;25:1023–33.

138. Greeven A, van Balkom A, van der Leeden R, Merkelbach J, van daen Heuvel O, Spinhoven P. Cognitive behavioral therapy versus paroxetine in the treatment of hypochondriasis: an 18-month naturalistic follow-up. J Behav Ther Exp Psychother. 2009;40(3):487–96.

139. Bouman TK, Visser S. Cognitive and behavioural treatment of hypochondriasis. Psychother Psychosom. 1998;67:214–21.

140. Bourgault-Fagnou MD, Hadjistavropoulos HD. A randomized trial of two forms of cognitive behaviour therapy for an older adult population with subclinical health anxiety. Cogn Behav Ther. 2013;42:31–44.

141. Clark DM, Salkovsis PM, Hackmann A, Wells A, Fennell M, Ludgate J, et al. Two psychological treatments for hypochondriasis: a randomized controlled trial. Br J Psychiatry. 1998;173:218–25.

142. Eilenberg T, Frostholm L, Schroder A, Jensen JS, Fink P. Long-term consequences of severe health anxiety on sick leave in treated and untreated patients: analysis alongside a randomized control trial. J Anxiety Disord. 2015;32:95–102.

143. Olantuji B, Kauffman BY, Meltzer S, Davis ML, Smits JA, Powers MB. Cognitive-behavioral therapy for hypochondriasis/health anxiety: a meta-analysis of treatment outcome and moderators. Behav Res Ther. 2014;58:65–74.

144. Sanatinia R, Wang D, Tyrer P, Tyrer H, Crawford M, Cooper S, et al. Impact of personality status on the outcomes and cost of cognitive behavioural therapy for health anxiety. Br J Psychiatry. 2016;209(3):244–50.

145. Salkovskis PM, Warwick HM, Deale AC. Cognitive-behavioral treatment for severe and persistent health anxiety (hypochondriasis). Brief Treat Crisis Interv. 2003;3:353–67.

146. Schrieber F, Witthoft M, Neng JM, Weck F. Changes in negative implicit evaluations in patients of hypochondriasis after treatment with cognitive therapy or exposure therapy. J Behav Ther Exp Psychiatry. 2016;50:139–46.

147. Seivewright H, Green J, Salkovskis P, Barret B, Nur U, Tyrer P. Cognitive-behavioural therapy for health anxiety in a genitourinary medicine clinic: randomised control trial. Br J Psychiatry. 2008;193:332–7.

148. Sorenson P, Birket-Smith M, Wattar U, Buemann I. A randomized clinical trial of cognitive behavioral therapy versus short-term psychodynamic psychotherapy versus no intervention for patients with hypochondriasis. Psychol Med. 2011;41(2):431–41.

149. Tyrer P, Cooper S, Salkovskis P, Tyrer H, Crawford M, Byford S, et al. Clinical and cost-effectiveness of cognitive behaviour therapy for health anxiety in medical patients: a multicentre randomized control trial. Lancet. 2014;383:219–25.

150. Visser S, Bouman TK. The treatment of hypochondriasis: exposure plus response prevention vs. cognitive therapy. Behav Res Ther. 2001;39:423–42.

151. Weck F, Neng JM. Response and remission after cognitive and exposure therapy for hypochondriasis. J Nerv Ment Dis. 2015;203(11):883–5.

152. Weck F, Neng JM, Richtberg S, Jakob M, Stangier U. Cognitive therapy versus exposure therapy for hypochondriasis (health anxiety): a randomized control trial. J Consult Clin Psychol. 2015;83(4):665–76.

153. Avia MD, Ruiz A, Olivaries ME, Cespo M, Guisado AB, Sandhez A, et al. The meaning of psychological symptoms: effectiveness of a group intervention with hypochondriacal patients. Behav Res Ther. 1996;34:23–31.

154. Hedman E, Ljotsson B, Andersson E, Ruck C, Andersson G, Lindefors N. Effectiveness and cost offset analysis of group CBT for hypochondriasis delivered in a psychiatric setting: an open trial. Cogn Behav Ther. 2010;39:239–50.

155. Hedman E, Anddersson G, Anderrsson E, Ljotsson B, Ruck C, Asmundson GJ, et al. Internet-based cognitive behavioural therapy for severe health anxiety: randomised controlled trial. Br J Psychiatry. 2011;198:230–6.

156. Weck F, Gropalis M, Hiller W, Bleichhardt G. Effectiveness of cognitive-behavioral group therapy for patients with hypochondriasis (health anxiety). J Anxiety Disord. 2015;30:1–7.

157. Hedman E, Andersson E, Linderfors N, Anderrson G, Ruck C, Ljotsson B. Cost-effectiveness and long-term effectiveness of internet-based cognitive behaviour therapy for severe health anxiety. Psychol Med. 2013;43(2):363–74.

158. Hedman E, Axelsson E, Andersson E, Lekander M, Liotsson B. Exposure-based cognitive-behavioural therapy via the internet and as bibliotherapy for somatic symptom disorder and Illness anxiety disorder: randomised control trial. Br J Psychiatry. 2016;209(5):407–13.

159. Hedman E, Exelsson E, Gorling A, Ritzman C, Ronnheden M, El Alaoui S, et al. Internet-delivered exposure-based cognitive-behavioural therapy and behavioral stress management for severe health anxiety: randomised control trial. Br J Psychiatry. 2014;205:307–14.

160. Nakao M, Shinozaki Y, Nolido N, Ahern DK, Barsky AJ. Responsiveness of hypochondriacal patients with chronic low back pain to cognitive-behavioral therapy. Psychosomatics. 2012;53:139–47.

161. Eilenberg T. Acceptance and Commitment Group Therapy (ACT-G) for health anxiety: a randomized, controlled trial. Dan J Med. 2015;63(10):85294.

162. Eilenberg T, Fink P, Jensen JS, Rief W, Frostholm L. Acceptance and Commitment Group Therapy (ACT-G) for health anxiety: a randomized controlled trial. Psychol Med. 2016;46(1):103–15.

163. Lovas DA, Barsky AJ. Mindfulness based cognitive therapy for hypochondriasis, or severe health anxiety: a pilot study. J Anxiety Disord. 2010;24:931–5.

164. McManus F, Surawy C, Muse K, Vazquez-Montes M, Williams JM. A randomized clinical trial of mindfulness-based cognitive therapy versus unrestricted services for health anxiety (hypochondriasis). J Consult Clin Psychol. 2012;80:817–28.

165. Stone J, Warlow C, Sharpe M. The symptom of functional weakness: a controlled study of 107 patients. Brain. 2010;133(5):1537–51.

166. Stone J, Aybek S. Functional limb weakness and paralysis. Handb Clin Neurol. 2016;139:213–28.

167. Thomas M, Vuong KD, Jankovic J. Long-term prognosis of patients with psychogenic movement disorders. Parkinsonism Relat Disord. 2006;12(6):382–7.

168. Cubo E, Hinson VK, Goetz CG, Ruiz PG, de Yebenes JG, Marti MJ, et al. Transcultural comparison of psychogenic movement disorders. Mov Disord. 2005;20(10):1343–5.

169. Jankovic J, Vuong KD, Thomas M. Psychogenic tremor: long term outcome. CNS Spectr. 2006;11:501–8.

170. Keane JR. Hysterical gait disorder: 60 cases. Neurology. 1989;39:586–9.

171. Lempert T, Dieterich M, Huppert D, Brandt T. Psychogenic disorders in neurology: frequency and clinical spectrum. Acta Neurol Scand. 1990;82:335–40.

172. Ng K, Lee J, Mui W. Aphonia induced by conversion disorder during a Cesarean section. Acta Anaesthesiol Taiwan. 2012;50(3):138–41.

173. Baslet G, Seshadri A, Bermeo-Ovalle A, Willment K, Myers L. Psychogenic non-epileptic seizures: an updated primer. Psychosomatics. 2016;51:1–17.

174. Ghaffar O, Staines R, Feinstein A. Unexplained neurologic symptoms: an fMRI study of sensory conversion disorder. Neurology. 2006;67(11):2036–8.

175. Rolak LA. Psychogenic sensory loss. J Nerv Ment Dis. 1988;176(11):686–7.

176. Tiihonen J, Kuikka J, Viinamki H, Lehtonen J, Partanen J. Altered cerebral blood flow during hysterical paresthesia. Biol Psychiatry. 1995;37(2):134–5.

177. Villegas RB, Ilsen PF. Functional visual loss: a diagnosis of exclusion. Optometry. 2007;78:523–33.

178. Breuer J. Fraulein Anna O. In: The complete works of Sigmund Freud, vol. II. standard ed. London: Hogarth Press; 1895/1974. p. 21–47.

179. Mott AE, Grushka M, Sessle BJ. Diagnosis and management of taste disorders and burning mouth syndrome. Dent Clin N Am. 1993;37(1):33–71.

180. Austen S, Lych C. Non-organic hearing loss redefined: understanding, categorizing, and managing non-organic behavior. Int J Audiol. 2004;43(8):449–57.

181. Dwyer J, Reid S. Ganser's syndrome. Lancet. 2004;364:471–3.

182. Delis DC, Wetter SR. Cogniform disorder and cogniform condition: proposed diagnosis for excessive cognitive symptoms. Arch Clin Neuropsychol. 2007;22(5):589–604.

183. Stone J, Reuber M, Carson A. Functional symptoms in neurology: mimics and chameleons. Pract Neurol. 2013;13:104–13.

184. Ganos C, Edwards MJ, Bhatia KP. Posttraumatic functional movement disorders. Handb Clin Neurol. 2016;139:499–507.

185. Stone J, Carson A, Aditya H, Prescott R, Zaubi M, Warlow C, et al. The role of physical injury in motor and sensory conversion symptoms: a systematic and narrative review. J Psychosom Res. 2009;66(5):383–90.

186. Daum C, Hubschmid M, Aybek S. The value of 'positive' clinical signs for weakness, sensory and gait disorders in conversion disorder: a systematic and narrative review. J Neurol Neurosurg Psychiatry. 2014;85:180–90.

187. Avbersek A, Sisodiya S. Does the primary literature provide support for clinical signs used to distinguish psychogenic nonepileptic

seizures from epileptic seizures? J Neurol Neurosurg Psychiatry. 2010;81:719–25.

188. Vossler DG, Haltiner AM, Schlepp SK, Friel PA, Caylor LM, Morgan JD, Dohery MJ. Ictal stuttering: a sign suggestive of psychogenic nonepileptic seizures. Neurology. 2004;63(3):516–9.

189. Factor SA, Podskalny GD, Molho ES. Psychogenic movement disorders: frequency, clinical profile, and characteristics. J Neurol Neurosurg Psychiatry. 1995;59:406–12.

190. Stone J, Smyth R, Carson A, Warlow C, Sharpe M. La belle indifference in conversion symptoms and hysteria: systematic review. Br J Psychiatry. 2006;188:204–9.

191. Hoerth MT, Wellik KE, Demaerschalk BM. Clinical predictors of psychogenic nonepileptic seizures: a critically appraised topic. Neurologist. 2008;14:266–70.

192. Boissy AR, Ford PJ. A touch of MS – therapeutic mislabeling. Neurology. 2012;78:1981–5.

193. Paulson GW. Pseudo-multiple sclerosis. South Med J. 1996;89(3):301–4.

194. Merwick A, Sweeney BJ. Functional symptoms in clinically definite MS—pseudo-relapse syndrome. Int MS J. 2008;15(2):47–51.

195. Nicolson R, Feinstein A. Conversion, dissociation, and multiple sclerosis. J Nerv Ment Dis. 1994;182(11):668–9.

196. Pavlou M, Stefoski D. Development of somatizing responses in multiple sclerosis. Psychother Psychosom. 1983;39:236–43.

197. Stone J, Carson A, Duncan R, Coleman R, Roberst R, Warlow C, et al. Symptoms 'unexplained by organic disease' in 1144 new neurology outpatients: how often does the diagnosis change at follow-up? Brain. 2009;132(1):2878–88.

198. Williams DT, Ford B, Fahn S. Phenomenology and psychopathology related to psychogenic movements disorders. Adv Neurol. 1995;65:231–57.

199. Benbadis SR, O'Neill E, Tatum WO, Heriaud L. Outcome of prolonged video-EEG monitoring at a typical referral epilepsy center. Epilepsia. 2004;45:1150–3.

200. LaFrance WC, Benbadis SR. Differentiating frontal lobe epilepsy from psychogenic nonepileptic seizures. Neurol Clin. 2011;29:149–62.

201. Matin N, Young SS, Williams B, LaFrance WC Jr, King JN, Caplan D, et al. Neuropsychiatric associations with gender, illness duration, work disability, and motor subtype in a US functional neurological disorders clinic population. J Neuropsychiatr Clin Neurosci. 2017;29:375–82.

202. McKenzie PS, Oto M, Graham CD, Duncan R. Do patients whose psychogenic non-epileptic seizures resolve, 'replace' them with other medically unexplained symptoms? Medically unexplained symptoms arising after a diagnosis of psychogenic non-epileptic seizures. J Neurol Neurosurg Psychiatry. 2011;82(9):967–9.

203. Carson A, Ludwig L, Welch K. Psychologic theories in functional neurologic disorders. Handb Clin Neurol. 2016;139:105–20.

204. Perez DL, Barsky AJ, Daffner K, Silbersweig DA. Motor and somatosensory conversion disorder: a functional unawareness syndrome? J Neuropsychiatr Clin Neurosci. 2012;24(2):141–51.

205. Demartini B, Goeta D, Romito L, Anselmetti S, Bertelli S, D'Agostino A, et al. Anorexia nervosa and functional motor symptoms: two faces of the same coin? J Neuropsychiatr Clin Neurosci. 2017;29:383–90.

206. Carson A, Stone J, Hibberd C, Murray G, Duncan R, Coleman R, et al. Disability, distress and unemployment in neurology outpatients with symptoms 'unexplained by disease'. J Neurol Neurosurg Psychiatry. 2011;82:810–3.

207. Crimlisk HL, Bhatia K, Cope H, et al. Slater revisited: 6 year follow up study of patients with medically unexplained motor symptoms. BMJ. 1998;316(7131):582–6.

208. Feinstein A, Stergiopoulos V, Fine J, Lang AE. Psychiatric outcome in patients with a psychogenic movement disorder: a prospective study. Neuropsychiatry Neuropsychol Behav Neurol. 2001;14(3):169–76.

209. Diprose W, Sundram F, Menkes DB. Psychiatric comorbidity in psychogenic nonepileptic seizures compared with epilepsy. Epilepsy Behav. 2016;56:123–30.

210. Ekanayake V, Kranick S, LaFaver K, Naz A, Webb AF, LaFrance WC Jr, et al. Personality traits in psychogenic non-epileptic seizures (PNES) and psychogenic movement disorder (PMD): neuroticism and perfectionism. J Psychosom Res. 2017;97:23–9.

211. Anderson KE, Gruber-Baldini AL, Vaughan CG, Reich SG, Fishman PS, Weiner WJ, et al. Impact of psychogenic movement disorders versus Parkinson's on disability, quality of life, and psychopathology. Mov Disord. 2007;22(15):2204–9.

212. Simon G, Gater R, Kisely S, Piccinelli M. Somatic symptoms of distress: an international primary care study. Psychosom Med. 1996;58(5):481–8.

213. Stone J, Hewett R, Carson A, Warlow C, Sharpe M. The 'disappearance' of hysteria: historical mystery or illusion? J R Soc Med. 2008;101(1):12–8.

214. Binzer M, Kullgren G. Motor conversion disorder. A prospective 2- to 5-year follow-up study. Psychosomatics. 1998;39:519–27.

215. Ewald H, Rogne T, Ewald K, Fink P. Somatization in patients newly admitted to a neurological department. Acta Psychiatr Scand. 1994;89:174–9.

216. Folks DG, Ford CV, Regan WM. Conversion symptoms in a general hospital. Psychosomatics. 1984;25:285.

217. Gelauff J, Stone J, Edwards M, Carson A. The prognosis of functional (psychogenic) motor symptoms: a systematic review. J Neurol Neurosurg Psychiatry. 2014;85(2):220–6.

218. Roy A. Hysteria: a case note study. Can J Psychiatry. 1979;24:157–60.

219. Feinstein A, Stergiopoulos V, Fine J, Lang AF. Psychiatric outcome in patients with a psychogenic movement disorder: a prospective study. Neuropsychiatry Neuropsychol Behav Neurol. 2001;14(3):169–76.

220. Stefansson JG, Messina JA, Meyerowitz S. Hysterical neurosis, conversion type: clinical and epidemiological considerations. Acta Psychiatr Scand. 1976;53:119–38.

221. Sharpe M, Stone J, Hibberd C, Warlow C, Duncan R, Coleman R, et al. Neurology out-patients with symptoms unexplained by disease: illness beliefs and financial benefits predict 1-year outcome. Psychol Med. 2010;40(4):689–98.

222. Dallocchio C, Arbasino C, Klersy C, Marchioni E. The effects of physical activity on psychogenic movement disorders. Mov Disord. 2010;25(4):421–5.

223. Kompoliti K, Wilson B, Stebbins G, Bernard B, Hinson V. Immediate vs. delayed treatment of psychogenic movement disorders with short term psychodynamic psychotherapy: randomized clinical trial. Parkinsonism Relat Disord. 2014;20(1):60–3.

224. Sharma VD, Jones R, Factor SA. Psychodynamic psychotherapy for functional (psychogenic) movement disorders. J Mov Disord. 2017;10(1):40–4.

225. Goldstein LH, Chalder T, Chigwedere C, Kondoker MR, Moriarty J, Toone BK, et al. Cognitive behavioral therapy for psychogenic non-epileptic seizures: a pilot RCT. Neurology. 2010;74(24):1986–94.

226. LaFrance CW Jr, Baird GL, Barry JJ, Blum AS, Webb AF, Keitner GI, et al. Multicenter pilot treatment trial for psychogenic nonepileptic seizures: a randomized clinical trial. JAMA Psychiat. 2014;71(9):997–1005.

227. Baslet G, Dworetzky B, Perez DL, Oser M. Treatment of psychogenic nonepileptic seizures: updated review and findings from a

mindfulness-based intervention case series. Clin EEG Neurosci. 2015;46(1):54–64.

228. Bullock KD, Mirza N, Forte C, Trockel M. Group dialectical-behavior therapy skills training for conversion disorder with seizures. J Neuropsychiatr Clin Neurosci. 2015;27:240–3.

229. Metin SZ, Ozmen M, Metin B, Talasman S, Yeni SN, Ozkara C. Treatment with group psychotherapy for chronic psychogenic nonepileptic seizures. Epilepsy Behav. 2013;28(1):91–4.

230. Barry JJ, Wittenberg D, Bullock KD, Michaels JB, Classen CC, Fisher RS. Group therapy for patients with psychogenic nonepileptic seizures: a pilot study. Epilepsy Behav. 2008;13(4):624–9.

231. Baslet G. Psychogenic nonepileptic seizures: a treatment review. What have we learned since the beginning of the millennium? Neuropsychiatr Dis Treat. 2012;8:585–98.

232. Zaroff CM, Myers L, Barr WB, Luciano D, Devinsky O. Group psychoeducation as treatment for psychological nonepileptic seizures. Epilepsy Behav. 2004;5(4):587–92.

233. Bravo TP, Hoffman-Snyder CR, Wellik KE, Martin KA, Hoerth MT, Demaerschalk BM, et al. The effect of selective serotonin reuptake inhibitors on the frequency of psychogenic nonepileptic seizures: a critically appraised topic. Neurologist. 2013;19(1):30–3.

234. LaFrance WC Jr, Keitner GI, Papandonatos GD, Blum AS, Machan JT, Ryan CE, et al. Pilot pharmacologic randomized controlled trial for psychogenic nonepileptic seizures. Neurology. 2010;75(13):1166–73.

235. Nicholson TRJ, Voon V. Transcranial magnetic stimulation and sedation as treatment for functional neurologic disorders. Handb Clin Neurol. 2016;139:619–29.

236. Deeley Q. Hypnosis as therapy for functional neurologic disorders. Handb Clin Neurol. 2016;139:585–95.

237. Heruti RJ, Levy A, Adunsi A, Ohry A. Conversion motor paralysis disorder: overview and rehabilitation. Spinal Cord. 2002;40:327–34.

238. Neilsen G, Stone J, Matthews A, Brown M, Spankes C, Farmer R, et al. Physiotherapy for functional motor disorders: a consensus recommendation. J Neurol Neurosurg Psychiatry. 2015;86(10):1113–9.

239. Ness D. Physical therapy management for conversion disorder: case series. JNPT. 2007;31:30–9.

240. McCormack R, Moriarty J, Mellers JD, Shotbolt P, Pastena R, Landes N, et al. Specialist inpatient treatment for severe motor conversion disorder: a retrospective comparative study. J Neurol Neurosurg Psychiatry. 2014;85(8):895–900.

241. Shapiro AP, Teasell RW. Behavioural interventions in the rehabilitation of acute v. chronic non-organic (conversion/factitious) motor disorders. Br J Psychiatry. 2004;185(2):140–6.

242. Williams DT, Lafaver K, Carson A, Fahn S. Inpatient treatment for functional neurologic disorders. Handb Clin Neurol. 2016;139:631–41.

243. Jirsch JD, Ahmed SN, Maximova K, Gross DW. Recognition of psychogenic nonepileptic seizures diminishes acute care utilization. Epilepsy Behav. 2011;22(2):304–7.

244. Razvi S, Mulhern S, Duncan R. Newly diagnosed psychogenic nonepileptic seizures: health care demand prior to and following diagnosis at a first seizure clinic. Epilepsy Behav. 2012;23(1):7–9.

245. Hall-Patch L, Brown R, House A, Howlett S, Kemp S, Lawton G, NEST collaborators, et al. Acceptability and effectiveness of a strategy for the communication of the diagnosis of psychogenic nonepileptic seizures. Epilepsia. 2010;51(1):70–8.

246. Stone J, Carson A, Hallett M. Explanation as treatment for functional neurologic disorders. Handb Clin Neurol. 2016;139:543–53.

247. Shen W, Bowman ES, Markand ON. Presenting the diagnosis of pseudoseizure. Neurology. 1990;40(5):756–9.

248. Bass C, Halligan P. Factitious disorders and malingering in relation to functional neurologic disorders. Handb Clin Neurol. 2016;139:509–20.

249. Yates GP, Feldman MD. Factitious disorder: a systematic review of 455 cases in the professional literature. Gen Hosp Psychiatry. 2016;41:20–8.

250. Heimbach D, Bruhl P. Urological aspects of Munchausen's syndrome. Eur Urol. 1997;31(3):371–5.

251. Hamre MC, Nguyen PH, Shepard SE, Caplan JP. Factitious mastectomy: the importance of staying abreast of the medical record. Psychosomatics. 2014;55:186–90.

252. Pessina AC, Bisogni V, Fassina A, Rossi GP. Munchausen syndrome: a novel cause of drug resistant hypertension. J Hypertens. 2013;31(7):1473–6.

253. Fliegner JR. Munchausen's syndrome and self-induced illness in gynaecology. Med J Aust. 1983;2(12):666–7.

254. Fliege H, Grimm A, Eckhardt-Henn A, Gieler U, Martin K, Klapp BF. Frequency of ICD-10 factitious disorder: survey of senior hospital consultants and physicians in private practice. Psychosomatics. 2007;48(1):60–4.

255. Ucmak D, Harman M, Akkurt ZM. Dermatitis artefacta: a retrospective analysis. Cutan Ocul Toxicol. 2014;33(1):22–7.

256. Tomas-Aragones L, Consoli SM, Consoli SG, Poot F, Taube K, Linder MD, et al. Self-inflicted lesions in dermatology: a management and therapeutic approach- a position paper from the European society for dermatology and psychiatry. Acta Derm Venereol. 2017;97:159–72.

257. Krahn L, Bostwick J, Stonnington C. Looking towards DSM-5: should factitious disorder become a subtype of somatoform disorder? Psychosomatics. 2008;49:277–82.

258. Kanaan RA, Wessely SC. Factitious disorders in neurology: an analysis of reported cases. Psychosomatics. 2010;51(1):47–54.

259. Bass C, Halligan P. Factitious disorders and malingering: challenges for clinical assessment and management. Lancet. 2014;383(9926):142–1432.

260. Krahn L, Honghzhe L, O'Connor K. Patients who strive to be ill: factitious disorder with physical symptoms. Am J Psychiatr. 2003;160:1163–8.

261. Hamilton JC, Eger M, Razzak S, Feldman MD, Hallmark N, Cheek S. Somatoform, factitious, and related diagnosis in the national discharge survey: addressing the proposed DSM-5 revision. Psychosomatics. 2013;54:142–8.

262. Goldstein AB. Identification and classification of factitious disorders: an analysis of cases reported during a ten year period. Int J Psychiatry Med. 1998;28(2):221–41.

263. Yates G, Bass C. The perpetrators of medical child abuse (Munchausen Syndrome by Proxy) – a systematic review of 796 cases. Child Abuse Negl. 2017;72:45–53.

264. Jones TW, Delplanche ML, Davies NP, Rose CH. Factitious disorder by proxy simulating fetal growth restriction. Obstet Gynecol. 2015;125(3):732–4.

265. Hoertel N, Lavaud P, Le Strat Y, Gorwood P. Estimated cost of a factitious disorder with 6-year follow-up. Psychiatry Res. 2012;200:107–8.

266. Vaduganathan M, McCullough SA, Fraser TN, Stern TA. Death due to Munchausen syndrome: a case of idiopathic recurrent right ventricular failure and a review of the literature. Psychosomatics. 2014;55(6):668–72.

267. Bass C, Taylor M. Recovery from chronic factitious disorder (Munchausen's syndrome): a personal account. Personal Ment Health. 2013;7(1):80–3.

268. Feldman M. Recovery from Munchausen's syndrome. South Med J. 2006;99:1398–9.

269. Higgins P. Temporary Munchausen's syndrome. Br J Psychiatry. 1990;157:613–6.

270. Axelsson E, Andersson E, Ljotsson B, Wallhed Finn D, Hedman E. The health preoccupation diagnostic interview: inter-rater reliability of a structured interview for diagnostic assessment of DSM-5 somatic symptom disorder and illness anxiety disorder. Cogn Behav Ther. 2016;45(4):259–69.

271. Brown TA, Barlow D. Anxiety and related disorder interview schedule for DSM-5 (ADIS-5). New York: Oxford University Pres; 2014.

272. Barsky AJ, Cleary PD, Wyshak G, Spitzer RL, Williams JB, Klerman GL. A structured diagnostic interview for hypochondriasis. A proposed criterion standard. J Nerv Ment Dis. 1992;180(1):20–7.

273. Hinson VK, Cubo E, Comella CL, Goetz CG, Leurgans S. Rating scale for psychogenic movement disorders: scale development and clinimetric testing. Mov Disord. 2005;20(12):1592–7.

274. Salkovskis P, Rimes K, Warwick H, Clark D. The health anxiety inventory: development and validation of scales for the measurement of health anxiety and hypochondriasis. Psychol Med. 2002;32:843–53.

275. Greeven A, Spinhoven P, van Balkom AJLM. Hypochondriasis Y-BOCS: a study of the psychometric properties of a clinician administered semi-structured interview to assess hypochondriacal thoughts and behaviors. Clin Psychol Psychother. 2009;16:431–43.

276. Wright KD, Asmundson GJ. Health anxiety in children: development and psychometric properties on the childhood illness attitudes scales. Cogn Behav Ther. 2003;32:194–202.

277. McElroy E, Shevlin M. The development and initial validation of the cyberchondria severity scale (CSS). J Anxiety Disord. 2014;28(2):259–65.

278. Kroenke K, Spitzer RI, Williams JBW. The PHQ-15: validity of a new measure for evaluating the severity of somatic symptoms. Psychosom Med. 2002;64:258–66.

279. Barsky AJ, Wyshak G, Klerman GL. The somatosensory amplification scale and its relationship to hypochondriasis. J Psychiatr Res. 1990;24:323–34.

280. Nijenhuis ERS, Spinhoven P, Van Dyck R, Van der Hart O, Vanderlinden J. The development and the psychometric characteristics of the Somatoform Dissociation Questionnaire (SDQ-20). J Nerv Ment Dis. 1996;184:688–94.

281. Shields SS, Mallory ME, Simon A. The body awareness questionnaire: reliability and validity. J Pers Assess. 1989;53(4):802–15.

282. Schmidt NB, Lerew DR, Trakowski JH. Body vigilance in panic disorder: evaluating attention to bodily perturbations. J Consult Clin Psychol. 1997;65(2):214–20.

283. Price CJ, Thompson EA. Measuring dimensions of body connection: body awareness and bodily dissociation. J Altern Complement Med. 2007;13(9):945–53.

284. Barsky A. Hypochondriasis and panic disorder: boundary and overlap. Arch Gen Psychiatry. 1994;51:918–25.

285. McGilchrist I, Cutting J. Somatic delusions in schizophrenia and the affective psychoses. Br J Psychiatry. 1995;167(3):350–61.

286. Greeven A, van Balkom AJ, van Rood YR, van Oppen P, Spinhoven P. The boundary between hypochondriasis and obsessive-compulsive disorder: a cross-sectional study from the Netherlands. J Clin Psychiatry. 2006;67(11):1682–9.

287. Katon W, Kleinman A, Rosen W. Depression and somatization: a review, part I. Am J Med. 1982;72:127–35.

288. Katon W, Kleinman A, Rosen W. Depression and somatization: a review, part II. Am J Med. 1982;72:241–7.

289. Van der Kolk BA, Pelcovitz D, Roth S, Mandel FS, McFarlane A, Herman JL. Dissociation, somatization, and affect dysregulation: the complexity of adaptation to trauma. Am J Psychiatr. 1996;153(7):83–93.

290. Tasca C, Rappetti M, Carta MG, Fadda B. Women and hysteria in the history of mental health. Clin Pract Epidemiol Ment Health. 2012;8:110–9.

291. Fahrenberg J. Somatic complaints in the German population. J Psychosom Res. 1995;39:809–17.

292. Haavio-Mannila E. Inequalities in health and gender. Soc Sci Med. 1991;32:579–90.

293. Ladwig KH, Marten-Mittag B, Formanek B. Gender differences of symptom reporting and medical health care utilization in the German population. Eur J Epidemiol. 2000;16:511–8.

294. Kandrack MA, Grant KR, Segall A. Gender differences in health related behavior: some unanswered questions. Soc Sci Med. 1993;36:21–32.

295. Kroenke K, Spitzer RL. Gender differences in the reporting of physical and somatoform symptoms. Psychosom Med. 1998;60:150–5.

296. Popay J, Bartley M, Owen C. Gender inequalities in health: social position, affective disorders, and minor physical morbidity. Soc Sci Med. 1993;36:21–32.

297. Verbrugge LM, Wingard DL. Sex differentials in health and mortality. Women Health. 1982;12:103–45.

298. Fink P, Toft T, Hansen MS, Ornbol E, Olesen F. Symptoms and syndromes of bodily distress: an exploratory study of 978 internal medical, neurological, and primary care patients. Psychosom Med. 2007;69(1):30–9.

299. Bujoreanu S, Randall E, Thomson K, Ibeziako P. Characteristics of medically hospitalized pediatric patients with somatoform diagnoses. Hosp Pediatr. 2014;4(5):283–90.

300. Cloninger SR, Martin RL, Guze SB, Clayton PJ. A prospective follow-up and family study of somatization in men and women. Am J Psychiatry. 1986;143:873–8.

301. Faravelli C, Solvatori S, Galassi F, Aiazzi L, Drei C, Cavras P. Epidemiology of somatoform disorders: a community survey in Florence. Soc Psychiatry Psychiatr Epidemiol. 1997;32:24–9.

302. Furnham A, Kirkcald B. Age and sex differences in health beliefs and behaviours. Psychol Rep. 1991;80:63–6.

303. Golding JM, Smith GR, Kashner TM. Does somatization disorder occur in men? Clinical characteristics of women and men with multiple unexplained somatic symptoms. Arch Gen Psychiatry. 1991;48:231–5.

304. Kellner R. Hypochondriasis and somatization. JAMA. 1987;258:2718–22.

305. Ladwig KH, Marten-Mittag B, Erazo N, Gundel H. Identifying somatization disorder in a population-based health examination survey: psychosocial burden and gender differences. Psychosomatics. 2001;42:511–78.

306. Smith GR, Monson RA, Ray DC. Patients with multiple unexplained symptoms: their characteristics, functional health, and health care utilization. Arch Intern Med. 1986;146:69–72.

307. Silverstein B. Gender differences in the prevalence of clinical depression: the role played by depression associated with somatic symptoms. Am J Psychiatry. 1999;156:480–2.

308. Silverstein B, Edwards T, Gamma A, Ajdacic-Gross V, Rossler W, Angst J. The role played by depression associated with somatic symptomology in accounting for the gender difference in the prevalence of depression. Soc Psychiatry Psychiatr Epidemiol. 2013;48:257–63.

309. Drossman DA, Whitehead WE, Camilleri M. Irritable bowel syndrome: a technical review for practice guideline development. Gastroenterology. 1997;112:212902137.

310. Payne CK, Joyce GF, Wise M, Clemens JQ. Interstitial cystitis and painful bladder syndrome. J Urol. 2007;177:2042–9.

311. Wolfe F, Ross K, Anderson J, Ressell IJ, Hebert L. The prevalence and characteristics of fibromyalgia in the general population. Arthritis Rheum. 1995;38(1):19–28.

312. Bush FM, Harkins SW, Harrington WG, Pricc DD. Analysis of gender effects on pain perception and symptom perception in temporomandibular pain. Pain. 1993;53:73–80.

313. Collin SM, Bakken IJ, Nazareth I, Crawley E, White PD. Trends in the incidence of chronic fatigue syndrome and fibromyalgia in the UK, 2001–2013: a clinical practice research datalink study. J R Soc Med. 2017;110(6):231–44.

314. Brunahl C, Dybowski C, Albrecht R, Riegel B, Hoink J, Fisch M, et al. Mental disorders in patients with chronic pelvic pain syndrome (CPPS). J Psychosom Res. 2017;98:19–26.

315. Farina B, Mazzotti E, Pasquini P, Mantione MG. Somatoform and psychoform dissociation among women with orgasmic and sexual pain disorders. J Trauma Dissoc. 2011;12:526–34.

316. Berkley KJ. Sex differences in pain. Behav Brain Sci. 1997;20:371–80.

317. Chang L, Heitkemper MM. Gender differences in irritable bowel syndrome. Gastroenterology. 2002;123:1686–701.

318. Derbyshire SWG. Sources of variation in assessing male and female responses to pain. New Ideas Psychol. 1997;15:83–95.

319. Fillingim RB, Maixner W. Gender differences in the response to noxious stimuli. Pain Forum. 1995;4:209–21.

320. Fillinghim RB, Maixner W, Girdler SS, et al. Ischemic but not thermal pain sensitivity varies across the menstrual cycle. Psychosom Med. 1997;59:512–20.

321. Ladwig KH, Marten-Mittag B, Formanek B, Dammann G. Gender differences of symptom reporting and medical health care utilization in the German population. Eur J Epidemiol. 2000;16:511–8.

322. Piccinelli M, Simon G. Gender and cross-cultural differences in somatic symptoms associated with emotional distress: an international study in primary care. Psychol Med. 1997;27:433–44.

323. Wool CA, Barsky AJ. Do women somatize more than men? Gender differences in somatization. Psychosomatics. 1994;35:445–52.

324. Kaminsky MJ, Slavney PR. Methodology and personality in Briquet's syndrome: a reappraisal. Am J Psychiatry. 1976;133:85–8.

325. Doghor ON, Haimovici F, Mathias D, Knudson-Gonzalez D, Freid C. A determined woman: anxiety, unresolved mourning, and capacity assessment in recurrent pregnancy loss. Harv Rev Psychiatry. 2017;25(1):39–45.

326. Greene JA, Querques J, Barksy AJ, Notman M. Somatic preoccupations of future pregnancy. Harv Rev Psychiatry. 2011;19:86–94.

327. Kenner WD, Nicolson SE. Psychosomatic disorders of gravida status: false and denied pregnancies. Psychosomatics. 2015;56:119–28.

328. Gijsbers Van Wijk CMT, Kolk AM. Sex differences in physical symptoms: the contribution of symptom perception theory. Soc Sci Med. 1997;45(2):231–46.

329. Otto MW, Dougher MJ. Sex differences in personality factors in responsivity to pain. Percept Mot Skills. 1985;61:383–90.

330. Jamison RN, Sbrocco T, Parris WCV. The influence of physical and psychosocial factors on accuracy of memory for pain in chronic pain patients. Pain. 1989;37:289–94.

331. Porzelius J. Memory for pain after nerve block injections. Clin J Pain. 1995;11:112–20.

332. Gove W, Hughes M. Possible causes of the apparent sex differences in physical health: an empirical investigation. Am Sociol Rev. 1979;44:126–46.

333. Scicchitano J, Lowell P, Pearce R, Marley J, Pilowsky I. Illness behavior and somatization in general practice. J Psychosom Res. 1996;41:247–54.

334. Klonoff EA, Landrine H, Brown M. Appraisal and response to pain may be a function of its bodily location. J Psychosom Res. 1993;37(6):661–70.

335. Nathanson CA. Sex, illness, and medical care: a review of data, theory, and method. Soc Sci Med. 1977;11:13–26.

336. Unruh AM. Gender variations in clinical pain experience. Pain. 1996;65:123–67.

337. Hall EG, Davies S. Gender differences in perceived intensity and affect of pain between athletes and nonathletes. Percept Mot Skills. 1991;73:779–86.

338. Klonoff EA, Landrine H. Sex roles, occupational roles, and symptom-reporting: a test of competing hypotheses on sex differences. J Behav Med. 1992;15(4):355–64.

339. Myers CD, Robinson ME, Riley JL, Sheffield D. Sex, gender, and blood pressure: contributions to experimental pain report. Psychosom Med. 2001;63:545–50.

340. Cloninger CR, Martin RL, Guze SG, Clayton PJ. A prospective follow-up and family study of somatization in men and women. Am J Psychiatry. 1986;143:873–8.

341. Cloninger CR, Sigvardsson S, von Knorring A, Bohman M. An adoption study of somatoform disorders II: identification of two discrete somatoform disorders. Arch Gen Psychiatry. 1984;41:863–71.

342. Cloninger CR, von Knorring A, Sigvardsson S, Bohman M. Symptom patterns and causes of somatization in men, part II: genetic and environmental independence from women. Genet Epidemiol. 1986;3:171–85.

343. Duncan R, Oto M, Martin E, Pelosi A. Late onset psychogenic nonepileptic attacks. Neurology. 2006;66:1644–7.

344. Bonvanie IJ, van Gila A, Janssens KAM, Rosmalen JGM. Sexual abuse predicts functional somatic symptoms: and adolescent population study. Child Abuse Negl. 2015;46:1–7.

345. Say GN, Tasdemir HA, Ince H. Semiological and psychiatric characteristics of children with psychogenic nonepileptic seizures: gender related differences. Seizure. 2015;31:144–8.

346. Thomas AA, Preston J, Scott RC, Bujarski KA. Diagnosis of probable psychogenic nonepileptic seizures in the outpatient clinic: does gender matter? Epilepsy Behav. 2013;29(2):295–7.

347. Mcfarlane AC, Atchison M, Rafalowicz E, Papay P. Physical symptoms in post-traumatic stress disorder. J Psychosom Res. 1994;38(7):715–26.

348. Kaiser M, Kuwert P, Braehler E, Glaesmer H. Depression, somatization, and posttraumatic stress disorder in children born of occupation after World War II in comparison with a general population. J Nerv Ment Dis. 2015;203:742–8.

349. Morina N, Kuenberg A, Schnyder U, Bryant RA, Nickerson A, Schick M. The association of post-traumatic and postmigration stress with pain and other somatic symptoms: an explorive analysis in traumatized refuges and asylum seekers. Pain Med. 2017;0:1–10.

350. Myers L, Perrine K, Lancman M, Fleming M, Lancman M. Psychological trauma in patients with psychogenic nonepileptic seizures: trauma characteristics and those who develop PTSD. Epilepsy Behav. 2013;28:121–6.

351. Fiszman A, Alves-Leon SV, Nunes RG, D'Andrea I, Figueira I. Traumatic events and posttraumatic stress disorder in patients with psychogenic nonepileptic seizures: a critical review. Epilepsy Behav. 2004;5(6):818–25.

352. Ibeziako P, Rohan JM, Bujoreanu S, Choi C, Hanrahan M, Freizinger M. Medically hospitalized patients with eating disorders and somatoform disorders in pediatrics: what are their similarities and differences and how can we improve their care? Hosp Pediatr. 2016;6(12):730–7.

353. Yamada K, Matsudaira K, Tanaka E, Oka H, Katsuhira J, Iso H. Sex-specific impact of early-life adversity on chronic pain: a large population based study in Japan. J Pain Res. 2017;10:427–33.

354. Paivi M, Tanskanen A, Haatainen K, Koivumaa-Honkanen H, Hintikka J, Viinamaki H. Somatoform dissociation and adverse childhood experiences in the general population. J Nerv Ment Dis. 2004;192(5):337–42.

355. Saxe GN, Chinman G, Berkowitz R, Hall K, Lieberg G, Schwartz J, et al. Somatization in patients with dissociative disorders. Am J Psychiatry. 1994;151:1329–34.

356. Bernstein B, Kane R. Physicians' attitudes towards female patients. Med Care. 1981;19(6):600–8.. (362)

357. Colameco S, Becker LA, Simpson M. Sex bias in the assessment of patient complaints. J Fam Pract. 1983;16(6):1117–21.. (363)

358. Verbrugge LM, Steiner RP. Physician treatment of men and women patients: sex bias or appropriate care? Med Care. 1981;19(6):609–32.

359. Hawkins CF, Cockel R. The prognosis and risk of missing malignant disease in patients with unexplained and functional diarrhea. Gut. 1971;12:208–11.

360. Kroenke K, Wood DR, Mangelsdorff AD, Meier NJ, Powell JB. Chronic fatigue in primary care: prevalence, patent characteristics, and outcome. JAMA. 1988;260:929–34.

361. Kroenke K, Lucas CA, Rosenberg ML, Scherokman B, Herbers JE, Wehrle PA, et al. Causes of persistent dizziness: a prospective study of 100 patients in ambulatory care. Ann Intern Med. 1992;117:898–904.

362. Stone J, Smyth R, Carson A, Lewis S, Prescott R, Warlow C, et al. Systematic review of misdiagnosis of conversion symptoms and "hysteria". Br Med J. 2005;331:989.

363. Sox HC, Margulies I, Sox CH. Psychologically mediated effects of diagnostic tests. Ann Intern Med. 1981;95:680–5.

Anxiety Disorders

Madeleine A. Becker, Nazanin E. Silver, Ann Chandy, and Subani Maheshwari

Anxiety Disorders in Women

Anxiety disorders are the most common class of psychiatric disorder [1]. Hormonal, societal and reproductive factors are known to contribute to an increased risk of anxiety disorders in women [2, 3]. Women have a higher prevalence rate of anxiety disorders including panic disorder (PD), agoraphobia, specific phobia, social anxiety disorder and generalized anxiety disorder (GAD) [4]. Women are twice as likely to have PD, post-traumatic stress disorder (PTSD) and GAD. Social anxiety disorder and obsessive compulsive disorder (OCD) are also more common in women although their differences in prevalence from males is less pronounced. Panic disorder (PD) in women is associated with more severe symptoms and higher rates of significant comorbidities of agoraphobia, GAD and somatization disorder [4]. Rates of PTSD in men and women are similar following exposure to a natural disaster but it is higher in women (21.3%) vs men (1.8%) following a personal attack. This suggests that women are more vulnerable to PTSD than men after an assaultive trauma [5, 6].

Gender roles may also affect differences in the reporting of anxiety. Identification with male gender role may lead to underreporting of anxiety symptoms resulting in reporting bias [7]. It is also known that during formative years, male children are encouraged to confront feared objects resulting in greater extinction of fear response [8]. Bem's gender role theory describes that expression of anxiety or fear is less acceptable in the male gender. Males are expected to be more assertive while anxious behavior in females is considered more acceptable [9].

Hormonal Influences

Estrogen has anxiolytic properties. Studies show that women may be more vulnerable to anxiety and fear related disorders than men. Estrogens are the primary female sex hormones and include estrone (E1), estradiol (E2), estriol (E3) and estetrol (E4). E1 is predominant during menopause, E2 is the most active estrogen produced by the ovaries before menopause. E3 and E4 are predominant during pregnancy. Low E2 levels in women have been linked with elevated levels of anxiety [10].

Allopregnanolone is a neuroactive metabolite of progesterone. It is a potent positive modulator at GABA-A receptors and is known to have anxiolytic properties [11–13]. Reduced levels of allopregnanolone have been associated with depression, anxiety disorder, premenstrual dysphoric disorder and Alzheimer's disease [14].

Hormonal changes during menstrual cycle have also been associated with increased anxiety among women. Anxiety is higher during the late luteal phase of the menstrual cycle and pregnancy. Cortisol level among women is elevated to levels similar to men during the luteal phase of menstrual cycle [8]. Elevated cortisol level during pregnancy has been associated with adverse fetal outcomes such as low birth weight, reduced fetal size and premature birth [15].

M. A. Becker (✉) · A. Chandy
Department of Psychiatry and Human Behavior, Thomas Jefferson University Hospital, Philadelphia, PA, USA
e-mail: madeleine.becker@jefferson.edu; ann.chandy@jefferson.edu

N. E. Silver
Division of Women's Behavioral Health, Department of Obstetrics and Gynecology, University of Pittsburg Medical Center Pinnacle, Camp Hill, PA, USA

S. Maheshwari
Department of Psychiatry, Wilmington Hospital, Christiana Care Health System, Wilmington, DE, USA
e-mail: subani.maheshwari@christianacare.org

© Springer Nature Switzerland AG 2019
M. A. O'Neal (ed.), *Neurology and Psychiatry of Women*, https://doi.org/10.1007/978-3-030-04245-5_7

Gender Differences in Specific Anxiety Disorders

Generalized Anxiety Disorder (GAD)

Risk factors associated with GAD are family history and personal history of other psychiatric disorders. However, biological factors such as genetics and hormonal fluctuations, as well as differing social roles and environmental factors, may also play a role and contribute to females being more likely to develop anxiety compared to men [16]. One study showed an association between GAD and stressful life events and personality traits such as behavioral inhibition which is characterized by shyness or withdrawal from distressing and unfamiliar situations. Other personality traits associated with GAD are high harm avoidance and reward dependence, social sensitivity and craving social acceptance [16, 17].

Panic Disorder (PD)

Panic disorder (PD) has also been associated with comorbid and family history of psychiatric disorders such as depression and anxiety. Several epidemiological studies have indicated a higher prevalence of PD in women. Women are more likely to experience respiration-related somatic symptoms such as difficulty breathing, feelings of choking and feeling faint [18]. A study by Papp et al. demonstrated that female patients with PD have greater CO_2 sensitivity resulting in higher respiratory rate. Their study also indicated that panicking and non-panicking female patients have a significantly lower end-tidal CO_2 as a result of hyperventilation [19].

Obsessive Compulsive Disorder (OCD)

Obsessive Compulsive Disorder (OCD) can be manifested in a number ways. It can present as concerns regarding (1) germs and contamination, (2) symmetry, completeness or "perfect" (3) unacceptable thoughts such as sexual or religious in nature and (4) thoughts regarding harming others or bad luck. A study looking at gender differences in OCD symptoms showed that males with OCD may report symptoms across a broad range of symptom clusters, whereas a female more often report symptoms from a specific symptoms cluster. This difference could be due to tendency to an earlier age of onset in males resulting in a broader presentation [20].

Phobias

Prevalence rate of phobias such as agoraphobia, specific phobia and social anxiety disorder is also greater in females [21].

A review indicated that women are more likely to have social anxiety disorder and report greater clinical severity. Men, however, are more likely to seek treatment [22].

Post-Traumatic Stress Disorder (PTSD)

Women are less likely to experience traumatic events, however, they are more vulnerable to sexual assault and childhood abuse [6, 23]. Risk factors for developing PTSD include: previous history of mental health disorder such as depression or anxiety, family psychiatric history and additional social stressors [24]. Saxe et al. described two different pathways to PTSD – the anxiety pathway, also known as the "fight or flight" response, or the dissociative pathway also known as a "freeze" response. The fight or flight response is regulated by the sympathetic system and more commonly observed in men in response to stress. Women more commonly demonstrate an additional form of reaction to stress -"tend and befriend"; when faced with a threat, women tend to care for their children or seek protection from others. In support of this hypothesis, it has been documented that men generally display hyperarousal or aggressive behavior during a traumatic event whereas women tend to group together and seek support from others, especially from other women. Women also tend to use more dissociative mechanisms [25]. Men are exposed to more traumatic events but the development of PTSD after trauma is more common in women than in men. This difference may be due to the fact that women are exposed to more toxic, violative trauma such as sexual abuse and rape [25].

Intimate Partner Violence (IPV) is very closely related to PTSD and anxiety. According to a 2011 survey in US, 36% of women and 29% of men reported lifetime IPV with more serious injuries reported among women. Prevalence of IPV in both ambulatory and hospitalized psychiatric patients is more than 30%. Women who are victims of IPV are at a higher risk of depressive disorder (Odds ratio [OR] 2.77), anxiety disorders (OR 4.08) and PTSD (OR 7.34) [26].

Anxiety Disorders Associated with Obstetric and Gynecologic Conditions

Pregnancy and Postpartum

Anxiety disorders are more common in women and tend to peak during the reproductive years. Many biological, psychological, and sociocultural changes occur during pregnancy and the postpartum period. Early pregnancy and then the postpartum period are times of great hormonal fluctuation, sleep disruption and physical changes, which are some of the biological factors increasing propensity for depression and anxiety. The psychological challenges that occur with pregnancy include transition to parenthood which can be frightening and stressful [27]. Postpartum anxiety disorders are common ranging between 4% and 15% [28]. A history of anxiety disorder is associated with postpartum anxiety disorders. Other factors contributing to the risk of developing postpartum anxiety disorders are hormonal and physiological changes, the stress and responsibility of caring for a baby and being a new mother. There has been much less research focus on anxiety disorders in the perinatal period compared with depressive disorders [29].

Risks Associated with Untreated Anxiety Disorders

Untreated mood and anxiety disorders affect both the mother and the fetus. For the mother, risks associated with untreated mood and anxiety disorders include poor self-care, sleep disturbances, inadequate nutrition, emotional instability, illicit drug and/or alcohol use, and smoking. However, many of the studies looking at risks are confounded with the use anxiolytic medication and other factors. Pre- and post-natal anxiety may impair the mother infant bond and the mother's ability to interact with the child [30]. Untreated anxiety during the perinatal period has also been found to be a risk for adverse outcomes for both the mother and fetus including postpartum depression, low birth weight, bonding difficulties, and poorer child development [31]. Elevated maternal cortisol has also been linked to prematurity and lower birth weight [32, 33]. Other studies have found that anxiety itself is not associated with adverse neonatal outcomes [34].

Generalized Anxiety Disorder (GAD)

To diagnose GAD, symptoms need to be present for a least 6 months, so new onset symptoms may not meet criteria within the course of pregnancy or postpartum periods. In addition it may be difficult to distinguish GAD from normal and common anxiety during the periods of pregnancy and postpartum [35]. GAD may be differentiated from normal perinatal concerns when it is excessive and interferes with day-to-day functioning [36], or when a women cannot be reassured or cannot control the worry [35]. When anxiety becomes pervasive and affects functioning, it may rise to the level of meeting criteria for GAD [34]. Preexisting anxiety is a more significant risk factor for postpartum depression than a history of depression itself [37].

In addition to the usual symptoms of GAD, pregnant women may find themselves paying more attention to fetal movements and seeing their obstetrician more often to check on fetal well-being [37]. The impact of maternal anxiety during pregnancy has not been well clarified. However over-activity of the maternal neuroendocrine system has been associated with negative impact on the child's subsequent development and health. Examples include effects on

attention regulation, cognitive and motor development, fearful temperament, negative reactivity to novelty during the 1st year of life, behavioral and emotional problems and decreased gray matter density in childhood, and impulsivity, externalizing, and processing speed in adolescents [35].

Postpartum generalized anxiety disorder (PPGAD) occurs in 4–8% of new mothers. Symptoms are similar to those in GAD [38]. GAD can be pervasive, and in the postpartum period, the worries may be more specifically related to appearance, motherhood, household responsibilities and the baby [35].

Panic Disorder

The rate of panic disorder (PD) in pregnancy is comparable to its rates outside of pregnancy. Many epidemiological studies for panic disorder in women have reported prevalence rates of 1–3.8% with a mean age of onset before or during the reproductive years. Epidemiological research on the prevalence of PD in pregnancy has reported rates of 0.2–5.2% [34, 39].

Panic disorder may occur in about 1–2% of new mothers [35]. The disorder may be a recurrence of a pre-existing disorder or present itself for the first time in the perinatal period. Symptoms are similar to non-postpartum panic disorder including avoidance of situations due to the anticipation of anxiety making it challenging for a mother to care for or be alone with her child for fear of having a panic attack. Women may interpret panic attacks as problems with the pregnancy/fetus. There have also been reports showing a relationship between lactation and time of weaning to panic symptoms in the mother [35].

Post-traumatic Stress Disorder

A history of previous traumatic birth or early life trauma such as sexual abuse may cause post-traumatic stress disorder (PTSD) symptoms to recur. This can be particularly related to the anticipated gynecologic procedures and pain during labor and delivery. A woman can feel helpless and not in control of her body resulting in flashbacks, hyperarousal, and avoidance [39].

In the postpartum period, PTSD rates of 1–6% have been reported in the medical literature [6]. Symptoms can be triggered by a traumatic labor and delivery or medical interventions during the labor and delivery in women who have previously been the victims of sexual abuse [40, 41].

Obsessive-Compulsive Disorder

Obsessive-Compulsive Disorder (OCD) is highly associated with anxiety disorders. It may present for the first time during pregnancy or more commonly, in the postpartum period [35, 38]. The prevalence of OCD during the post-partum period is in the range of 2–3% [42]. Women with a history of major depressive disorder (MDD), premenstrual dysphoric disorder (PMDD), or OCD have an increased risk of developing postpartum (PPOCD). Studies of new-onset perinatal OCD report that as many as 40% of childbearing OCD patients have onset during pregnancy and up to 30% during the postpartum period [43].

Common obsessions include Intrusive thoughts of harm occurring to the fetus or inadvertently or intentionally harming one's baby. These thoughts are perceived as intrusive and frightening and it is very rare for pregnant and postpartum women with OCD to act on these thoughts. Compulsions tend to be less common in the postpartum period, but may have to do with hand washing or cleaning behaviors to avoid the fear of contamination of the infant [35].

It is important to differentiate OCD obsessions from infanticidal thoughts that may present in postpartum psychosis. Psychosis be treated as high risk as these patients require emergent psychiatric care [35]. Women with OCD have more insight that their fears are unreasonable. Women with postpartum psychosis do not show this insight, and generally do not have anxiety related to these thoughts. Impulsivity and co-occurring mood disorders can increase the risk for this concern [39]. Postpartum OCD has a high relapse rate in subsequent pregnancies and may be more difficult to treat than other postpartum anxiety disorders [44].

Treatment of perinatal anxiety disorders may include cognitive behavioral therapy [45], serotonin reuptake inhibitors (SSRIs) and benzodiazepines. The risks and benefits of the use of medications should be weighed with each patient. The SSRIs have been associated with preterm birth [46], hypertension diseases of pregnancy [34], neonatal adaptation syndrome and persistent pulmonary hypertension of the newborn [47, 48]. Maternal benzodiazepine use has been associated with low birth weight, cesarean delivery, need for respiratory support [34], and floppy infant syndrome [49, 50].

Pregnancy Loss

Miscarriage

Approximately 12–24% of clinically recognized pregnancies result in miscarriage, predominantly in the first trimester [51]. It is estimated that at least 30–60% of all conceptions (recognized and unrecognized) will end within the first 12 weeks of gestation. Many women experience feelings of grief, depression or anxiety following a pregnancy loss, and symptoms may last up to 2 years. A large number of miscarriages are due to unknown causes and women may blame themselves for the loss. Many women report increased anxiety up to 6 months post-miscarriage putting them at an increased risk for OCD and PTSD [52]. Women with a history of miscarriages more often suffer from pregnancy-specific anxieties during the first trimester of a new pregnancy than those without. It is imperative to validate women's feel-

ings and counsel them regarding the gradual course of improvement of typical grief. If a woman's symptoms are prolonged or excessive the grieving may be accompanied by major depressive and/or anxiety disorders and will need treatment [53, 54].

Stillbirth

Stillbirth is the death of a fetus after 20 weeks' gestation or after a weight of 14 oz. Half of stillbirths occur in uncomplicated pregnancies with most parents being unprepared for this loss. Loss of a desired pregnancy can result in complicated grief (CG) CG reactions after perinatal loss can be generally specified within the existing diagnostic criteria, but they differ from grief after other significant losses in a number of key aspects. These differences are: a consistent feeling of guilt, self-blame, failure of their bodies, undermining of their femininity, child envy, reluctance to make contact with friends or family members who have children or who are at the same stage of pregnancy as that at which the loss was suffered, poor coping, avoidance, and isolation [55]. One study found that mothers who held their stillborn babies had higher rates of depression than women who had just seen their babies or those who had had no contact [56]. Women who are pressured into seeing their stillborn babies had higher rates of anxiety and PTSD up to 7 years post-stillbirth [57]. The best current approach to responding to this loss is to allow the parents to choose to whether or not to see and/or hold the stillborn child [57]. After a stillbirth, a woman should be monitored closely for signs and symptoms of depression, anxiety and trauma related disorders.

Infertility

Infertility is defined as the inability to conceive after 12 months of regular, appropriate and unprotected intercourse, or therapeutic donor insemination [58]. Fertility rates worldwide have decreased since 1970 [59], and according to the CDC, an estimated 12% of women aged 15–44 years in the United States now have difficulty getting pregnant or carrying a pregnancy to term. Reasons cited for decreasing fecundity include obesity, smoking, substance abuse, exposure to environmental pollutants, sexually transmitted diseases and delay in childbearing due to career choices [60].

In many societies, the role of motherhood is expected to form an integral part of a woman's identity. Infertility can consequently precipitate feelings of failure, inadequacy, guilt, isolation, anger and jealousy of other women who are pregnant [61–63]. In some cultures, infertile women are stigmatized [61]. Not surprisingly, infertility significantly increases the risk of anxiety and mood disorders [64]. One study done on infertile couples found that 54% of the females had psychiatric morbidity, and the two most common diagnoses among them were Major Depressive Disorder (18%) and Generalized Anxiety Disorder (16%) [65]. Infertility has been compared to cancer and heart disease in its psychological impact [66]. Artificial reproductive therapies undertaken for the treatment of infertility may also precipitate anxiety and/or depressive disorders, due to associated hormonal effects, severe financial burden, multiple surgical procedures and frequent doctor appointments, among other stressors [67–69].

The relationship between psychological stress and infertility appears to be bidirectional, and can thus enter a vicious cycle. Studies show that chronically high levels of hormones such as cortisol and norepinephrine, and circulating inflammatory mediators (as seen in chronic stress, anxiety or depression), are associated with suppression of the female gonadal axis and increasing risk of unsuccessful reproductive outcomes [70–73]. This is further suggested by a 2015 meta-analysis that searched databases from 1978 to 2014, and found that larger reductions in anxiety via psychosocial interventions, in particular cognitive behavioral therapy and mindfulness-based interventions, were associated with greater chances of pregnancy, among couples in treatment for infertility [74].

Psychological distress may lead to substance use such as smoking, marijuana use or alcohol use. These substances have also been shown to impair infertility, in addition to other harmful effects on health [75–81].

Some studies have shown no impairment in fecundability secondary to psychotropics [82]. Other studies, that show a negative impact of psychotropics on fertility rates, are often subject to confounding by indication, in which a disease is associated with both use of a medication and the outcome [83, 84]. Certain medications, however, like valproic acid and carbamazepine [85] are clearly teratogenic and should be avoided in the reproductive age group. Others can have adverse effects that negatively impact fertility rates, for example hyperprolactinemia and/or metabolic syndrome caused by some antipsychotics [86, 87].

Gynecologic Pain

Vulvar Pain

Chronic vulvar pain is defined as pain lasting 3–6 months and affects about 16–28% of women. It can occur in any age group with the most common onset occurring between the ages of 16 and 25 years old. It is divided into pains caused by specific disorders or unknown etiology called vulvodynia. Known causes include: infections (i.e. candidiasis, Herpes simplex), inflammation (i.e. lichen sclerosis), neoplasms, and neurologic disorders (i.e. multiple sclerosis) [88]. Vulvar pain has a huge impact on a woman's quality of life leading to decreased sexual pleasure resulting in impaired sexual relationships and hence feelings of guilt

and depression and anxiety from living with chronic pain. In the absence of visible abnormalities, many women are labelled as having a psychological illness, which can contribute to further anxiety and mood disorders [89].

Bladder Pain Syndrome (Interstitial Cystitis)

Bladder pain syndrome (BPS), the preferred nomenclature over interstitial cystitis (IC), is defined as discomfort and pain associated with the lower urinary tract for more than 6 weeks in the absence of infection or other identifiable causes [88, 90]. Discomfort may also be felt in the suprapubic area, urethra, vulva, vagina, pelvis, or lower back. Symptoms include urinary urgency, frequency (up to every 5–10 min), nocturia, and dyspareunia are very common and distressing [91]. The pain occurs during bladder filling and is relieved with voiding. This condition can progress to chronic symptoms with frequent exacerbations and remissions. It can be difficult to differentiate from recurrent urinary tract infections (UTIs), an overactive bladder, chronic pelvic pain, or vulvodynia [91, 92]. Urinary tract infections are frequently diagnosed even in the absence of a positive urine culture and may be the initiating stressor for the development of BPS/IC [88, 90].

Symptoms of IC/BPS can severely impair a woman's quality of life and are associated with an increased prevalence of mental health disorders such as depression, anxiety, and panic disorder [93]. Chung et al. found that the prevalence of anxiety disorder was higher in BPS/IC than the control in women [94]. Additionally, some studies have reported that patients with IC/PBS have a higher reported prevalence of sexual abuse than those without it [92].

Serotonergic pathways are linked with the regulation of voiding and depression. In PBS/IC, pain modulation may be altered due to a deficit in endogenous pain inhibitory systems [91]. SNRIs have also been shown to be effective in both PBS/IC as well as anxiety/depression. Due to the chronic nature of BPS/IC, it is recommended that urogynecologists/urologists and psychiatrists work together in an integrative approach to treat patients with these conditions.

Chronic Pelvic Pain

Chronic pelvic pain (CPP) is defined as pain in the pelvis for 6 months or longer without evidence of infection or other local pathology that may cause the pain, with incomplete relief from treatments, impaired function at home or work, and signs of depression [95]. Its prevalence worldwide is estimated at 4–10% [95]. CPP in women is devastating and a challenging clinical issue to manage due to its complexity in presentation, adequate treatments, and impact on patients' lives. Many disorders such as endometriosis, adenomyosis, pelvic inflammatory disease, and bladder pain syndrome can result in CPP [96]. CPP is frequently comorbid with depression, anxiety, sleep disturbances, previous or current physical or sexual abuse, psychological stress, and substance abuse [96].

Urogynecology

Incontinence

Urinary incontinence, defined by the International Continence Society Standardization Committee, is an involuntary loss of urine that causes social and hygienic problems, has a prevalence of 15–55% in women and can result in social isolation, sexual dysfunction, and worsen quality of life for those affected [97]. This can in turn contribute to disorders such as depression and anxiety [97, 98]. Asoglu et al. found that patients with urge incontinence symptoms, especially those with both urge and stress incontinence, had an increased risk of having anxiety disorders and worse quality of life than those with only stress urinary incontinence. Patients with stress urinary incontinence reported worse sexual lives than those with urge or mixed incontinence [97]. One study found that those with mixed urinary incontinence had higher anxiety scores than those with pure stress urinary incontinence [98].

Pelvic Organ Prolapse

Pelvic organ prolapse (POP) is defined as the descent of the pelvic organs into or outside of the vaginal canal. Symptoms related to POP may affect psychological, social, occupational, physical, sexual, and domestic aspects of a woman's life [99]. Approximately 30% of women, more than half of whom are over age 50 have POP, which is a common indication for gynecological surgery [99, 100].

POP can have a considerable impact on a women's quality of life. Women's psychological well-being is intimately related to their pelvic floor disorders. However, despite its prevalence, very little research has been conducted to study the association of psychiatric symptoms and POP. Ghetti et al. demonstrated that anxiety and depressive symptoms in patients with POP were varied. Some women had fears of having cancer, while others were most worried about the significant effect this condition had on their daily lives and routine. Other emotions experienced included being alone, isolated, broken, defective, and ashamed [100]. Another study which looked at body image related to pelvic floor disorders, identified similar findings of varied worries as stated above [101].

Conclusion

Factors such as biology, socialization and gender roles may contribute to the higher prevalence of anxiety disorders in females. There are many circumstances that are unique to women's' health and lifecycle that carry a increased risk for developing anxiety disorders. Pregnancy, pregnancy loss, post-partum, infertility, have all been associated with a risk of anxiety. Gynecological disorders impact both women's physical and also mental health. Anxiety disorders should be recognized and treated to optimize health in our patients.

References

1. Kessler RC, Chiu WT, Demler O, Walters EE. Prevalence, severity, and comorbidity of 12-month DSM-IV disorders in the national comorbidity survey replication. Arch Gen Psychiatry. 2005;62(6):617–27.
2. Pigott TA. Anxiety disorders in women. Psychiatry Clin N Am. 2003;26(3):621–72.
3. Altemus M, Sarvaiya N, Neill Epperson C. Sex differences in anxiety and depression clinical perspectives. Front Neuroendocrinol. 2014;35(3):320–30.
4. Pigott TA. Gender differences in the epidemiology and treatment of anxiety disorders. J Clin Psychiatry. 1999;60(18):4–15.
5. Breslau N. Gender differences in trauma and posttraumatic stress disorder. J Gend Specif Med. 2002;132(6):959–92.
6. Kessler RC. Posttraumatic stress disorder in the national comorbidity survey. Arch Gen Psychiatry. 1995;52(12):1048.
7. Pierce KA, Kirkpatrick DR. Do men lie on fear surveys? Behav Res Ther. 1992;30(4):415–8.
8. McLean CP, Anderson ER. Brave men and timid women? A review of the gender differences in fear and anxiety. Clin Psychol Rev. 2009a;29(6):496–505.
9. Bem SL. Gender schema theory: a cognitive account of sex typing. Psychol Rev. 1981;88(4):354–64.
10. Cover KK, Maeng LY, Lebrón-Milad K, Milad MR. Mechanisms of estradiol in fear circuitry: implications for sex differences in psychopathology. Transl Psychiatry. 2014;4:e422. https://doi.org/10.1038/tp.2014.67.
11. Nillni YI, Toufexis DJ, Rohan KJ. Anxiety sensitivity, the menstrual cycle, and panic disorder: a putative neuroendocrine and psychological interaction. Clin Psychol Rev. 2011;31(7):1183–91.
12. Yoshizawa K, Okumura A, Nakashima K, Sato T, Higashi T. Role of allopregnanolone biosynthesis in acute stress-induced anxiety-like behaviors in mice. Synapse. 2017;71(8):e21978.
13. Zhang LM, Qiu ZK, Chen XF, Zhao N, Chen HX, Xue R, Zhang YZ, Yang RF, Li YF. Involvement of allopregnanolone in the anti-PTSD-like effects of AC-5216. J Psychopharmacol. 2016;30(5):474–81.
14. Takei Y, Ando H, Tsutsui K. Handbook of hormones: comparative endocrinology for basic and clinical research. Oxford: Academic; 2015.
15. Kendall-Tackett K, Hale TW. The use of antidepressants in pregnant and breastfeeding women: a review of recent studies. J Hum Lact. 2010;26(2):187–95.
16. Remes O, Wainwright N, Surtees P, Lafortune L, Khaw KT, Brayne C. Sex differences in association between area deprivation and generalized anxiety disorder: British population study. Br J Med Open. 2017;7(5):e013590.
17. Beesdo K, Pine DS, Lieb R, Wittchen HU. Incidence and risk patterns of anxiety and depressive disorders and categorization of generalized anxiety disorder. Arch Gen Psychiatry. 2010;67(1):47–57.
18. Sheikh JI, Leskin GA, Klein DF. Gender differences in panic disorder: findings from the National Comorbidity Survey. Am J Psychiatry. 2002;159(1):55–8.
19. Papp LA, Martinez JM, Klein DF, Coplan JD, Norman RG, Cole R, de Jesus MJ, Ross D, Goetz R, Gorman JM. Respiratory psychophysiology of panic disorder: three respiratory challenges in 98 subjects. Am J Psychiatry. 1997;154(11):1557–65.
20. Raines AM, Oglesby ME, Allan NP, Mathes BM, Sutton CA, Schmidt NB. Examining the role of sex differences in obsessive-compulsive symptom dimensions. Psychiatry Res. 2018;259:265–9. https://doi.org/10.1016/j.psychres.2017.10.038.
21. McLean CP, Asnaani A, Litz BT, Hofmann SG. Gender differences in anxiety disorders: prevalence, course of illness, comorbidity and burden of illness. J Psychiatr Res. 2011;45(8):1027–35. https://doi.org/10.1016/j.jpsychires.2011.03.006.

22. Asher M, Asnaani A, Aderka IM. Gender differences in social anxiety disorder: a review. Clin Psychol Rev. 2017;56:1–12. https://doi.org/10.1016/j.cpr.2017.05.004.

23. Tolin DF, Foa EB. Sex differences in trauma and posttraumatic stress disorder: a quantitative review of 25 years of research. Psychol Bull. 2006;132(6):959–92.

24. Brewin CR, Andrews B, Valentine JD. Meta-analysis of risk factors for posttraumatic stress disorder in trauma-exposed adults. J Consult Clin Psychol. 2000;68(5):748–66.

25. Christiansen DM, Elklit A. Risk factors predict post-traumatic stress disorder differently in men and women. Ann General Psychiatry. 2008;8(7):24.

26. Stewart DE, Vigod SN. Mental health aspects of intimate partner violence. Psychiatr Clin N Am. 2017;40(2):321–34.

27. Figueiredo B, Conde A. Anxiety and depression symptoms in women and men from early pregnancy to 3-months postpartum: parity differences and effects. J Affect Disord. 2011;132(1–2):146–57.

28. Heron J, O'Connor TG, Evans J, Golding J, Glover V. The course of anxiety and depression through pregnancy and the postpartum in a community sample. J Affect Disord. 2004;80(1):65–73.

29. Dennis C, Brown HK, Falah-Hassani K, Marini FC, Vigod SN. Identifying women at risk for sustained postpartum anxiety. J Affect Disord. 2017;213:131–7.

30. Feldman R, Greenbaum CW, Mayes LC, Erlich SH. Change in mother-infant interactive behavior: relations to change in the mother, the infant, and the social context. Infant Behav Dev. 1997;20(2):151–63.

31. Skouteris H, Wertheim EH, Rallis S, Milgrom J, Paxton SJ. Depression and anxiety through pregnancy and the early postpartum: an examination of prospective relationships. J Affect Disord. 2009;113(3):303–8.

32. Field T, Hernandez-Reif M, Diego M, Figueiro B, Schanberg S, Kuhn C. Prenatal cortisol, prematurity and low birth weight. Infant Beh Dev. 2006;29:268–75.

33. Orr ST, Reiter JP, Blazer DG, James SA. Maternal prenatal anxiety and spontaneous birth in Baltimore Maryland. Psychosom Med. 2007;69:566–70.

34. Yonkers K, Gilstad-Hayden K, Forray A, Lipind HS. Association of panic disorder, generalized anxiety disorder, and benzodiazepine treatment during pregnancy with a risk of adverse birth outcomes. J Am Med Assoc Psychiatry. 2017;74(11):1145–52.

35. Ross LE, McLean LM. Anxiety disorders during pregnancy and the postpartum period. J Clin Psychiatry. 2006;67(08):1285–98.

36. Figueiredo B, Costa R. Mother's stress, mood and emotional involvement with the infant: 3 months before and 3 months after childbirth. Arch Womens Ment Health. 2009;12(3):143–53.

37. Matthey S, Barnett B, Howie P, Kavanagh DJ. Diagnosing postpartum depression in mothers and fathers: whatever happened to anxiety? J Affect Disord. 2003;74(2):139–47.

38. Altshuler LL, Hendrick V, Cohen LS. Course of mood and anxiety disorders during pregnancy and the postpartum period. J Clin Psychiatry. 1998;59(Suppl 2):29–33.

39. Meschino DC, Dalfen A, Robinson GE. Pregnancy and postpartum (Ch. 68). In: Psychiatric care of the medical patient. New York: Oxford University Press; 2015. p. 1354–64.

40. Wenzel A, Haugen EN, Jackson LC, Brendle JR. Anxiety symptoms and disorders at eight weeks postpartum. J Anxiety Disord. 2005;19(3):295–311.

41. Wenzel A, Haugen EN, Jackson LC, Robinson K. Prevalence of generalized anxiety at eight weeks postpartum. Arch Womens Ment Health. 2003;6(1):43–9.

42. Brandes M, Soares CN, Cohen LS. Postpartum onset obsessive-compulsive disorder: diagnosis and management. Arch Womens Ment Health. 2004;7(2):99–110.

43. Timpano KR, Abramowitz JS, Mahaffey BL, Mitchell MA, Schmidt NB. Efficacy of a prevention program for postpartum obsessive-compulsive symptoms. J Psychiatr Res. 2011;45(11):1511–7.

44. Sichel DA, Cohen LS, Rosenbaum JF, Driscoll J. Postpartum onset of obsessive-compulsive disorder. Psychosomatics. 1993;34(3):277–9.

45. Marchesi C, Ossola P, Amerio A, Daniel BD, Tonna M, De Panfilis C. Clinical management of perinatal anxiety disorders: a systematic review. J Affect Disord. 2016;190:543–50. https://doi.org/10.1016/j.jad.2015.11.004. Epub 2015 Nov 4.

46. Eke AC, Saccone G, Berghella V. Selective serotonin re-uptake inhibitor (SSRI) use during pregnancy and preterm birth: a systemic review and meta-analysis. BJOG. 2016;123(12):1900–7.

47. Ross LE, Grigoriadis S, Mamisashvili L, VonderPorten EH, Roerecke M, Rehm J, et al. Selected pregnancy and delivery outcomes after exposure to antidepressant medication: a systematic review and meta-analysis. JAMA Psychiatry. 2013;70:436–43.

48. Byatt N Deligiannidis KM, Freeman MP. Antidepressant use in pregnancy: a critical review focused on risks and controversies. Acta Psychiatr Scand. 2013;127:94–114.

49. McElhatton PR. The effects of benzodiazepine use during pregnancy and lactation. Reprod Toxicol. 1994;8(6):461–75.

50. Iqbal MM, Sobhan T, Ryals T. Effects of commonly used benzodiazepines on the fetus, the neonate and the nursing infant. Psychiatr Serv. 2002;53(1):39–49.

51. Robinson GE. Infertility, pregnancy loss, and abortion. In: Psychiatric care of the medical patient. New York: Oxford University Press; 2015. p. 1336–43.

52. Bergner A, Beyer R, Klapp BF, Rauchfuss M. Pregnancy after early pregnancy loss: a prospective study of anxiety, depressive symptomatology and coping. J Psychosom Obstet Gynecol. 2008;29(2):105–13.

53. Nikcevic AV, Tinkel SA, Kuczmierczyk AR, Nicolaides KH. Investigation of the cause of miscarriage and its influence on women's psychological distress. BJOG Int J Obstet Gynaecol. 1999;106(8):808–13.

54. Brier N. Grief following miscarriage: a comprehensive review of the literature. J Women's Health. 2008;17(3):451–64.

55. Bennett SM, Litz BT, Sarnoff Lee B, Maguen S. The scope and impact of perinatal loss: current status and future directions. Prof Psychol Res Pract. 2005;36(2):180–7.

56. Hughes P, Turton P, Hopper E, Evans CDH. Assessment of guidelines for good practice in psychosocial care of mothers after stillbirth: a cohort study. Lancet. 2002;360(9327):114–8.

57. Turton P, Evans C, Hughes P. Long-term psychosocial sequelae of stillbirth: phase II of a nested case-control cohort study. Arch Womens Ment Health. 2009;12(1):35–41.

58. Practice Committee of American Society for Reproductive Medicine. Definitions of infertility and recurrent pregnancy loss: a committee opinion. Fertil Steril. 2013;99(1):63.

59. Skakkebæk NE, Jørgensen N, Main KM, Rajpert-De Meyts E, Leffers H, Andersson A, Juul A, Carlsen E, Mortensen GK, Jensen TK, Toppari J. Is human fecundity declining? Int J Androl. 2006;29(1). Blackwell Publishing Ltd:2–11.

60. Petraglia F, Serour GI, Chapron C. The changing prevalence of infertility. Int J Gynaecol Obstet. 2013;123(2):S4–8.

61. Batool SS, de Visser RO. Experiences of infertility in British and Pakistani women: a cross-cultural qualitative analysis. Health Care Women Int. 2016;37(2):180–96.

62. Hinton L, Kurinczuk JJ, Ziebland S. Infertility; isolation and the internet: a qualitative interview study. Patient Educ Couns. 2010;81(3):436–41.

63. Kirkman M. Thinking of something to say: public and private narratives of infertility. Health Care Women Int. 2001;22(6):523–35.

64. Klemetti R, Raitanen J, Sihvo S, Saarni S, Koponen P. Infertility, mental disorders and well-being: a nationwide survey. Acta Obstet Gynecol Scand. 2010;89(5):677–82.

65. Sethi P, Sharma A, Devi Goyal L, Gurmeet K. Prevalence of psychiatric morbidity in females amongst infertile couples: a hospital based report. J Clin Diagn Res. 2016;10(7):VC04–7.

66. Domar AD, Zuttermeister PC, Friedman R. The psychological impact of infertility: a comparison with patients with other medical conditions. J Psychosom Obstet Gynaecol. 1993;14:45–52.

67. Maroufizadeh S, Karimi E, Vesali S, Omani Samani R. Anxiety and depression after failure of assisted reproductive treatment among patients experiencing infertility. Int J Gynaecol Obstet:Off Organ Int Fed Gynaecol Obstet. 2015;130(3):253–6.

68. Domar AD. Impact of psychological factors on dropout rates in insured infertility patients. Fertil Steril. 2004;81(2):271–3.

69. Olivius C, Friden B, Borg G, Bergh C. Why do couples discontinue in vitro fertilization treatment? A cohort study. Fertil Steril. 2004;81(2):258–61.

70. Lynch CD, Sundaram R, Maisog JM, Sweeney AM, Buck Louis GM. Preconception stress increases the risk of infertility: results from a couple-based prospective cohort study—the LIFE study. Hum Reprod. 2014;29(5). Oxford University Press:1067–75.

71. Li X, Ma Y, Geng L, Qin L, Hu H, Li S. Baseline psychological stress and ovarian norepinephrine levels negatively affect the outcome of in vitro fertilisation. Gynecol Endocrinol. 2011;27(3):139–43.

72. Kalantaridou SN, Zoumakis E, Makrigiannakis A, Lavasidis LG, Vrekoussis T, Chrousos GP. Corticotropin-releasing hormone, stress and human reproduction: an update. J Reprod Immunol. 2010;85(1):33–9.

73. Ebbesen SMS, Zachariae R, Mehlsen MY, Thomsen D, Højgaard A, Ottosen L, Petersen T, Ingerslev HJ. Stressful life events are associated with a poor in-vitro fertilization (IVF) outcome: a prospective study. Human Reprod. 2009;24(9):2173–82.

74. Frederiksen Y, Farver-Vestergaard I, Grønhøj Skovgård N, Jakob Ingerslev H, Zachariae R. Efficacy of psychosocial interventions for psychological and pregnancy outcomes in infertile women and men: a systematic review and meta-analysis. BMJ Open. 2015;5(1):e006592.

75. Alvarez S. Do some addictions interfere with fertility? Fertil Steril. 2015;103(1):22–6.

76. Wdowiak A, Sulima M, Sadowska M, Grzegorz B, Bojar I. Alcohol consumption and quality of embryos obtained in programmes of in vitro fertilization. Ann Agric Environ Med. 2014;21(2):450–3.

77. Wang H, Dey SK, Maccarrone M. Jekyll and Hyde: two faces of cannabinoid signaling in male and female fertility. Endocr Rev. 2006;27(5):427–48.

78. Park B, McPartland JM, Glass M. Cannabis, cannabinoids and reproduction. Prostaglandins Leukot Essent Fat Acids. 2004;70(2):189–97.

79. Klonoff-Cohen H, Lam-Kruglick P, Gonzalez C. Effects of maternal and paternal alcohol consumption on the success rates of in vitro fertilization and gamete intrafallopian transfer. Fertil Steril. 2003;79(2):330–9.

80. Augood C, Duckitt K, Templeton AA. Smoking and female infertility: a systematic review and meta-analysis. Hum Reprod. 1998;13(6):1532–9.

81. Mendelson JH, Mello NK, Ellingboe J, Skupny AS, Lex BW, Griffin M. Marihuana smoking suppresses luteinizing hormone in women. J Pharmacol Exp Ther. 1986;237(3):862–6.

82. Nillni YI, Wesselink AK, Gradus JL, Hatch EE, Rothman KJ, Mikkelsen EM, Wise LA. Depression, anxiety, and psychotropic medication use and fecundability. Am J Obstet Gynecol. 2016;215(4):453.e1–8.

83. Hemels MEH, Einarson A, Koren G, Lanctôt KL, Einarso TR. Antidepressant use during pregnancy and the rates of spontaneous abortions: a meta-analysis. Ann Pharmacother. 2005;39(5):803–9.

84. Casilla-Lennon MM, Meltzer-Brody S, Steiner AZ. The effect of antidepressants on fertility. Am J Obstet Gynecol. 2016;215(3):314.e1–5.

85. Isojärvi J. Disorders of reproduction in patients with epilepsy: antiepileptic drug related mechanisms. Seizure J Br Epilepsy Assoc. 2008;17(2):111–9.

86. Misra M, Papakostas GI, Klibanski A. Effects of psychiatric disorders and psychotropic medications on prolactin and bone metabolism. J Clin Psychiatry. 2004;65(12):1607–18.

87. Haddad PM, Hellewell JSE, Wieck A. Antipsychotic induced hyperprolactinaemia: a series of illustrative case reports. J Psychopharmacol. 2001;15(4):293–5.

88. Danby CS, Margesson LJ. Approach to the diagnosis and treatment of vulvar pain. Dermatol Ther. 2010;23(5):485–504.

89. Burrows LJ, Creasey A, Goldstein AT. The treatment of vulvar lichen sclerosus and female sexual dysfunction. J Sex Med. 2011;8(1):219–22.

90. Hanno PM, Erickson D, Moldwin R, Faraday MM, American Urological Association. Diagnosis and treatment of interstitial cystitis/bladder pain syndrome: AUA guideline amendment. J Urol. 2015;193(5):1545–53.

91. Chuang YC, Weng SF, Hsu YW, Lung-Cheng Huang C, Wu MP. Increased risks of healthcare-seeking behaviors of anxiety, depression and insomnia among patients with bladder pain syndrome/intersitital cystitis: a nationwide population-based study. Int Urol Nephrol. 2014;47:275–81.

92. Nickel JC, Tripp DA, Pontari M, Moldwin R, Mayer R, Carr LK, Doggweiler R, Yang C, Mishra N, Nordling J. Childhood sexual trauma in women with interstitial cystitis/bladder pain syndrome: a case control study. Can Urol Assoc J. 2011;5(6):410–5.

93. Watkins KE, Eberhart N, Hilton L, Suttorp MJ, Hepner KA, Clemens JQ, Berry SH. Depressive disorders and panic attacks in women with bladder pain syndrome/interstitial cystitis: a population-based sample. Gen Hosp Psychiatry. 2011;33(2):143–9.

94. Chung KH, Liu SP, Lin HC, Chung SD. Bladder pain syndrome/interstitial cystitis is associated with anxiety disorder. Neurourol Urodyn. 2014;33:101–5.

95. Brunahl C, Dybowski C, Albrecht R, Riegel B, Hoink J, Fisch M, Lowe B. Mental disorders in patients with chronic pelvic pain syndrome (CPPS). J Psychol Res. 2017;98:19–26.

96. Jarrell JA, Vilos GA, Allaire C, Burgess S, Fortin C, Gerwin R, et al., Society of Obstetrics and Gynaecologists of Canada. Consensus guidelines for the management of chronic pelvic pain. J Obstet Gynaecol Can. 2005;27(8):781–801.

97. Asoglu MR, Selcuk S, Cam C, Cogendez E, Karateke A. Effects of urinary incontinence subtypes on women's quality of life (including sexual life) and psychosocial state. Eur J Obstet Gynecol Reprod Biol. 2011;176:187–90.

98. Lim JR, Bak CW, Back CW, Lee JB. Comparison of anxiety between patients with mixed incontinence and those with stress urinary incontinence. Scand J Urol Nephrol. 2007;41:403–6.

99. Ghetti C, Lowder JL, Ellison R, Krohn MA, Maolli P. Depressive symptoms in women seeking surgery for pelvic organ prolapse. Int Urogynecol J. 2010;21:855–60.

100. Ghetti C, Skoczylas LC, Oliphant SS, Nikolajski C, Lowder JL. The emotional burden of pelvic organ prolapse in women seeking treatment: a qualitative study. Female Pelvic Med Reconstr Surg. 2015;21(6):323–38.

101. Lowder JL, Ghetti C, Nikolajski C, Oliphant SS, Zyczynski HM. Body image perceptions in women with pelvic organ prolapse: a qualitative study. Am J Obstet Gynecol. 2011;204(5):441.e1–5.

Neuro-inflammatory Disorders in Women

Ivana Vodopivec

Introduction

Inflammatory reactions within the CNS differ substantially from those of other tissues in several ways. This has led to the introduction of the term *neuro-inflammation* to distinguish inflammatory reactions in the CNS from inflammation in other tissues [1]. The term *neuro-inflammatory disorders* encompasses all conditions that are caused or dominated by adaptive and innate immune responses to self-antigens and pathogens. The components of the immune system, including cells, cytokines, and complement do not only have neurodestructive properties but are required for neuroaxonal growth, survival, and plasticity [2, 3].

Autoimmune diseases are defined as conditions in which the adaptive immune system erroneously targets self-antigens (autoantigens), resulting in tissue damage. Autoantigens recruit an immune response not only in *autoimmune* but also in *paraneoplastic* disorders. In neurological paraneoplastic disorders, the immune response is typically directed against neuronal antigens that are inadvertently expressed by benign or malignant neoplasms (e.g. teratoma-induced anti-NMDA [NMDAR] receptor limbic encephalitis). *Parainfectious* conditions are believed to be mediated by an abnormal or enhanced immune response triggered by an infectious antigen (e.g., Guillain-Barré syndrome, post-herpes simplex anti-NMDAR encephalitis [4]). Unlike paraneoplastic disorders that respond to treatments focused on removal of an underlying neoplasm, and parainfectious disorders that have a limited course, autoimmune conditions are chronic with relapsing-remitting or progressive disease activity. Remissions and adequate disease control rely on chronic immunosuppressive therapy.

There are many differences between men and women in their susceptibility not only to neuro-inflammatory disorders

but also to adverse effects of the chronic immunosuppression. Women of childbearing age, who are most commonly affected by autoimmune conditions, represent a population that requires particularly high vigilance. Immunosuppressants may have embryotoxic, teratogenic, and/or fetotoxic properties and, therefore, require contraception. Their use during pregnancy or postpartum period in women with active disease should always be weighed against potential risks. Implementation of safety strategies is a key to successful management of women affected by neuro-inflammatory conditions. This chapter covers these areas in detail.

Sex-Related Differences in Neuro-inflammatory Disorders

Many but not all autoimmune diseases, ranging from systemic disorders, such as systemic lupus erythematosus (SLE), to organ-specific diseases, such as neuromyelitis optica (NMO), are characterized by a greater prevalence in women than in men (Table 1) [5, 6]. Overall, estimates indicate that about 75% of the people affected with autoimmune diseases are women. Sex hormones are among the most-studied factors contributing to this sex bias [7]. Recent discoveries support the role of sex hormone-independent mechanisms in promoting female-biased autoimmunity. These include epigenetic and genetic factors, including expression of a transcription factor VGLL3 ('vestigial-like family member 3') and genes on the X chromosome [7, 8]. Together or independent one of another, these factors modulate both cellular and humoral components of innate and adaptive immune systems as well as their signaling molecules (cytokines, including chemokines and interleukins). For example, the female-biased VGLL was reported to influence type I interferon responses and to promote the expression of several inflammatory molecules, including IL-7, matrix metallopeptidase MMP9, cell adhesion molecule ICAM-1, and B-cell activating factor (BAFF) [8]. The expression of BAFF, a cytokine critical for B cell maturation,

I. Vodopivec (✉)
Department of Neurology, Brigham and Women's Hospital, Harvard Medical School, Boston, MA, USA
e-mail: ivodopivec@partners.org

Table 1 Sex distribution of the most common autoimmune disorders affecting the nervous system

Autoimmune diseases	Female-to-male ratio
Neuromyelitis optica	5–10:1
Sjögren's syndrome	9:1
Anti-NMDAR encephalitis	4:1 (2.5:1 in patients without ovarian teratoma)
Susac syndrome	3.5:1
Multiple sclerosis, relapsing-remitting	3:1
Myasthenia gravis	Bimodal distribution (2:1 <50 years)
Behçet's disease	2:1 in the US and northern Europe
Giant cell arteritis	2:1
ADEM	1:1.25–1.8 (pediatric population)
Guillain-Barré syndrome	1:1.25–2
CIDP	1:1.6
IgG4-related disease	Variable, 1:2.8 for pancreatitis
Sarcoidosis	1:1, younger age at onset in men compared with women
Myasthenia gravis	Bimodal distribution (1:1.5–2 >50 years)
Primary angiitis of CNS	1:1

selection, and survival, is also upregulated by estrogen [9]. Further studies are needed to address all aspects of the sex-related susceptibility to autoimmunity on the molecular level.

Multiple sclerosis (MS), the most common neuro-inflammatory condition, is characterized by higher incidence, prevalence, and relapse rate in women. However, it is important to note that female sex is not associated with worse outcomes. There are no overall sex-related differences in survival. Women are less likely to have progressive onset of MS compared to men; they also have lower rates of cognitive impairment and slower disability progression from symptom onset in relapsing-onset MS, including a longer time to secondary progression and disability requiring an assistive device to walk (EDSS 6; reviewed in [10]). Complex hormonal, genetic and epigenetic sex-related factors are thought to account for the sex differences [11]. Recently, it has been shown that testosterone favors astrocyte recruitment and spontaneous oligodendrocyte-mediated remyelination in CNS through androgen receptors [12]. The state of pregnancy has a substantial protective effect on disease activity in MS, as discussed later.

Similar to MS, female sex is associated with a higher risk of relapse in acute disseminated encephalomyelitis (ADEM) [13], a demyelinating condition with established male predominance [14].

About 80% of patients with anti-NMDAR encephalitis, the second most common type of autoimmune encephalitis after ADEM [15, 16], are women. The condition is more prevalent in women, even when not associated with ovarian teratoma, but this female-to-male ratio remains unexplained.

Adaptive Immune Responses and Autoimmune Disease Activity during Pregnancy

Successful pregnancy depends on immunologic alterations resulting in an immunotolerant state, which promotes survival of the semiallogeneic fetus. The same immune alterations that regulate immune responses to provide a secure niche for fetal development hinder the development of certain types of autoimmunity. The immunological changes coincide with increase in estrogen and progesterone levels, but are also known to be regulated by many other non-hormonal factors, including local changes at the maternal–fetal interface [17]. These adaptations include expression of HLA and other regulatory molecules by the trophoblast cells, shifts in lymphocyte populations, macrophage polarization, and changes in cytokine profiles. More specifically, pregnancy is characterized by expression of tolerogenic non-classical HLA-G [18], expansion of decidual type 2 (M2) macrophages, uterine regulatory natural killer (NK) cells (CD16-CD56+), Tregs, production of immunoregulatory cytokines, including IL-10, and suppression of T helper (Th) 17 cells, all of which guarantee fetal survival [17, 19–21]. There is a parallel switch from a Th1- to Th2-type cytokine profile, which, unlike previously listed factors, does not seem crucial for maintenance and completion of pregnancy [22, 23] but is relevant for modulation of autoimmune inflammation during pregnancy.

It has been recognized that common neuro-inflammatory conditions, including MS, NMO, and myasthenia gravis (MG), have increased relapse rates in the first 3 months of the postpartum period compared to the relapse rate during pregnancy or prior to pregnancy (Table 2) [24–30]. Since

Table 2 Interaction between disease activity, pregnancy and postpartum state in most common autoimmune conditions of the nervous system

	Adverse pregnancy and fetal outcomes	Disease activity during pregnancy	Disease activity during postpartum period
Multiple sclerosis	Slightly decreased birth weight and rates of cesarean delivery	Decreased, especially in the 3rd trimester	Increased
Neuromyelitis optica	Increased risk of miscarriage, preeclampsia	Unchanged	Increased
Myasthenia gravis	Risk of arthrogryposis and transient neonatal myasthenia gravis	Unpredictable; improves in 30–40%, unchanged in 30–40%, worsens in 20–30%	Increased

similar observations were made in many other autoimmune conditions [31, 32], this temporal relationship between termination of pregnancy and increased disease activity is thought to reflect the loss of pregnancy-induced immunotolerance. The relapse rate in patients with MS is lower during pregnancy and reaches a nadir in the third trimester, which is a pattern recognized in several other autoimmune conditions, such as rheumatoid arthritis (RA) [33] and autoimmune hepatitis [34]. The decrease in MS activity coincides with and has been attributed to all the listed modifications, including expansion of regulatory NK cells and increased Treg:Th17 and Th2:Th1 ratios during pregnancy [35]. Unlike MS, disease activity in the antibody-mediated neurological conditions NMO and MG may worsen during pregnancy. Similar observations with variable rates of flares during pregnancy have been made in other antibody-mediated disorders, including SLE (reviewed in [36]). There are multiple molecular and cellular mechanisms induced by pregnancy-related factors, particularly estrogen, that may account for the increased autoantibody production and pathogenicity, including enhanced immunoglobulin IgM-to-IgG isotype switching, enhanced glycosylation of immunoglobulins, increased synthesis of BAFF that promotes plasmablast survival, and the aforementioned shift to Th2 cytokine production, among others [37–39]. Recognizing the disease course and risks of exacerbations during and after pregnancy should translate into closer monitoring during these critical periods and possible use of immunosuppressants that are deemed safe and compatible with healthy pregnancy and breastfeeding.

Immunosuppressants and Their Non-infectious Adverse Effects in Women

Neuro-inflammatory disorders are treated with immunomodulating or immunosuppressive agents (known as disease-modifying therapies [DMTs] in MS or disease-modifying antirheumatic drugs [DMARD] in RA), which are associated with various infectious and non-infectious adverse effects. Adverse effects that are prevalent in or specific for women include glucocorticoid-induced osteoporosis (GIOP); certain malignancies, such as cervical cancer; cyclophosphamide- and mitoxanthrone-induced infertility; as well as adverse pregnancy outcomes and potential toxicity in nursing infants.

Glucocorticoid-Induced Osteoporosis and Fractures

Glucocorticoids are the leading cause of secondary, including iatrogenic, osteoporosis [40]. The pathogenesis of GIOP is linked to direct inhibition of bone formation and increase in bone resorption caused by supraphysiologic doses of glucocorticoids (reviewed in [40, 41]). Bone is lost more rapidly with glucocorticoid therapy than in any other condition, including postmenopausal osteoporosis and hyperparathyroidism. GIOP also differs from other causes of osteoporosis with its higher risk of vertebral than hip fractures and the fact that bone density does not fully reflect the risk of fracture in GIOP due to bone micro-architectural changes that are undetectable using conventional bone densitometry [42]. Bone loss and the fracture risk are highest during the first 3–6 months after the start of treatment, slow down after about a year of therapy and decrease after stopping therapy [42]. According to a recent Cochrane review of the benefits of bisphosphonates for GIOP, 8% of patients receiving long-term (≥90 days) steroid treatment who were untreated with bisphosphonates experienced incidental vertebral fractures within the first 12–24 months, and about 6% developed non-vertebral fractures within the same period [43]. There is conflicting evidence regarding the minimum dose and duration of glucocorticoid treatment required to produce bone loss and result in fractures, with reports of increased fracture rates on daily doses as low as 2.5–7.5 mg of prednisolone equivalent [42]. It should be noted that the risk of GIOP is not influenced by sex; however, significantly more postmenopausal women than men at or over age of 50 years are at high risk of GIOP-associated fracture and require management with antiosteoportic agents [44].

The American College of Rheumatology (ACR) recommendations for treatment and prevention of GIOP summarized risk assessment steps, monitoring strategies, lifestyle modifications, and pharmacologic recommendations [45]. All patients should introduce lifestyle modifications including smoking cessation, avoidance of excessive alcohol (>2 drinks/day), and regular weight-bearing exercises (≥3–5 times weekly). Adequate calcium (1200–1500 mg/day) and vitamin D (vitamin D3 800–2000 IU/day) supplementation is an important but insufficient measure in patients on long-term (≥3 months) glucocorticoid therapy. Bisphosphonates are first-line medications for prevention and treatment of GIOP, especially in postmenopausal women and men at or over age of 50 years. Younger patients, patients receiving doses lower than 7.5 mg of prednisone a day, or those treated for shorter periods of time can be risk stratified to determine whether they should receive pharmacologic therapy [45]. While there is high-certainty evidence for a reduction in new vertebral fractures and increase in vertebral and femoral neck bone density with bisphosphonates, the medications make little or no difference in the reduction of new non-vertebral fractures [43]. Data are still lacking for denosumab, a monoclonal antibody to an osteoclast differentiation factor receptor activator of nuclear factor kappa-B ligand (RANKL), which has been approved for osteoporosis with high risk of fractures and men undergoing androgen deprivation therapy for prostate cancer [46].

Immunosuppressants and Cervical Cancer

Available data suggest that immunocompromised populations, including patients on chronic immunosuppressive therapy, are at higher risks for human papilloma virus (HPV)-related infections, pre-cancerous and cancerous lesions [47, 48]. The increased risk is associated with decreased rates of clearance of HPV infection. Currently, there have been no studies or major society recommendations to guide cervical cancer screening in women who are immunocompromised because of non-HIV causes. Annual cytology (Pap test) has been traditionally performed in these women.

Immunosuppressants, Fertility, Pregnancy, and Breastfeeding

Cyclophosphamide is a well-known gonadotoxic agent that can cause premature ovarian failure (primary ovarian insufficiency) in women and impaired spermatogenesis (azoospermia) and reduced testosterone levels in men, thus leading to permanent infertility. Mitoxantrone frequently leads to permanent amenorrhea and typically causes transient azoospermia. All women of childbearing age and men who express desire to preserve fertility should be referred to a reproductive endocrinologist for evaluation and management prior to instituting therapy with the two agents. Cryopreservation of sperm, oocytes, or embryos is the first line fertility-preserving measure, as gonadal suppression with gonadotropin-releasing hormone (GnRH) analogue in women or supraphysiologic doses of testosterone in men has had unclear efficacy.

When immunosuppressants are given, their risks on fertility and birth outcomes should always be outweighed by their potential benefits. Evidence-based recommendations for contraceptive use by women with MS, SLE, and RA were included in 2016 US Medical Eligibility Criteria for Contraceptive Use [49]. These recommendations can be reasonably applied in women with other neuro-inflammatory conditions. Contraception is mandatory in women taking the teratogenic medications methotrexate, mycophenolate mofetil, cyclophosphamide, and DMTs mitoxantrone and teriflunomide. Effective contraception should be maintained for a certain period of time after discontinuation of these medications (Table 3) [50, 51]. The same medications may adversely affect pregnancy by causing genetic mutations in spermatozoa and/or by being excreted in seminal fluid and thus warrant contraception in couples in which a man is treated with such a medication (Table 3).

A decision on drug therapy during pregnancy and breastfeeding should be made by a drug prescriber, who may be a neurologist, internist, rheumatologist, maternal-fetal medicine specialist, or pediatrician, and by the patient, who brings in her own sets of values and beliefs.

To optimize maternal and fetal outcomes, pregnancy should be planned during times of inactive disease. In women with a history of progressive or highly active disease off immunomodulation, continuous use of treatment regimens compatible with pregnancy may be required. In women who experience disease exacerbation during pregnancy or breastfeeding while untreated, pregnancy-compatible therapies with a rapid onset of action should be provided (Table 3).

To date, there have been no prospective studies of disease-modifying agents for multiple sclerosis or immunomodulators for other conditions during pregnancy and lactation. Based on systematic literature review and pregnancy exposure data from several registries, a European League Against Rheumatism (EULAR) task force reached expert consensus on the compatibility of these agents with pregnancy and lactation [51]. Agents that are deemed relatively safe and thus compatible with pregnancy and lactation include hydroxychloroquine used in patients with SLE, azathioprine up to 2 mg/kg/day, DMTs glatiramer acetate (the only medication classified as FDA category B), interferon-β, natalizumab, as well as therapies with rapid onset of action used for management of disease exacerbation including non-fluorinated glucocorticoids, preferably given intravenously, and intravenous immunoglobulins (Table 3). Plasmapheresis, used for the same purpose, is also considered reasonably safe during pregnancy and lactation. TNFα inhibitors are considered reasonably safe in the first and second trimester and in breastfeeding women.

Decision-making in postpartum women regarding reinstitution of immunotherapy is driven by expected risk of worsening disease activity or relapses, effect of breastfeeding on disease activity, and patients' desire to breastfeed. A recent study in women with relapsing-remitting MS followed during pregnancy and for the first postpartum year suggested that exclusive breastfeeding was modestly effective in lowering the risk of relapse [52]. Similar conclusions were reached in a meta-analysis of 12 studies, all of which, however, had several limitations [53]. In women with MS, breastfeeding is deemed safe and potentially even beneficial for disease activity. Breastfeeding patients should continue off immunomodulators until weaning. In women who do not breastfeed, immunomodulators should be initiated as soon as it is feasible after delivery.

Genetic Risk and Reproductive Counseling

The only condition with defined genetic risk of disease development is MS. The age adjusted risk in children with one parent with MS is 2% [54], which is 20-fold higher than expected in the general population from Western countries. The risk still remains low and should not discourage MS patients from having a child.

Table 3 Approved therapies for neuro-inflammatory disorders and pregnancy, washout, and breastfeeding recommendations

Therapeutic agents and modalities	FDA category	Washout period before conception in women	Washout period before conception in men	Breastfeeding
Medications incompatible with pregnancy (teratogenic)				
Methotrexate	X	6 months	3 months	Avoid (contraindicated)
Mycophenolate mofetil	D	6 weeks	3 months	Avoid (contraindicated)
Mitoxantrone	D	6 months	3 months	Avoid (contraindicated)
Cyclophosphamide	D	3 months	Insufficient data: 3–9 or 12 months	Avoid (contraindicated)
Teriflunomide and leflunomide	X	2 years or washout protocol (completed in ≤11 days)	2 years or washout protocol (completed in ≤11 days)	Avoid (no data)
Insufficient documentation				
Biologics (monoclonal antibodies)				
Rituximab	C	12 months	N/A	Avoid (no data)[a]
Alemtuzumab	C	4 months	N/A	Avoid (no data)[a]
Daclizumab	C	4 months	N/A	Avoid (no data)[a]
Dimethyl fumarate	C	A few days or weeks (short half-life)	N/A	Avoid (no data)
Fingolimod	C	2 months	N/A	Avoid (no data)
Medications compatible with 1st and 2nd trimester of pregnancy and breastfeeding				
TNF-α inhibitors	B	Adalimumab, certulizumab: 5 months. Infliximab, golimumab: 6 months	N/A	Compatible[a]
Therapies compatible with pregnancy and breastfeeding				
Hydroxychloroquine	C	Should be continued throughout pregnancy and during breastfeeding	N/A	Compatible
Azathioprine up to 2 mg/kg/day	D	3 months	N/A	Compatible
Glatiramer acetate	B	1–2 months	N/A	Compatible
IFNβ	C	0 or 2 months	N/A	Compatible
Natalizumab	C (consider as rescue medication in 3rd trimester)	Probably not necessary (0–2 months)	N/A	Avoid (no data)[a]
Intravenous immunoglobulin	C	N/A	N/A	Safe
Glucocorticoids, non-fluorinated (prednisone, methylprednisolone)	C (safe in the 2nd and 3rd trimester)	None	N/A	Compatible[b]
Plasmapheresis (plasma exchange)	N/A	N/A	N/A	Safe

Abbreviation: N/A non-applicable
[a]Large protein molecule, absorption unlikely
[b]Pump and discard milk within 4 h after each steroid infusion

Take Home Points
- Many neuro-inflammatory disorders, including multiple sclerosis, predominantly affect women.
- Optimal management decisions both in women with neuroinflammatory disorders and their offspring require knowledge of the expected disease activity during pregnancy and the postpartum period and understanding of potential adverse effects of immunosuppressants.
- Equally important are screening evaluations, preventative measures, and long-term monitoring for chronic adverse effects that are unrelated to reproductive issues, such as osteoporosis and cancer.

References

1. Xanthos DN, Sandkuhler J. Neurogenic neuroinflammation: inflammatory CNS reactions in response to neuronal activity. Nat Rev Neurosci. 2014;15(1):43–53.

2. Hohlfeld R, Kerschensteiner M, Meinl E. Dual role of inflammation in CNS disease. Neurology. 2007;68(22 Suppl 3):S58–63; discussion S91–6.

3. Schafer DP, Lehrman EK, Kautzman AG, Koyama R, Mardinly AR, Yamasaki R, et al. Microglia sculpt postnatal neural circuits in an activity and complement-dependent manner. Neuron. 2012;74(4):691–705.

4. Armangue T, Moris G, Cantarin-Extremera V, Conde CE, Rostasy K, Erro ME, et al. Autoimmune post-herpes simplex encephalitis of adults and teenagers. Neurology. 2015;85(20):1736–43.

5. Beeson PB. Age and sex associations of 40 autoimmune diseases. Am J Med. 1994;96(5):457–62.

6. Whitacre CC. Sex differences in autoimmune disease. Nat Immunol. 2001;2(9):777–80.

7. Fish EN. The X-files in immunity: sex-based differences predispose immune responses. Nat Rev Immunol. 2008;8(9):737–44.

8. Liang Y, Tsoi LC, Xing X, Beamer MA, Swindell WR, Sarkar MK, et al. A gene network regulated by the transcription factor VGLL3 as a promoter of sex-biased autoimmune diseases. Nat Immunol. 2017;18(2):152–60.

9. Panchanathan R, Choubey D. Murine BAFF expression is upregulated by estrogen and interferons: implications for sex bias in the development of autoimmunity. Mol Immunol. 2013;53(1–2):15–23.

10. Bove R, McHenry A, Hellwig K, Houtchens M, Razaz N, Smyth P, et al. Multiple sclerosis in men: management considerations. J Neurol. 2016;263(7):1263–73.

11. Bove R, Chitnis T. The role of gender and sex hormones in determining the onset and outcome of multiple sclerosis. Mult Scler. 2014;20(5):520–6.

12. Bielecki B, Mattern C, Ghoumari AM, Javaid S, Smietanka K, Abi Ghanem C, et al. Unexpected central role of the androgen receptor in the spontaneous regeneration of myelin. Proc Natl Acad Sci U S A. 2016;113(51):14829–34.

13. Koelman DL, Chahin S, Mar SS, Venkatesan A, Hoganson GM, Yeshokumar AK, et al. Acute disseminated encephalomyelitis in 228 patients: a retrospective, multicenter US study. Neurology. 2016;86(22):2085–93.

14. Tenembaum S, Chitnis T, Ness J, Hahn JS, International Pediatric MSSG. Acute disseminated encephalomyelitis. Neurology. 2007;68(16 Suppl 2):S23–36.

15. Granerod J, Ambrose HE, Davies NW, Clewley JP, Walsh AL, Morgan D, et al. Causes of encephalitis and differences in their clinical presentations in England: a multicentre, population-based prospective study. Lancet Infect Dis. 2010;10(12):835–44.

16. Gable MS, Sheriff H, Dalmau J, Tilley DH, Glaser CA. The frequency of autoimmune N-methyl-D-aspartate receptor encephalitis surpasses that of individual viral etiologies in young individuals enrolled in the California Encephalitis Project. Clin Infect Dis. 2012;54(7):899–904.

17. Svensson-Arvelund J, Mehta RB, Lindau R, Mirrasekhian E, Rodriguez-Martinez H, Berg G, et al. The human fetal placenta promotes tolerance against the semiallogeneic fetus by inducing regulatory T cells and homeostatic M2 macrophages. J Immunol. 2015;194(4):1534–44.

18. Tilburgs T, Evans JH, Crespo AC, Strominger JL. The HLA-G cycle provides for both NK tolerance and immunity at the maternal-fetal interface. Proc Natl Acad Sci U S A. 2015;112(43):13312–7.

19. Fu B, Li X, Sun R, Tong X, Ling B, Tian Z, et al. Natural killer cells promote immune tolerance by regulating inflammatory TH17 cells at the human maternal-fetal interface. Proc Natl Acad Sci U S A. 2013;110(3):E231–40.

20. Santner-Nanan B, Peek MJ, Khanam R, Richarts L, Zhu E, Fazekas de St Groth B, et al. Systemic increase in the ratio between Foxp3+ and IL-17-producing CD4+ T cells in healthy pregnancy but not in preeclampsia. J Immunol. 2009;183(11):7023–30.

21. Arck PC, Hecher K. Fetomaternal immune cross-talk and its consequences for maternal and offspring's health. Nat Med. 2013;19(5):548–56.

22. Zenclussen AC. Adaptive immune responses during pregnancy. Am J Reprod Immunol. 2013;69(4):291–303.

23. Saito S, Nakashima A, Shima T, Ito M. Th1/Th2/Th17 and regulatory T-cell paradigm in pregnancy. Am J Reprod Immunol. 2010;63(6):601–10.

24. Confavreux C, Hutchinson M, Hours MM, Cortinovis-Tourniaire P, Moreau T. Rate of pregnancy-related relapse in multiple sclerosis. Pregnancy in Multiple Sclerosis Group. N Engl J Med. 1998;339(5):285–91.

25. Fabian M. Pregnancy in the setting of multiple sclerosis. Continuum (Minneap Minn). 2016;22(3):837–50.

26. Kim W, Kim SH, Nakashima I, Takai Y, Fujihara K, Leite MI, et al. Influence of pregnancy on neuromyelitis optica spectrum disorder. Neurology. 2012;78(16):1264–7.

27. Fragoso YD, Adoni T, Bichuetti DB, Brooks JB, Ferreira ML, Oliveira EM, et al. Neuromyelitis optica and pregnancy. J Neurol. 2013;260(10):2614–9.

28. Shimizu Y, Fujihara K, Ohashi T, Nakashima I, Yokoyama K, Ikeguch R, et al. Pregnancy-related relapse risk factors in women with anti-AQP4 antibody positivity and neuromyelitis optica spectrum disorder. Mult Scler. 2016;22(11):1413–20.

29. Norwood F, Dhanjal M, Hill M, James N, Jungbluth H, Kyle P, et al. Myasthenia in pregnancy: best practice guidelines from a U.K. multispecialty working group. J Neurol Neurosurg Psychiatry. 2014;85(5):538–43.

30. Boldingh MI, Maniaol AH, Brunborg C, Weedon-Fekjaer H, Verschuuren JJ, Tallaksen CM. Increased risk for clinical onset of myasthenia gravis during the postpartum period. Neurology. 2016;87(20):2139–45.

31. Gayed M, Gordon C. Pregnancy and rheumatic diseases. Rheumatology (Oxford). 2007;46(11):1634–40.

32. Andersen SL, Olsen J, Carle A, Laurberg P. Hyperthyroidism incidence fluctuates widely in and around pregnancy and is at variance with some other autoimmune diseases: a Danish population-based study. J Clin Endocrinol Metab. 2015;100(3):1164–71.

33. de Man YA, Dolhain RJ, van de Geijn FE, Willemsen SP, Hazes JM. Disease activity of rheumatoid arthritis during pregnancy: results from a nationwide prospective study. Arthritis Rheum. 2008;59(9):1241–8.

34. Buchel E, Van Steenbergen W, Nevens F, Fevery J. Improvement of autoimmune hepatitis during pregnancy followed by flare-up after delivery. Am J Gastroenterol. 2002;97(12):3160–5.

35. Airas L, Saraste M, Rinta S, Elovaara I, Huang YH, Wiendl H, et al. Immunoregulatory factors in multiple sclerosis patients during and after pregnancy: relevance of natural killer cells. Clin Exp Immunol. 2008;151(2):235–43.

36. Lateef A, Petri M. Management of pregnancy in systemic lupus erythematosus. Nat Rev Rheumatol. 2012;8(12):710–8.

37. Davoudi V, Keyhanian K, Bove RM, Chitnis T. Immunology of neuromyelitis optica during pregnancy. Neurol Neuroimmunol Neuroinflamm. 2016;3(6):e288.

38. Shosha E, Pittock SJ, Flanagan E, Weinshenker BG. Neuromyelitis optica spectrum disorders and pregnancy: interactions and management. Mult Scler. 2017;23(14):1808–17.

39. Jones BG, Penkert RR, Xu B, Fan Y, Neale G, Gearhart PJ, et al. Binding of estrogen receptors to switch sites and regulatory elements in the immunoglobulin heavy chain locus of activated B cells suggests a direct influence of estrogen on antibody expression. Mol Immunol. 2016;77:97–102.

40. Weinstein RS. Clinical practice. Glucocorticoid-induced bone disease. N Engl J Med. 2011;365(1):62–70.
41. Compston J. Management of glucocorticoid-induced osteoporosis. Nat Rev Rheumatol. 2010;6(2):82–8.
42. van Staa TP, Leufkens HG, Cooper C. The epidemiology of corticosteroid-induced osteoporosis: a meta-analysis. Osteoporos Int. 2002;13(10):777–87.
43. Allen CS, Yeung JH, Vandermeer B, Homik J. Bisphosphonates for steroid-induced osteoporosis. Cochrane Database Syst Rev. 2016;10:CD001347.
44. Overman RA, Toliver JC, Yeh JY, Gourlay ML, Deal CL. United States adults meeting 2010 American College of Rheumatology criteria for treatment and prevention of glucocorticoid-induced osteoporosis. Arthritis Care Res (Hoboken). 2014;66(11):1644–52.
45. Grossman JM, Gordon R, Ranganath VK, Deal C, Caplan L, Chen W, et al. American College of Rheumatology 2010 recommendations for the prevention and treatment of glucocorticoid-induced osteoporosis. Arthritis Care Res (Hoboken). 2010;62(11):1515–26.
46. Mok CC, Ho LY, Ma KM. Switching of oral bisphosphonates to denosumab in chronic glucocorticoid users: a 12-month randomized controlled trial. Bone. 2015;75:222–8.
47. Santana IU, Gomes Ado N, Lyrio LD, Rios Grassi MF, Santiago MB. Systemic lupus erythematosus, human papillomavirus infection, cervical pre-malignant and malignant lesions: a systematic review. Clin Rheumatol. 2011;30(5):665–72.
48. Nguyen ML, Flowers L. Cervical cancer screening in immunocompromised women. Obstet Gynecol Clin N Am. 2013;40(2):339–57.
49. Curtis KM, Tepper NK, Jatlaoui TC, Berry-Bibee E, Horton LG, Zapata LB, et al. U.S. medical eligibility criteria for contraceptive use, 2016. MMWR Recomm Rep. 2016;65(3):1–103.
50. Vukusic S, Marignier R. Multiple sclerosis and pregnancy in the 'treatment era'. Nat Rev Neurol. 2015;11(5):280–9.
51. Gotestam Skorpen C, Hoeltzenbein M, Tincani A, Fischer-Betz R, Elefant E, Chambers C, et al. The EULAR points to consider for use of antirheumatic drugs before pregnancy, and during pregnancy and lactation. Ann Rheum Dis. 2016;75(5):795–810.
52. Hellwig K, Rockhoff M, Herbstritt S, Borisow N, Haghikia A, Elias-Hamp B, et al. Exclusive breastfeeding and the effect on postpartum multiple sclerosis relapses. JAMA Neurol. 2015;72(10):1132–8.
53. Pakpoor J, Disanto G, Lacey MV, Hellwig K, Giovannoni G, Ramagopalan SV. Breastfeeding and multiple sclerosis relapses: a meta-analysis. J Neurol. 2012;259(10):2246–8.
54. Westerlind H, Ramanujam R, Uvehag D, Kuja-Halkola R, Boman M, Bottai M, et al. Modest familial risks for multiple sclerosis: a registry-based study of the population of Sweden. Brain. 2014;137(Pt 3):770–8.

Catamenial Epilepsy

P. Emanuela Voinescu

Definition

Catamenial epilepsy is defined by a monthly (Greek *katamenios*, monthly: *kata-*, according to, per; *men-*, month) seizure clustering pattern, encountered in both focal and generalized epilepsy patients who have a twofold or greater increase in their seizure frequency during the different phases of their periodic hormonal cycling (see Fig. 1, Table 1): C1, perimenstrual phase (days −3 to +3); C2 periovulatory phase (days +10 to −13); C3, luteal phase (days +10 to +3 of the next cycle for anovulatory cycles with inadequate luteal phase), where day +1 is considered to be the 1st day of the menstrual flow and day −14 is 14 days prior to the onset of the menstrual cycle and corresponds to ovulation [1, 2]. Experts in the area have labelled this as a "complex neuroendocrine condition" and because of a lack for personalized treatment, women with catamenial epilepsy are frequently refractory to traditional anti-epileptic medications [3, 4].

For a diagnosis of catamenial epilepsy to be made, the patient needs to keep a diary for at least 3 months, charting both seizures and menses. Theoretically, to be able to distinguish a C3 pattern, a mid-luteal phase serum progesterone concentration needs to be checked to differentiate between ovulatory and anovulatory cycles [3, 5].

Epidemiology

It is estimated that approximately one third of women have a catamenial pattern to their epilepsy, but numbers in the literature go as low as 10% [6] and as high as 70% [7, 8], because differences in assessing for and diagnosing catamenial seizures. Among the three catamenial patterns, the perimenstrual type (C1) is the most frequently observed [4, 9], though the prevalence may be higher for the C3 pattern [5].

P. E. Voinescu (✉)
Brigham and Women's Hospital, Harvard Medical School, Boston, MA, USA
e-mail: pevoinescu@bwh.harvard.edu

Pathophysiology

Hypothalamic-Pituitary-Ovarian Axis

The pathophysiology of the hypothalamic-pituitary-ovarian axis and of the ovarian cycle is well established. The arcuate nucleus of the hypothalamus produces the gonadotropin releasing-hormone (GnRH) which triggers the pulsatile secretion of the follicle stimulating hormone (FSH) and luteinizing hormone (LH) by the pituitary gland, essential for a healthy ovarian/menstrual cycle (Fig. 2a).

The menstrual cycle lasts 24–35 (average 28) days; the 1st day of menses marks its onset and end, and the ovulation occurring mid-cycle (day 14 or day −14 for cycles longer than 28 days) divides it in two major phases: the follicular phase (variable duration: days 1–14, longer when the cycle is longer than 28 days) and the luteal phase (fixed length of 14 days: days 15–28 or −14 to −1 for cycles longer than 28 days). During the follicular phase, the ovarian follicles mature, with one follicle becoming the dominant one that is released on day −14 (ovulation). During the luteal phase, the dominant follicle forms the progesterone-producing corpus luteum (Fig. 2b). Inadequate FSH secretion leads to poor follicular development, lack of ovulation and poor development and functioning of the corpus luteum with low production of progesterone during the luteal phase [4, 10]. Figure 1 shows the time course of fluctuations in the female sex hormone concentrations during a normal menstrual cycling (1A), as well as in anovulatory menstrual cycling with an inadequate luteal phase (1B).

Sex Hormones and Epileptogenesis

The pathophysiology of how sex hormones influence epileptogenesis is less well understood. Seizure clustering is not an uncommon phenomenon [11], but observations that in a large percentage of women, this clustering is most likely to occur at certain times of the menstrual cycling, led to the

Fig. 1 Patterns of catamenial epilepsy. Day 1 is the 1st day of menstrual flow and day −14 is the day of ovulation. (**a**) Normal cycle with normal ovulation. C1 pattern is associated with exacerbation of seizures in the perimenstrual phase (day −3 to day +3 of next cycle), and C2 pattern is associated with exacerbation of seizures in the periovulatory phase (day +10 to day −13). (**b**) Inadequate luteal phase cycle with anovulation. The C3 pattern is associated with exacerbations during the entire inadequate luteal phase (day +10 to day +3 of the next cycle). C catamenial seizure pattern, F follicular phase, O periovulatory phase, L luteal phase, M perimenstrual phase. Practical guideline: calculate the daily seizure frequency during the specified C1, C2, or C3 time windows and compare to the daily seizure frequency for the rest of the menstrual cycle. (From Harden and Pennell [4] as modified from Herzog et al. [1]. Reproduced with automatic permission from Elsevier through the STM signatory guidelines and with permission from John Wiley and Sons)

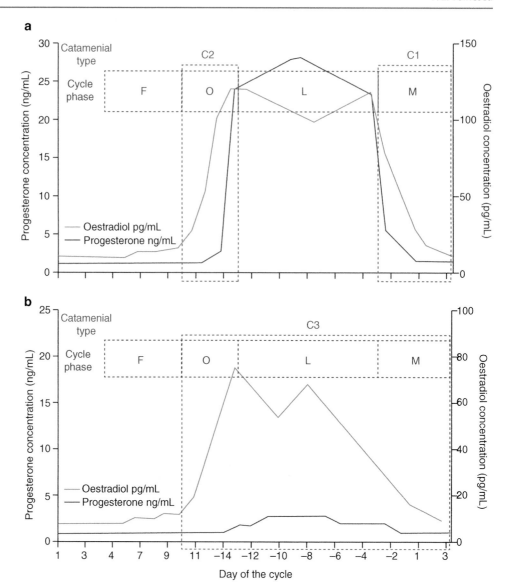

hypothesis that sex hormones modulate cortical excitability. It was shown that they act through both genomic and non-genomic pathways [3, 4]. They bind to steroid-receptors and form complexes that interact with or directly act as a transcription factors on hormone-responsive elements in the gene promoter regions and, thus modulate gene expression. There are several non-genomic pathways described, but the most important one for the nervous system is through neurosteroids, sex hormone metabolites (e.g. allopregnanolone), that can directly modulate ion channel receptors and membrane excitability (Fig. 3).

A simplified explanation is that progesterone has definite antiepileptic properties, promoting inhibition, while estrogen's role is complex, but possibly neuroexcitatory in certain circumstances. This seems to explain why the rapid decline in progesterone concentration on day −3 may be responsible for perimenstrual seizure worsening, while

some women might be susceptible to the proconvulsant effects of estrogen during the rapid estrogen surge on day −15 and have periovulatory seizure worsening [4].

Animal studies have shown that progesterone, through its metabolite allopregnanolone, promotes neuroinhibition primarily through modulation of GABA type A receptor. Reddy et al. showed that neurosteroids binding to extrasynaptic δ subunit of GABA-A receptors promote tonic inhibition and that there is plasticity in the expression level and compositions of these receptors throughout the menstrual cycle that may trigger a fluctuation in membrane excitability to justify catamenial seizures [12]. Estrogen, on the other hand, may have dual actions depending on dose, route of administration, acute versus chronic administration, natural hormonal environment, and estrogenic species. Work by Velíšková et al. revealed that estradiol within the physiological concentration range can protect hippocampal neurons against

Table 1 Patterns of catamenial epilepsy and suggested therapeutic methods

Menstrual cycle phases	Follicular	(Peri) Ovulatory	Luteal	(Peri) Menstrual
Days	+3 to +10	+10 to −13	−13 to −3	−3 to +3
Estradiol (E) and Progesterone (P) concentrations				
Ovulatory cycle	Low E & P values	E rising sooner than P	High values of both E & P	P declines before E
Anovulatory cycle	Low E & P values	Rising E with low P	High E and low P	E declines and low P
Phase with increased seizure frequency during this catamenial pattern:				
Ovulatory cycles				C1
		C2		
Anovulatory cycles		C3		
Treatment options and timing of treatment based on the catamenial type:				
C1 (peri-menstrual seizure frequency worsening)	≥ 3-fold increase			Progesterone lozenges
	< 3-fold increase			Cyclic acetazolamide, clobazam, increased patient's AED dose[a]
All catamenial patterns	Continuous hormonal treatment with MPA or COCs, allowing for the withdrawal week only every few months[b]			

Color-coded catamenial pattern based on the phase of the menstrual cycle and hormonal changes (C1, red, peri-menstrual; C2, green, peri-ovulatory; C3, yellow, luteal phase for anovulatory cycles only). Day 1 is the 1st day of menstrual flow and day −14 is the day of ovulation

Abbreviations: E Estradiol, *P* Progesterone, *MPA* medroxyprogesterone acetate, *COCs* continuous oral contraceptives (no placebo week), *AED* antiepileptic drug

[a]No control trials to support use of acetazolamide, clobazam or increasing the patient's medication in the perimenstrual period

[b]No specific treatment options for C2 and C3 catamenial epilepsy patterns; some providers use clobazam or increase the patient's medication for the period of seizure worsening, but no clinical data is available to support this practice

seizure-induced damage; its anticonvulsant effects possibly involve regulation of gene expression since the beneficial effects depend on treatment duration [13, 14]. Prior work, however, has reported increased density of NMDA receptors on the dendritic spines of hippocampal cells, and thus increase neuronal excitability, detected 2 days after the start of exogenous estradiol treatment [15].

Besides animal studies, clinical studies in women with epilepsy also associated both estrogen and progesterone cycling with catamenial seizure. In one report, progesterone concentrations were lower and estrogen/progesterone ratio higher in patients with catamenial epilepsy [16], while other studies found little variation in progesterone concentration, but larger variations in estrogen concentrations correlating with a catamenial seizure pattern [17, 18].

Antiepileptic Medication Clearance Changes

Sex hormones may also have an impact on antiepileptic medication disposition and thus the hormonal cyclic fluctuations may trigger differences in the medication pharmacokinetics and serum concentrations. Studies on this topic showed variable results: in women with catamenial seizures, end-cycle phenytoin serum concentrations were significantly lower while phenobarbital concentrations did not change [19], phenobarbital concentrations did not change significantly [19], and neither did valproate concentrations [20]; lamotrigine concentrations remained stable in one study [21], but declined by 31% during the mid-luteal phase in another [20]. One observational study on seven patients on phenytoin, phenobarbital and carbamazepine found no correlation between the plasma estradiol or progesterone and the serum

the anti-epileptic drug concentrations [22]. Therefore, larger studies are needed, but the pathophysiology of catamenial epilepsy cannot be explained only by the alterations in the concentrations of antiepileptic drugs.

Effects of the Menstrual Cycle on Other Neurological and Non-neurological Disorders

Exacerbation of certain medical conditions at specific menstrual cycle phases is a well-recognized phenomenon [23]. Numerous other conditions are reported to display menstrual fluctuations: some common (migraine, asthma, rheumatoid arthritis, irritable bowel syndrome, pneumothorax, acute appendicitis) others more rare (endocrine allergy and anaphylaxis, hereditary angioedema, erythema multiforme, urticaria, aphthous ulcers, Behçet syndrome, acute intermittent porphyria, paroxysmal supraventricular tachycardia, glaucoma, and multiple sclerosis). The underlying pathophysiology is not very well understood in either of these disorders, but some of

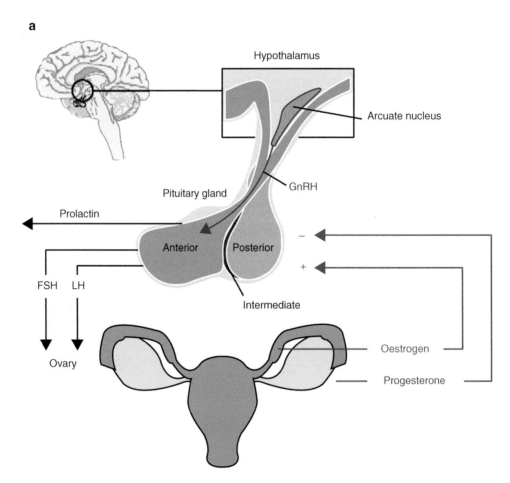

Fig. 2 Anatomical structures and physiologic changes underlying the menstrual cycle. (**a**) Hypothalamic-pituitary-ovarian axis in women. FSH follicle-stimulating hormone, LH luteinizing hormone, GnRH gonadotropin-releasing hormone. (**b**) The menstrual cycle. The physiologic changes associated with the follicular development and endometrial cycle as related to the pituitary (FSH, LH) and ovarian (estrogen, progesterone) hormone concentrations. (**a** is reproduced from Harden and Pennell [4] with automatic permission from Elsevier through the STM signatory guidelines)

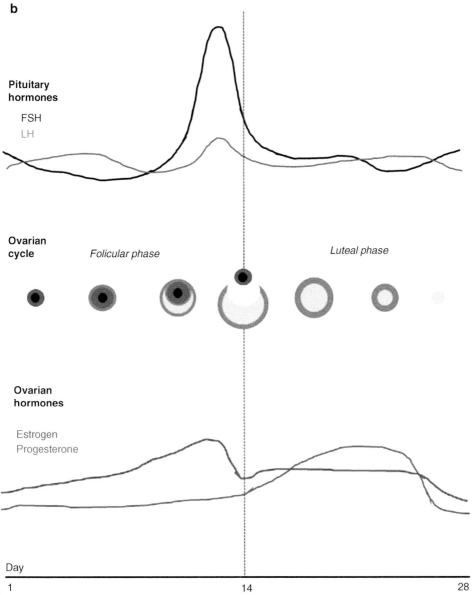

b

Pituitary hormones

FSH
LH

Ovarian cycle   *Folicular phase*   *Luteal phase*

Ovarian hormones

Estrogen
Progesterone

Day

1   14   28

Fig. 2 (continued)

the pathways are likely to be common. The main hypothesis is that the fluctuations in the plasma concentrations of sex steroids are central and trigger cyclic specific alterations in each of the organ/system affected, as well as changes in the perceptions of disease severity brought about by premenstrual alterations in mood, as seen in premenstrual syndrome.

Management

Determining that a woman's epilepsy has a catamenial pattern may have significant practical implications for her therapeutic management. With a working hypothesis that it is a neurosteroid-sensitive form of epilepsy, one would expect that the seizure control would vary as sex

hormone concentrations change with the patient's biological stage. In particular, the raising hormone concentrations during pregnancy and the erratic fluctuations at menopause are expected to have an impact on the seizure control. Indeed, most studies suggest that women with catamenial epilepsy experience better control during pregnancy, but worsening disease during the perimenopausal period. One may speculate further that they are more likely to experience seizure worsening during the postpartum period and, in contrast, seizure reduction during the postmenopausal years. Cagnetti et al. [24] demonstrated that women with a C1 catamenial epilepsy have better seizure control (higher rate of seizure freedom or reduced seizure frequency) during pregnancy when compared with women who do not have catame-

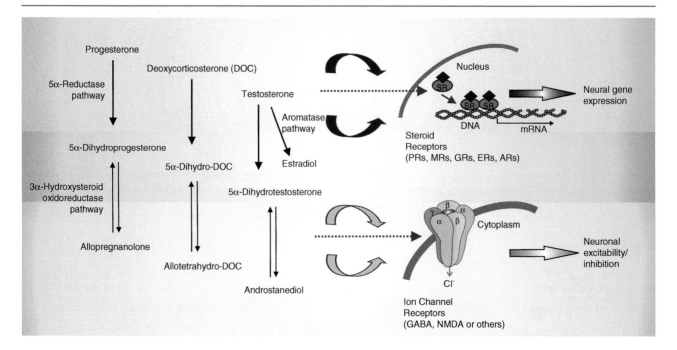

Fig. 3 Potential neuroendocrine basis of neuronal excitability and seizure susceptibility. There are at least two distinct mechanisms by which steroid hormones, such as progesterone, deoxycorticosterone, testosterone and estrogens, affect neuronal excitability and seizure susceptibility: (i) binding to intracellular steroid receptors (SRs) – progesterone receptors (PRs), estrogen receptors (ERs), androgen receptors (ARs), glucocorticoid receptors (GCs) and mineralocorticoid receptors (MRs) (top panel) and (ii) metabolism to neuroactive steroids that can modulate ion channel receptors – for example, allopregnanolone binding and potentiating GABA-A receptor function (bottom panel). (Reproduced from Reddy [3] with automatic permission from Elsevier through the STM signatory guidelines)

nial epilepsy. No prospective information is available on the course of epilepsy for women undergoing menopausal transition.

The awareness of these clinical details may influence the consideration for surgical options, tailoring the aggressiveness of treatment for different biological states, planning for times of possible seizure worsening, selection of contraceptive methods, consideration for hormonal treatments. Because of the ease of diagnosis and the ease to determine the period of seizure worsening, the interventions presented in this chapter have been tested mostly for a perimenstrual (C1) seizure pattern.

Hormonal Treatments

The only evidence-based therapeutic guidance for specific treatment comes from a double-blind, placebo-controlled, randomized multi-center trial that showed a benefit for progesterone lozenges during menstrual days 14–28, but only in the subgroup of women with epilepsy who had a threefold or greater seizure frequency increase during the C1 phase [25].

Prior to this clinical trial, the same investigators had run two small, open-label studies which suggested that natural progesterone (administered as a vaginal suppository or oral lozenge) from ovulation until the onset of menses was efficacious for the treatment of epilepsy [2, 26]. Therefore, the NIH Progesterone Treatment clinical trial and follow-up open-label extension phases, were designed to add to an already optimized antiepileptic agent either natural progesterone 200 mg lozenges or placebo taken three times daily starting at ovulation (on day −14), with the option of a decremented taper (to 100 mg three times daily on days 26–27, 50 mg three times on day 28), and then stopped at the onset of menses until day 14 of the next cycle. When comparing the proportion of ≥50% responders in seizure frequency between a 3-month baseline and 3-month treatment phase, there were no difference in seizure frequency when comparing the treatment arm or placebo [25]. However, isolating the patients with a strong C1 pattern – those who had three times more seizures during the cycle days −3 to +3 – the difference became significant: 37.8% were responders to progesterone versus 11.1% responders in the placebo group. Analyzing further this C1 group of patient, the benefit seemed to increase the more seizures were confined to the perimenstrual days, with 70% seizure frequency reduction in patients with a perimenstrual seizure frequency of ≥8-times compared to the rest of the menstrual cycle. No response was observed for subjects with catamenial patterns type 2 or 3 or for the enrolled subjects without a catamenial pattern, who comprised slightly more than 50% of the study population. Despite the beauty of the hypothesis, this study offers still no treatment options for C2 and C3 catamenial patterns and even for the majority of the patients who display a C1 seizure pattern.

The authors of the NIH Progesterone Treatment Trial went further with their analysis and tried to find an explanation for the difference in progesterone's efficacy observed among different catamenial epilepsy types. They measured the mid-luteal phase allopregnanolone and showed a significant correlation between reduction in seizure frequency and increases in the allopregnanolone concentrations for the C1 ≥3 group, supporting the idea that allopregnanolone mediates the changes in seizure threshold seen with progesterone withdrawal and that cyclic progesterone supplementation in the subset of C1 catamenial epilepsy may be beneficial [27].

The same authors had provided a case report proving a gain of function/loss of function example for the presumed hypothesis above. A 34-year-old woman with intractable focal epilepsy and an apparent C3 catamenial pattern of her seizures, was successfully treated with carbamazepine and cyclic progesterone, with an impressive decrease in her seizure frequency upon progesterone treatment initiation for several years. When started on finasteride for baldness years later, seizure frequency increased from none to 3–6/month despite no change in her antiseizure regimen and stable carbamazepine concentrations. The author's hypothesis is that finasteride, as a reductase enzyme inhibitor and would inhibit the metabolism of progesterone to its neurosteroid metabolite, allopregnanolone, the true mediator of treatment rather than the progesterone itself [28].

One small open-label study suggested that synthetic forms of progestogens, such as medroxyprogesterone acetate (MPA), may possibly provide beneficial treatment of catamenial epilepsy, likely through a suppression of menstrual cycling [29]. However, this finding has not been replicated in other studies, and the risk for bone density loss makes MPA an unattractive long-term treatment option. More commonly used are continuous combined (ethinyl-estradiol and synthetic progestin) oral contraceptive pills [COCs] without the placebo week in an attempt to minimize the cyclic variation of endogenous hormones and thus reduce seizure frequency, although no supportive evidence is available for this approach. With the same goal, gonadotropin releasing hormone (GnRH) analogues [30] have been tried in small case series and may be possibly beneficial, but the efficacy and safety of longer-term use have not been established in larger studies.

A related observation is that hormonal replacement therapy at perimenopause should be used with caution given clinical evidence for an increase in seizure frequency with the use of a combination of estrogen-medroxyprogesterone hormone replacement therapy in a dose-dependent manner [31]. Even in the absence of hormonal replacement therapy, women with epilepsy may experience fluctuations in seizure frequency during the perimenopausal transition period. During perimenopause, the cyclic progesterone elevations become less frequent with increased anovulatory cycles, but elevated FSH concentrations trigger erratic estrogen surges until the onset of menopause. The resulting elevated estrogen-to-progesterone ratio may explain why some women experience increased seizure frequency during the perimenopausal transition [32, 33]. Once they complete the menopause transition, some women with epilepsy experience decreased seizure frequency. Fluctuations in estrogen concentrations may trigger clearance changes and transiently alter the antiepileptic medication serum concentrations, yet such clearance changes during menopause are again poorly characterized [34]. A retrospective study suggested that almost two thirds of perimenopausal women with epilepsy reported an increase in their seizure frequency [32]; this represents more than the presumed "catamenial" epilepsy subset, reported to be ~30%.

Alternative Strategies

There are a few case reports or small open-label series exploring non-hormonal treatment options possibly helpful to further raise the seizure threshold when given during the time of exacerbation. Acetazolamide is perhaps the oldest strategy employed as a specific treatment for catamenial epilepsy, with the first reports in 1950s [35]. The algorithm has been mostly reported for C1 patterns, but employed in others as well: 250–500 mg daily from 3 to 7 days prior to menses [36]. Benzodiazepines are also frequently used in practice, with similar slim data, the most being available for clobazam – 20–30 mg daily, for 10 days starting 2 days before the period of seizure worsening [37]. Increasing the patient's antiepileptic medication dose, if allowed by the medication serum concentrations, side-effects and pharmacokinetics, is another option, but again there is no supportive evidence.

Case Example
Initial clinical history: A 30-year-old woman with a history of generalized tonic-clonic seizures in her 20s, with an apparent catamenial pattern, seizure free on the same doses of lamotrigine and levetiracetam dual therapy for 5 years, presents to the emergency room for a break through convulsive seizure. There are no apparent provoking factors: she missed no medication doses and there is no change in her lifestyle or health. Basic labs obtained at the time of her

presentation are within normal limits, her toxicology screen is normal. A pregnancy test is negative. Antiepileptic medication concentrations are tested and resulted 2 days later: levetiracetam concentration is stable when compared with her previous values, but her lamotrigine is lower. Upon further discussion with the patient, she reports being in a stable relationship now and starting oral contraceptive pills a few weeks prior to her breakthrough seizure. She had her first menstruation, since being on oral contraceptives, starting a day after her breakthrough seizure. She is convinced her catamenial epilepsy is worsened by oral contraceptive medications and is planning to transition to an IUD.

Explanation: There is no clinical data to support that oral contraceptive medications lead to seizure worsening, though exogenous hormones, similar to endogenous ones, may also influence neuronal excitability. There is however evidence that lamotrigine metabolism is influenced by sex hormones – both endogenous (dramatic clearance changes during pregnancy) and exogenous, with medication concentration dropping significantly 8 days after oral contraceptive pills have been initiated.

Therapeutic approach: We explained to the patient that despite her seizure occurring perimenstrually, it is more likely the lower lamotrigine concentration that triggered the seizure breakthrough and she could continue her current contraceptive method, but increase the lamotrigine dose to compensate for the OCP-triggered clearance changes. She remains skeptical and prefers to switch to a non-hormonal contraceptive method, so she gets an IUD inserted a couple of days afterwards and discontinues her oral contraceptive medications.

Clinical story continued (1): 6 month later she returns with another breakthrough seizure. She reports that there have been again no changes in her life-style or medical problems. She is on no additional medication or supplements. Regarding contraceptive methods, she is back to using barrier methods as she could not tolerate the IUD and had it removed a few weeks after its insertion. Her seizure happens again as she is due for her menstruation, though she reports that she may be about a week late. Her blood work is normal,

except that this time both lamotrigine and levetiracetam concentrations are low. A pregnancy test is now positive.

Explanation: Many medication have pregnancy-related pharmacokinetic changes and lamotrigine and levetiracetam are among those reported to have a significant increase in their clearance early in pregnancy. Therefore, although there is a study reporting an improvement in the seizure frequency of women with catamenial epilepsy, seizure worsening in pregnancy can occur in all women with epilepsy when the pregnancy-related clearance changes are not accounted for with an adequate dose increase. Several studies have shown that a decrease below 0.65 of the preconception concentration leads to seizure worsening.

Therapeutic approach: The patient was followed with therapeutic dose monitoring throughout her pregnancy: her antiepileptic serum concentrations were checked monthly and doses adjusted to maintain preconception values. She did well through her pregnancy, with no seizure recurrence.

Clinical story continued (2): At her 1-year postpartum visit, she reports she is worried about her disease progression: after years of seizure freedom, she had three generalized convulsive seizures in her 1st-year post-partum, despite further medication uptitration. She long stopped breastfeeding to make sure she gets adequate sleep per night, as sleep deprivation was initially thought to be a provoking factor. She reports feeling depressed for not being able to care for her baby the way she would like to. All of her seizures have occurred again at the time of her menstruation and she is asking whether there is a way to suppress hormonal cycling as she and her husband are not planning for another pregnancy in the near future.

Therapeutic approach: The patient was referred to the complex contraceptive clinic at our institution. Several options were presented: continuous combined oral contraceptive pills (no placebo week) intended to provide menstrual/cycle suppression, including progesterone-only pills, injections of DMPA, or the progestin-based subdermal implant. She chose a progestin-based implant, Nexplanon, and regained seizure freedom.

Take Home Points

1. Seizure diaries for at least three menstrual cycles, that also accurately track the 1st day of menses, are essential to determine the presence and type of catamenial epilepsy and to correctly schedule a therapeutic intervention

2. For patient with a strong C1 catamenial pattern (perimenstrual seizure frequency at least threefold the seizure frequency in the rest of the menstrual cycle), consider progesterone lozenges 200 mg three times daily on days 14–25, 100 mg three times daily on days 26–27, 50 mg three times daily on day 28, then stop (if menses begin prior to day 26, the tapering would begin on that day)

3. Disease course for patients with catamenial epilepsy
   (a) Possible improvement in seizure frequency during pregnancy
   (b) Possible worsening of the seizure frequency during perimenopause and improvement once menopause is achieved
   (c) Higher proportion of medically-refractory disease

4. For patients with any catamenial seizure patterns, alternative strategies can be considered:
   (a) Clobazam, 20–30 mg daily for 10 days, starting 2 days before predicted period of seizure worsening (if menses occur in a regular, predictable fashion)
   (b) Increase daily dose of patient's antiepileptic medications during the predicted period of seizure worsening (if menses occur in a regular, predictable fashion)
   (c) Acetazolamide, 250–500 mg/day, beginning day −7 to −3 until day 1 of the menstrual cycle (if menses occur in a regular, predictable fashion)
   (d) Consider suppression of the hormonal cycling (continuous oral contraceptive pills, medroxyprogesterone acetate)

References

1. Herzog AG, Klein P, Ransil BJ. Three patterns of catamenial epilepsy. Epilepsia. 1997;38(10):1082–8.
2. Herzog AG, Fowler KM, Sperling MR, Massaro JM. Distribution of seizures across the menstrual cycle in women with epilepsy. Epilepsia. 2015;56(5):e58–62.
3. Reddy DS. The neuroendocrine basis of sex differences in epilepsy. Pharmacol Biochem Behav sciencedirect. 2017;152:97–104.
4. Harden CL, Pennell PB. Neuroendocrine considerations in the treatment of men and women with epilepsy. Lancet Neurol. 2013;12(1):72–83.
5. Herzog A. Catamenial epilepsy: update on prevalence, pathophysiology and treatment from the findings of the NIH Progesterone Treatment Trial. Seizure. sciencedirect. 2015;28:18–25.
6. Duncan S, Read CL, Brodie M. How common is catamenial epilepsy? Epilepsia [Internet]. 1993. Available from: http://onlinelibrary.wiley.com/doi/10.1111/j.1528-1157.1993.tb02097.x/full.
7. Rosciszewska D. Analysis of seizure dispersion during menstrual cycle in women with epilepsy. Epilepsy [Internet]. 1980. Available from: https://www.karger.com/Article/Fulltext/387521.
8. Taubøll E, Lundervold A, Gjerstad L. Temporal distribution of seizures in epilepsy. Epilepsy Res [Internet]. 1991;8:153–65. Available from: https://www.sciencedirect.com/science/article/pii/092012119190084S.
9. Navis A, Harden C. A treatment approach to catamenial epilepsy. Curr Treat Options Neurol springer. 2016;18(7):30.
10. Jones GS. The luteal phase defect. Fertil Steril [Internet]. 1976. Available from: http://europepmc.org/abstract/med/1269800.
11. Haut S. Seizure clusters: characteristics and treatment. Curr Opin Neurol. 2015;28(2):143.
12. Reddy D. Catamenial epilepsy: discovery of an extrasynaptic molecular mechanism for targeted therapy. Front Cell Neurosci. frontiers. 2016;10:101.
13. Velíšková J, DeSantis K. Sex and hormonal influences on seizures and epilepsy. Horm Behav. 2013;63(2):267–77.
14. Velíšková J, Jesus G, Kaur R, Velíšek L. Females, their estrogens, and seizures. Epilepsia. 2010;51(s3):141–4.
15. Weiland N. Estradiol selectively regulates agonist binding sites on the N-methyl-D-aspartate receptor complex in the CA1 region of the hippocampus. Endocrinology [Internet]. 1992;131:662–8. Available from: https://academic.oup.com/endo/article-abstract/131/2/662/2496261.
16. Khayat H, Soliman N, Tomoum H, Omran M, Wakad A, Shatla R. Reproductive hormonal changes and catamenial pattern in adolescent females with epilepsy. Epilepsia. 2008;49(9):1619–26.
17. Herzog AG, Fowler KM, Sperling MR, Liporace JD, Kalayjian LA, Heck CN, Krauss GL, Dworetzky BA, Pennell PB, Progesterone Trial Study Group. Variation of seizure frequency with ovulatory status of menstrual cycles. Epilepsia. 2011;52(10):1843–8.
18. Quigg M, Fowler KM, Herzog AG, NIH Progesterone Trial Study Group. Circalunar and ultralunar periodicities in women with partial seizures. Epilepsia. 2008;49(6):1081–5.
19. Rościszewska D, Buntner B, Guz I, Zawisza L. Ovarian hormones, anticonvulsant drugs, and seizures during the menstrual cycle in women with epilepsy. J Neurol Neurosurg Psychiatry. 1986;49(1):47–51.
20. Herzog AG, Blum AS, Farina EL, Maestri XE, Newman J, Garcia E, Krishnamurthy KB, Hoch DB, Replansky S, Fowler KM, Smithson SD. Valproate and lamotrigine level variation with menstrual cycle phase and oral contraceptive use. Neurology. 2009;72(10):911–4.
21. Wegner I, Edelbroek PM, Bulk S, Lindhout D. Lamotrigine kinetics within the menstrual cycle, after menopause, and with oral contraceptives. Neurology. 2009;73(17):1388–93.

22. Bäckström T, Jorpes P. Serum phenytoin, phenobarbital, carbamazepine, albumin; and plasma estradiol, progesterone concentrations during the menstrual cycle in women with epilepsy. Acta Neurol Scand. Wiley Online Library. 1979;59(2):63–71.

23. Case AM, Reid R. Effects of the menstrual cycle on medical disorders. Arch Intern Med [Internet]. 1998;158:1405–12. Available from: https://jamanetwork.com/journals/jamainternalmedicine/fullarticle/208109.

24. Cagnetti C, Lattanzi S, Foschi N, Provinciali L, Silvestrini M. Seizure course during pregnancy in catamenial epilepsy. Neurology. 2014;83(4):339–44.

25. Herzog AG, Fowler KM, Smithson SD, Kalayjian LA, Heck CN, Sperling MR, et al. Progesterone vs placebo therapy for women with epilepsy: a randomized clinical trial. Neurology. 2012;78(24):1959–66.

26. Herzog A. Intermittent progesterone therapy and frequency of complex partial seizures in women with menstrual disorders. Neurology [Internet]. 1986;36:1607–10. Available from: http://www.neurology.org/content/36/12/1607.short.

27. Herzog AG, Frye C. Allopregnanolone levels and seizure frequency in progesterone-treated women with epilepsy. Neurol Int. 2014;83:345–8. Available from: http://www.neurology.org/content/83/4/345.short.

28. Herzog AG, Frye CA. Seizure exacerbation associated with inhibition of progesterone metabolism. Ann Neurol. 2003;53(3):390–1.

29. Mattson RH, Cramer JA, Caldwell BV, Siconolfi BC. Treatment of seizures with medroxyprogesterone acetate: preliminary report. Neurology. 1984;34(9):1255–8.

30. Bauer J, Wild L, Flügel D, Stefan H. The effect of a synthetic GnRH analogue on catamenial epilepsy: a study in ten patients. J Neurol [Internet]. 1992. Available from: https://link.springer.com/article/10.1007/BF00810354.

31. Harden CL, Herzog AG, Nikolov BG, Koppel BS, Christos PJ, Fowler K, et al. Hormone replacement therapy in women with epilepsy: a randomized, double-blind, placebo-controlled study. Epilepsia. 2006;47(9):1447–51.

32. Harden CL, Pulver MC, Ravdin L, Jacobs AR. The effect of menopause and perimenopause on the course of epilepsy. Epilepsia. 1999;40(10):1402–7.

33. Harden CL, Koppel BS, Herzog AG, Nikolov BG, Hauser WA. Seizure frequency is associated with age at menopause in women with epilepsy. Neurology. 2003;61(4):451–5.

34. Sveinsson O, Tomson T. Epilepsy and menopause: potential implications for pharmacotherapy. Drugs Aging. springer. 2014;31(9):671–5.

35. Ansell B, Clarke E. Acetazolamide in treatment of epilepsy. Br Med J [Internet]. 1956;1:650–4. Available from: https://www.ncbi.nlm.nih.gov/pmc/articles/PMC1979321/.

36. Lim LL, Foldvary N, Mascha E, Lee J. Acetazolamide in women with catamenial epilepsy. Epilepsia [Internet]. 2001. Available from: http://onlinelibrary.wiley.com/doi/10.1046/j.1528-1157.2001.33600.x/full.

37. Feely M, Calvert R, Gibson J. Clobazam in catamenial epilepsy. A model for evaluating anticonvulsants. Lancet. 1982;2(8289):71–3.

Neuro-oncological Disorders in Women

Na Tosha N. Gatson and Erika N. Leese

*In the front of **her** mind, from the bottom of **his** heart, underneath the cancer, and at the edge of what seems like an eternity, she remains the same woman, working to pull strength from the corners of the earth. **To live as well as possible, for as long as possible**. The time is N.O.W. for us to understand cancer issues in Women's Neurology.*

Introduction

Overview and Epidemiology

There exists a gap within the neuro-oncology community to address women's issues as they relate to clinical management, ethics/bioethics, and research development in the field. Neuro-oncologic disease includes primary and metastatic central nervous system (CNS) tumors as well as the neurologic complications that occur secondary to body cancer or cancer therapies. It has been estimated that upwards of 35% of cancer patients will have some CNS involvement over the course of their cancer history [1]. While there have been multiple research efforts aimed at uncovering environmental and behavioral risk factors for brain and CNS tumors, exposure to ionizing radiation is the single proven risk factor [2]. Interestingly, those that have a medical history of allergy or atopy such as eczema, asthma, and psoriasis have a reduced risk overall for brain cancer [3].

The Central Brain Tumor Registry of the United States (CBTRUS) statistical report estimates that nearly 79,000 persons will be diagnosed with brain or other CNS tumors in 2018 [4]. Based on data collected between 2009 in 2013, we could expect the majority (57.9%) of these tumors to be diagnosed in females [4]. Women are disproportionately impacted by certain neuro-oncologic conditions, and specific questions surrounding fertility and women's issues have gone unanswered or poorly researched. Subsequently, new and relevant guidelines have been difficult to integrate into clinical neuro-oncology. This chapter provides an update in the field and is structured to highlight common neuro-oncologic issues that impact women, outline specific pressing concerns by clinicians and patients, and offer next steps towards increasing awareness of women's neuro-oncology. The goal is to stimulate academic discussions that promote all levels of research, drive our understanding of the relevant issues, and ultimately lead to the development of clinical guidelines in Reproductive & Women's Neuro-Oncology.

Impact of Pregnancy and Menopause on Brain and Other CNS Tumors

An early 1990s study of 127 women with a history of meningiomas, gliomas, and acoustic schwannomas were compared to 233 age-matched healthy controls. In comparing their respective histories for number of pregnancies, menopausal status, and report of any gynecological surgeries the study demonstrated four interesting trends: (1) Menopausal women have a reduced risk for meningiomas. This could be secondary to the post-menopausal reduction in estrogen levels. (2) Menopausal woman had an increased trend toward gliomas and acoustic schwannomas. (3) Parity had no influence on these tumor trends. (4) Bilateral oophorectomy prior to menopause decreased the overall risk for all histologic brain tumor types studied [5]. This study supports the role for hormones either directly or indirectly in CNS tumors, however, targeting hormones in certain tumor types has not led to compelling evidence for anti-hormone based therapies in brain tumor. While parity in this study was not demonstrated to influence these tumors, the study design reviewed patient questionnaires and it is unclear if time of

N. T. N. Gatson (✉)
Geisinger Neuroscience Institute, Danville, PA, USA

Geisinger Cancer Institute, Danville, PA, USA
e-mail: ngatson@geisinger.edu

E. N. Leese
Geisinger Neuroscience Institute, Danville, PA, USA
e-mail: eleese@geisinger.edu

© Springer Nature Switzerland AG 2019
M. A. O'Neal (ed.), *Neurology and Psychiatry of Women*, https://doi.org/10.1007/978-3-030-04245-5_10

tumor diagnosis was matched with pregnancy or the post pregnancy period.

The incidence of pregnancy concurrent with all cancer types estimated at about 1 cancer per 1000 pregnancies, with breast cancer, cervical cancer, and malignant melanomas being most frequently diagnosed [6]. This number is likely a gross underestimation as it does not consider spontaneous abortion in women due to cancer/cancer treatment, elective abortions, and limited feasibility to capture all actual clinical cases. As patients live longer with improved therapeutics and earlier diagnosis in cancer, we will certainly see more cases of pregnancy in patients with a cancer diagnosis.

Newly diagnosed brain tumor during pregnancy is related to the increased frequency of clinical evaluation of pregnant women who in turn might complain of headaches, vomiting, vision changes, and seizures as these tumors develop or expand in size. Increased systemic immunosuppression during pregnancy further assists the tumor's evasion of the immune response – which is already reduced in the CNS. Some studies suggest vascular hemodynamic changes and pregnancy hormones also impact tumor aggressive behaviors [7]. The clinical decision to subject the pregnant woman to radiation (CT) versus contrast dye and high magnetism (contrasted MRI) is delayed when symptoms are presumed to be routine pregnancy-related changes. Imaging most commonly reveals meningiomas, gliomas, and pituitary tumors [6]. Importantly, the September 2016 issue of the *Journal of the American Medical Association* reported that while magnetic energy used in MRI is not found to be harmful in pregnancy, the gadolinium contrast dye in small number of cases crossed the placenta and accumulates in the fetus and potentially causes death or a host of immune and rheumatologic issues in the child long-term [8]. The recommendation since that time has been to avoid the use of gadolinium dye during pregnancy, and MRI is the preferred modality over CT due to radiation risks, when avoidable and especially during the first trimester.

Common Primary Brain/CNS Tumors Which Impact Women

Meningiomas

Meningiomas account for 37% of all CNS tumors and are the most frequently reported tumor type (Fig. 1a, b). Overall, meningiomas occur two times more frequently in females as compared to males. The rate increases to nearly three times more likely in women between the ages of 35 and 54 [4]. Almost 70% of meningiomas express progesterone receptors and 30% express estrogen receptors and have been targeted in therapeutic trials (discussed below). Meningioma cell proliferation is thought to be driven, in-part, by these hormones which might partially explain the noted sex-discrepancy toward a female predominance. While a few studies find that

progesterone receptor might be a favorable marker for tumor behavior [9], most studies have been inconclusive [10]. Other hormone receptors for androgen and growth hormone have also been identified and targeted in the treatment of refractory meningiomas [11, 12]. A large study by Claus et. al. 2014 collected responses from 1127 women with intracranial meningioma to evaluate personal history factors that might offer insight into potentially modifiable risk factors. Women ranged from 29-79 years of age. Based on their responses, the study concluded the following: (1) Increased risk in premenopausal women using oral contraceptives [odds ratio of 95%]; (2) Positive association for risk in patients with increased body mass index; (3) Reduced risk associated with breastfeeding for at least six months [odds ratio of 95%]; (4) Negative association with concurrent tobacco smoking; and (5) No association with age at menarche or menopause, and no clear association with parity [13].

Different hormonal stages for females throughout development from including puberty, pregnancy, menopause, post-menopause, and periods of exposure to exogenous hormones should be more closely monitored to evaluate for potential influence on tumor growth rates. The widest gap in sex-discrepancy for meningioma risk occurs between the mid-reproductive to perimenopausal period in women, whereby women become three times as likely as men to be diagnosed. Interestingly, there is no noted sex-difference for meningioma among children (ages 0–14). The overall incidence of meningioma increases steadily with age with the most significant increase being after age 65 [4]. This is partially attributable to the fact that males over age 60 have higher expression levels of estrogens due to conversion of testosterone, likely increasing their susceptibility to tumor changes and diagnosis. It is debated that there is a significant impact on the risk for development of meningioma for events such as the onset of puberty, menopause, first pregnancy, and with use of low dose oral contraceptives. However, a higher risk for diagnosis and tumor progression has been demonstrated in women on hormone replacement therapy (HRT), also during the post-menopausal stage, and for multiparous women [14, 15]. As this data can impact pregnancy planning and election for HRT, there is a need for increased discussion between the clinician and the patient about the risk for increased tumor aggressive behaviors and the potential for surgical or radiotherapy interventions. This clinical discussion should also potentially include a plan for closer clinical surveillance during certain life stages. Currently, there is no clear recommendation for such.

One clinical trial [NCT03015701] evaluated the use of an antiprogesterone therapy, mifepristone, in patients with meningioma, but did not demonstrate a significant difference in tumor control as compared to placebo therapy as reported in the *Journal of Clinical Oncology* in 2015 [16]. Review of the study outcomes noted that patients on mifepristone had more adverse events and shorter median overall survival as compared to placebo. In this study, the median age on the

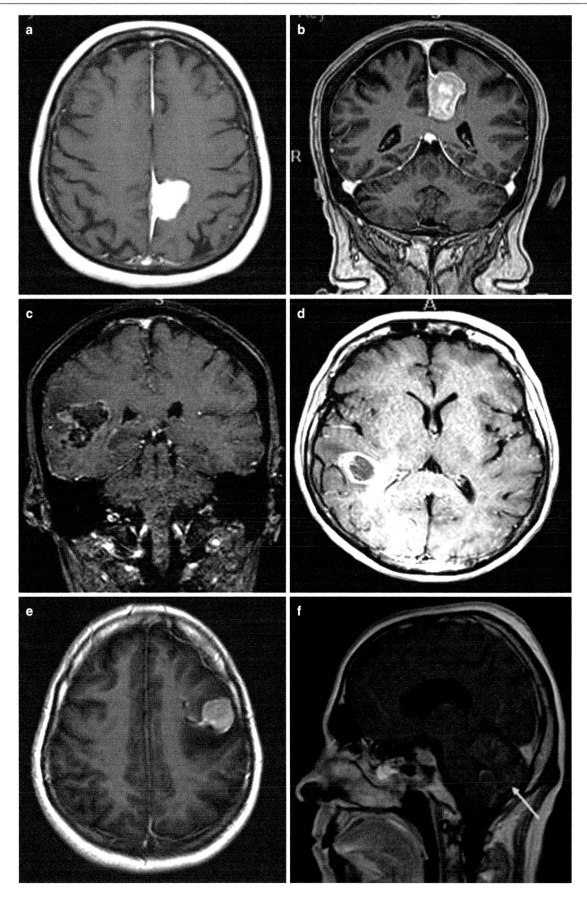

Fig. 1 (**a–f**) 63 year old female with left parasagittal meningioma axial view (**a**) coronal view (**b**) 56 year old female with right temporoparietal glioblastoma coronal view (**c**) axial view (**d**) 54 year old female left frontal breast cancer metastasis to brain parenchyma axial view (**e**) and metastasis to leptomeninges, yellow arrow demonstrates classic cerebellar region enhancement (**f**)

drug was about 60, and the majority were post-menopausal females with progressed or recurrent disease. These findings suggest that optimal meningioma control should be initiated prior to progression, and that we need to seek out better biological factors to target in this patient population. Another study, using tamoxifen, which targets estrogen, had a similar poorly efficacious response to treating meningiomas [17].

Identifying the true risk factors in women with meningioma is controversial, making it difficult to come up with a set of guidelines for women with meningiomas as it relates to pregnancy and use of hormone based supplements. There are no current clinical trials specifically studying the biological basis of meningiomas in post-pubertal women aimed to determine potential drivers of growth or tumor aggressiveness in this population, which is most commonly impacted.

Gliomas/Glioblastomas

Gliomas account for more than 30% of all brain tumors ranging from low to high grade, with glioblastoma (GBM) being the most frequent and most deadly histologic type (Fig. 1c, d). GBM is slightly more common in males as compared to females (1.6:1). However, pregnancy concurrent with even low-grade brain tumors has been found to increase risk for tumor transformation to a higher grade. This increased risk for aggressive tumor behavior has been reported most commonly in the second and third trimesters [18]. Admittedly, pregnancy concurrence with brain tumor is rare, but there might be important biological learning points to be gained through a better understanding of the reproductive immune processes that might influence driver oncogenes. Furthermore, as we work to extend the lives of brain tumor patients, we will inevitably have to address issues of fertility and high-risk pregnancy cancer treatment approaches.

Pituitary Tumors

Pituitary tumors occur primarily in females and account for about 16% of all primary brain tumors. These tumors are at highest incidence between ages 15 and 39 years of age [4]. Pituitary lesions, when pathologic, can present clinically as vision loss, headaches, or abnormal endocrine function. The most common of these, prolactinomas, are nearly 4.5 times as likely to occur in females as compared to males [4, 19]. Lesions of the anterior portion of the pituitary gland could lead to excess secretion of other hormones that cause clinical syndromes. Prolactinomas occur most commonly during the primary reproductive ages in women and can cause infertility. There exists an important window of opportunity for surgical intervention as the gold standard for treatment in symptomatic patients with early tumor detection. However, short-term medical therapy with a dopamine hormone agonists which regulates the synthesis of prolactin, is frequently used to help shrink the tumor [20]. Pregnancy planning in these patients usually prompts a discussion with their clinicians about indication for neurosurgery as pregnancy is known to accelerate the growth of these tumors [20].

Common Secondary Neuro-oncology Conditions Which Impact Women

Brain and Leptomeningeal Metastases

Breast cancer is the most common cancer in women among those ages 15–39 with an estimated 200,000 cases annually [4, 21]. Overall, 25–30% of women with breast cancer will be diagnosed with CNS metastasis (Fig. 1e) over the course of their disease [21]. Twenty-percent of all breast cancers have the aggressive tumor characteristic of being "triple negative", meaning the tumors do not express receptors for targetable markers such as estrogen, progesterone, or human epidermal growth factor receptor 2 (Her2) [21]. Triple negative breast cancers have a twofold increase in premenopausal women under age 40, and slightly increased risk for women who have had ≥3 pregnancies [22]. Nulliparous women were noted to have a trend toward a lower propensity for triple negative breast cancer [22]. Patients with triple negative breast cancer should be monitored carefully for increased propensity for late brain or leptomeningeal metastases (Fig. 1f). Breast cancer represents 50% of all solid tumor leptomeningeal metastases [23]. Other gynecological cancers have a lower risk for metastases to the brain.

Cancer Neurology and CNS Complication of Paraneoplastic Disease

Cancer neurology deals with a wide range of neurologic complications that are secondary to cancer or cancer treatment. Neurologic side-effects of cancer treatment are wide-ranging and include: (1) Radiation therapy induced nerve or muscle injury, cognitive decline, and brain tissue necrosis. (2) Intrathecal chemotherapy induced chemical meningitis, headaches, seizures, and cognitive decline due to leukoencephalopathy, (3) Oral or infused chemotherapy induced leukoencephalopathy, sensory or motor neuropathies, and thrombocytopenia – which could lead to intracranial hemorrhage. (4) Surgical removal of tumors can compromise special senses (vision, hearing, touch, etc.…), motor strength, cognition, and speech depending on the tumor location. These conditions are major concerns in the treatment of tumor conditions that impact women such as meningiomas of the brain or spine, pituitary tumors, and breast cancers [24, 25].

Neurologic symptoms can also occur secondary to direct cancer infiltration into extracranial locations, or cause stroke secondary to hypercoagulability. A common condition in breast cancer patients is brachial plexopathies. Tumor cells can infiltrate into these locations and lead to pain or motor weakness [24, 25]. Paraneoplastic encephalopathy, encephalitis, or other CNS degenerative processes have been noted in association with antibodies produced in association with breast and ovarian cancers [26].

Questions on Sex, Fertility, Partnership, and Therapies in Women's Neuro-oncology

Below are just seven of many critical questions commonly presented in the clinical setting either by patients, their family members, or by their providers. Information below is anecdotal for the most part, but offers some food for thought.

How Long Should I (or My Partner) Be Off All Chemotherapy Prior to Conception?

A quick GOOGLE search will yield answers anywhere from 6 months to 5 years! Of course, issues such as type and dose of chemotherapy, as well as gestational age at first exposure are important. An equally important question would be that of any remaining fertility after exposure to chemotherapy. Both males and females exposed to chemotherapy could experience damage to the DNA in the sperm or ova. While there is adequate literature about fetal developmental and fertility risks in women treated for cancer, the lapse in communication usually occurs at the initial clinical visit. Most often, pregnancy is discouraged in women with brain tumors, that is, if the subject is even broached in the clinical setting. When clinicians fail to have these discussions, despite excellent intentions, we risk having patients who feel robbed of their fertility.

Does Chemotherapy Get into Semen or Other Body Fluids? Are There Exposure Risks to Consider That Might Impact My Health or Fertility?

Chemotherapy can be excreted in body fluids including semen, vaginal secretions, urine, stool, vomitus, saliva, sweat, and blood for up to 7 days after last exposure. OncoLink provided a "Men's Guide to Sexuality During and After Cancer Treatment [June 20, 2017, https://www.onco-link.org/support/sexuality-fertility/sexuality/men-s-guide-to-sexuality-during-after-cancer-treatment] which covers a wide range of issues to address these concerns. Querying the internet about a woman's risk for chemotherapy in semen during oral or vaginal sex ranged from recommendations to use a barrier method, to no precautions needed due to the *low concentration* present in semen. Although, I am not sure that there are validated studies that provide a minimum toxic dose (or accumulated dose) for oral or cervical epithelial cells. I would recommend use of barrier protection, when reasonable, to minimize exposure to potential chemo-contaminated body fluids.

How Should Clinical Monitoring Be Modified During Pregnancy and in the Post-Partum Period in Patients with GBM?

A rare occurrence, until the patient is standing before you – pregnant. Dr. Yust-Katz et al. [18] published a series of pregnancy and glial brain tumors. The key conclusions drawn from this study suggest that indeed there is increased tumor aggressiveness during the late pregnancy and early post-partum period. This study recommends increased tumor surveillance of pregnant brain tumor patients. As a neuroimmunologist, I would also propose a benefit to closer evaluation of serum-based peripheral immune responses during the various trimesters. Sampling the fetal cord blood and placenta in these patients might yield a better understanding of putative immune factors without harm to the mother or child.

Glioma cells have been documented to circulate in peripheral blood – with the current knowledge about maternal and fetal cell microchimerism (exchange of cells between mother and fetus) is there an increased risk for my patient's children to develop brain cancer?

Fetal cells have been known to circulate in the maternal host since 1893 Dr. Georg Schmorl – we are only wondering 'What for?' and 'What else?' again in the twenty-first century. In 2014, scientist first reported the existence of circulating glioma cells in the peripheral blood of GBM patients [27, 28]. During pregnancy and for decades following delivery, fetal cells circulate in the mother and are thought to offer protection from injurious disease states [29]. Dr. J. Lee Nelson's Lab [30], of the Fred Hutchinson Cancer Research Center, is one of the leaders in the field of chimerism, and was first to identify the role for these exchanged of cells in maternal autoimmunity [30]. She and her colleagues offered details on both the good and the negative consequences of microchimerism – and in 2012 her lab was involved in research that demonstrated remnants of fetal cells in the maternal brain. So, if we agree that glioma cells circulate, and that there is an exchange of cells between mother and fetus during pregnancy that persist in their new host – we should consider the potential to evaluate offspring born to mothers with known prior glioma history.

Why Am I Discouraged from Using the Tumor Treating Fields (TTF) Device Shown to Be Beneficial in High Grade Gliomas During Pregnancy?

*"Do not use Optune if you are **pregnant**, you think you might be **pregnant** or are trying to get pregnant..."* This is captioned on the packaging insert inside for the NovoTTF device (Optune) by Novocure. Optune uses TTFs to deliver therapy via transducer arrays that are loaded within four adhesive patches placed on the shaved scalps of patients with high-grade gliomas. This out of the box therapy is one of the most well tolerated therapies in brain tumor – and is the first therapy with a significant survival impact in glioma patients since 2005 to be approved by the FDA [31]. As a matter-of-fact, use of Optune after standard of care surgery and chemoradiation therapy has been demonstrated to increase the overall 5-year-survival of GBM by 2.5 times that of those patients who follow standard of care alone [32]. So, why NOT use it during pregnancy – although pregnant patients have a limited few available treatment options and where pregnancy has been demonstrated to increased tumor growth? Well…it has not been tested.

I've Noticed My Patient is More Frequently Unaccompanied by Her Spouse at Out Follow-Up Visits, Should I Inquire About the Health of Their Marriage? Who is Caring for Her at Home?

Weak, she crosses the threshold of the front door after returning from her 4th week of chemoradiation therapy. Her pants are baggy with weight loss. Removing her headscarf, she reveals the surgical scar only sparsely encircled by tufts of hair – not yet targeted by the radiation. She stands over the bathroom sink to take her mid-day therapies, 'gulp'. A second's glance in the mirror before she's kneeling over the toilet only to spit them back up… again. Then, it's off to bed… again. She will lift her head for the evening meds and push through to tomorrow… again. Everything that could be said, has been, and will be… but can I do it all, over again?

In the front of *her* mind, from the bottom of *his* heart, underneath the cancer, and at the edge of what seems like an eternity, she remains the same woman working to pull strength from the corners of the earth. **To live as well as possible, for as long as possible.**

While the divorce rate among patients with serious illness is similar to that of the general population in the U.S., women with serious illnesses are more likely to be abandoned in divorce as compared to males [33]. A 2001 study completed at the University of Utah, Huntsman Cancer Institute evaluated patients with primary brain tumors, multiple sclerosis (MS), and systemic cancers who were married at diagnosis. This study evaluated 183 patients with gliomas and noted that women with gliomas were nearly ten times more likely to be abandoned than males with the same disease [33]. Women with MS and systemic cancers were found to be nearly seven and six times as likely as males with the disease to be abandoned, respectively [33]. Younger age and frontal lobe dysfunction were two other noted risk factors for divorce in brain tumor patients [33] – but we must agree that this is an alarming finding that demands attention and consideration from the first clinical visit. Interpreting these findings led to a number of speculations about how men versus women deal with the challenges of being the primary emotional, financial, and physical caregiver in a relationship. As clinicians, I think we worry about crossing certain boundaries – understanding, however, that quality of life issues in caring for our patients does extend to the psychosocial aspects of disease. Evaluating the relationship dynamics early and keeping all members of the care team in discussion and with maximal support is very important.

Conclusions

Women are more commonly diagnosed with brain and other CNS tumors, and are disproportionately affected by cancer neurology issues overall. In 1986 the National Institutes of Health (NIH) established a policy aimed to include women in clinical research. This policy has evolved over the years to be inclusive of women and minorities as subjects in clinical research and to offer guidance on reporting practices. It was not until 2014 (policy effective as of 2016) that the NIH required the consideration of sex as a relevant biological variable requiring consideration in both human and animal studies. Women's issues in neuro-oncology are covered under these research guidelines, but there remains a gap in the development of the appropriate research questions in this population. This is especially true as it pertains to issues of fertility, pregnancy, psychosocial/survivorship support, and application of therapies for women at various life phases in neuro-oncology. Promoting these issues among the leadership, organizing topic-workgroups, sections, and leading research or educational courses at the national and international subspecialty meetings such as the American Academy of Neurology (AAN), Society for Neuro-Oncology (SNO), American Society of Clinical Oncology (ASCO), American Association for Cancer Research (AACR), and other related organizations is important to furthering our understanding of the Neuro-Oncology of Women. Increased awareness of the issues represented in this book will help with the development of guidelines that improve clinical practice, increase collaborative research around reproductive and oncological immunology, and advance therapeutic design in Women's Neurology as a whole.

References

1. Murrell DH, Foster PJ. Brain metastasis: basic biology, clinical management, and insight from experimental model systems. In: Introduction to cancer metastasis. Aamir Ahmad. Elsevier UK. 2017. p. 317–333.
2. Braganza MZ, Kitahara CM, Berrington de Gonzalez A, Inskip PD, Johnson KJ, Rajaraman P. Ionizing radiation and the risk of brain and central nervous system tumors: a systematic review. Neuro-Oncology. 2012;14(11):1316–24.
3. Turner MC. Epidemiology: allergy history, IgE, and cancer. Cancer Immunol Immunother. 2012;61:1493–510.
4. Ostrom QT, Gittleman H, Xu J, Kromer C, Wolinsky Y, Kruchko C, et al. CBTRUS statistical report: primary brain and other central nervous system tumors diagnosed in the united states in 2009–2013. Neuro-Oncology. 2016;18(5):1–75.
5. Schlehofer B, Blettner M, Wahrendorf J. Association between brain tumors and menopausal status. J Natl Cancer Inst. 1992;84(17):1346–9.
6. Pavlidis NA. Coexistence of pregnancy and malignancy. Oncologist. 2002;7(4):279–87.
7. Simon RH. Brain tumors in pregnancy. Semin Neurol. 1988;8(3):214–21.
8. Ray JG, Vermeulen MJ, Bharatha A, Montanera WJ, Park AL. Association between MRI exposure during pregnancy and fetal and childhood outcomes. JAMA. 2016;316(9):952–61.
9. Markwalder TM, Zara DT, Goldhirsch A, Markwalder RV. Estrogen and progesterone receptors in meningiomas in relation to clinical and pathologic features. Surg Neurol. 1983;20:42–7.
10. Black PM. Meningiomas. Neurosurgery. 1993;32:643–57.
11. Chamberlain MC, Barnholtz JS. Medical treatment of recurrent meningiomas. Exp Rev Neurothera. 2014;11(10):1425–32.
12. Carroll RS, Zhang J, Dashner K, Sar M, Wilson EM, Black PM. Androgen receptor expression in meningiomas. J Neurosurg. 1995;82:453–60.
13. Claus EB, Calvocoressi L, Bondy ML, Wrensch M, Wiemels JL, Schildkraut JM. Exogenous hormone use, reproductive factors, and risk of intracranial meningioma in females. J Neurosurg. 2013;118(3):649–56.
14. Blitshteyn S, Cook JE, Jaeckle KA. Is there an association between meningioma and hormone replacement therapy? J Clin Oncol. 2008;26(2):279–82.
15. Qi Z, Shao C, Huang Y, Huo G, Zhou Y, Wang Z. Reproductive and exogenous hormone factors in relation to risk of meningioma in women: a meta-analysis. PLoS One. 2013;8(12):e83261.
16. Ji Y, Rankin C, Grunberg S, Sherrod AE, Ahmadi J, Townsend JJ, et al. Double-blind phase III randomized trial of the antiprogestin agent mifepristone in the treatment of unresectable meningioma: SWOG S9005. J Clin Oncol. 2015;33(34):4093–8.
17. Rubinstein AB, Loren D, Geier A, Reichenthal E, Gadoth N. Hormone receptors in initially excised versus recurrent intracranial meningiomas. J Neurosurg. 1994;81:184–7.
18. Yust-Katz S, de Groot JF, Liu D, Wu J, Yuan Y, Anderson MD, et al. Pregnancy and glial brain tumors. Neuro-Oncology. 2014;16(9):1289–94.
19. Thapar K, Laws ER. Pituitary tumors. In: Kaye AH, Laws ER, editors. Brain tumors. New York: Churchill Livingstone; 1995. p. 759–76.
20. Randall RV, Laws ER, Abboud CF, Ebersold MJ, Kao PC, Scheithauer BW. Transphenoidal microsurgical treatment of prolactin-producing pituitary adenomas. Results in 100 patients. Mayo Clin Proc. 1983;58:108–21.
21. Swain SM. Triple-negative breast cancer: metastatic risk and role of platinum agents. Paper presented at: 44th Annual Meeting of the American Society of Clinical Oncology; May 30–June 3, 2008; Chicago.
22. Glick RP, Penny D, Hart A. The pre-operative and post-operative management of the brain tumor patient. In: Morantz RA, Walsh JW, editors. Brain tumors. New York: Marcel Dekker; 1994. p. 345–66.
23. Phipps AI, Chlebowski RT, Prentice R, McTiernan A, Wactawski-Wende J, Kuller LH, et al. Reproductive history and oral contraceptive use in relation to risk of triple-negative breast cancer. J Natl Cancer Inst. 2011;103(6):470.
24. Forsyth PJ, Cascino TL. Neurological complications of chemotherapy. In: Wiley RG, editor. Neurological complications of cancer. New York: Marcel Dekker; 1995. p. 241–66.
25. Posner JB. Neurologic complications of cancer. Philadelphia: F. A. Davis Company; 1995.
26. Graus F, Vega F, Delattre JY, Bonaventura I, Rene R, Arbaiza D, et al. Plasmapharesis and antineoplastic treatment in central nervous system paraneoplastic syndromes with antineuronal autoantibodies. Neurology. 1992;42:536–40.
27. OncLink. Men's guide to sexuality during & after cancer treatment [Internet]. Philadelphia: The Abramson Cancer Center of the University of Pennsylvania. [updated 2017 June 20]. Available from: https://www.oncolink.org/support/sexuality-fertility/sexuality/men-s-guide-to-sexuality-during-after-cancer-treatment
28. Müller C, Holtschmidt J, Auer M, Heitzer E, Lamszus K, Schulte A, et al. Hematogenous dissemination of glioblastoma multiforme. Sci Transl Med. 2014;6(247):247.
29. Gao F, Cui Y, Jiang H, Dali S, Wang Y, Jiang Z, et al. Circulating tumor cell is a common property of brain glioma and promotes the monitoring system. Oncotarget. 2016;7(44):71330–40.
30. Khosrotehrani K, Johnson KL, Cha DH, Salomon RN, Bianchi DW. Transfer of fetal cells with multilineage potential to maternal tissue. JAMA. 2004;292(1):75–80.
31. Stupp R, Taillibert S, Kanner AA, Kesari S, Steinberg DM, Toms SA, et al. Maintenance therapy with tumor-treating fields plus temozolomide vs temozolomide alone for glioblastoma: a randomized clinical trial. JAMA. 2015;314(23):2535–43.
32. Chan WN, Gurnot C, Montine TJ, Sonnen JA, Guthrie KA, Nelson JL. Male microchimerism in the human female brain. PLoS One. 2012;7(9):e45592.
33. Carlson RH. Study: women with brain tumors have 10 times rate of divorce as men with brain tumors. Oncol Times. 2001;23(8):63.

Substance Use Disorders in Women

Whitney Peters, Connie Guille, and Leena Mittal

Introduction

The pathogenesis of substance use disorders is multifactorial and complex and is thought to involve the interplay of various genetic and environmental factors, including gender. This chapter will review the ways in which sex and gender influence the clinical manifestations, course and treatment of substance use disorders. However to provide a framework for discussion about specific substances, an overview of Substance Use Disorders in women is necessary.

Part I: Overview of Substance Use Disorders in Women

Epidemiology

In adults, Substance Use Disorders (SUD) are more prevalent in males than females, though rates are equal in adolescents [1]. The difference in adults is narrowing over time owing in part to the increased prevalence in adolescents.

Disease Course and Pathogenesis [2]

Studies on substances including alcohol, cannabis and opioids have shown that women tend to have a pattern of more rapid disease progression from the time of first substance use

W. Peters
Department of Psychiatry, Beth Israel Deaconess Medical Center, Boston, MA, USA

C. Guille
Medical University of South Carolina, Institute of Psychiatry, Charleston, SC, USA
e-mail: guille@musc.edu

L. Mittal (✉)
Department of Psychiatry, Brigham and Women's Hospital, Boston, MA, USA
e-mail: lmittal@bwh.harvard.edu

to the time of diagnosis of substance use disorder and the time of first treatment, a phenomenon referred to as telescoping [3]. In other words, although the overall incidence and prevalence of substance use disorders is lower in women, women are prone to develop more severe substance use disorders more quickly compared to men. Table 1 contains a summary of the diagnostic criteria for substance use disorder.

Interpersonal and relationship factors can impact the course of SUD for women as well. Interpersonal conflict with a partner can increase the risk of consuming alcohol for women more than for men, and having a partner who abuses or relapses with alcohol or drugs is more strongly related to relapse for women than for men [4]. Additionally, residing with and retaining custody of children during treatment can have a positive impact on treatment retention and duration of recovery for women [5].

Biological differences between women and men impact the course and outcomes of SUDs. Despite often using relatively smaller quantities of substances for a shorter amount of time than their male counterparts, women are just as much at risk of developing medical consequences of substance use disorders and in some instances are vulnerable to increased and additional risks related to biological sex differences. For example, because women have larger stores of body fat, they

Table 1 Summary of the diagnostic criteria for substance use disorder

Problematic substance use leading impairment or distress
Requires two of the following over 12 months:
Hazardous use
Social or interpersonal problems related to use
Neglect of major roles due to use
Withdrawal for those substances that have a withdrawal syndrome
Tolerance
Using larger amounts or for longer duration
Making repeated attempts to quit or control use
Spending more time using
Physical or mental health problems due to use
Giving up activities in order to use
Cravings

metabolize lipid soluble medications, such as benzodiaze-pines more slowly, which may put them at increased risk of side effects such as falls, especially because the proportion of fat to water (and volume of distribution) increases with age. Similarly, slower rates of gastric absorption of alcohol are related to more rapid progression of liver disease in women with alcohol use disorders [6]. There is a higher mortality associated with SUD for women as compared to men such that women with SUD have a 5× greater mortality risk than the general population while men with SUD have a 3× greater mortality risk [7].

Hormonal fluctuations across the reproductive life cycle spanning menstruation, pregnancy, and menopause have implications related to all aspects of substance use disorders in women, including onset of substance use, disease course and treatment. As an example, women find cocaine more rewarding during the follicular compared to the luteal phase of the menstrual cycle [8]. Alternatively, substance abuse may influence women's hormonal milieu, impacting fertility and the menstrual cycle. For example, smoking cigarettes and use of opioids are associated with menstrual irregularity and early menopause [6].

In pregnancy and lactation, ongoing substance use and treatments for substance use carry risks to both mother and fetus, and these risks need to be weighed when considering the appropriate treatment plan. However, pregnancy also offers a unique treatment opportunity, often serving as a strong motivator for change. Data from epidemiologic survey show that rates of past month use for all substances decreases among pregnant women as compared to reproductive aged women who are not pregnant. Women with substance use disorders often present later to prenatal care, thus narrowing the window of time in which to assess and engage them in discussions about treatment. Amongst women entering substance abuse treatment, pregnant women are most likely to identify marijuana as their primary problem substance, whereas non-pregnant women most commonly identify alcohol as their primary problem [9]. Concerns regarding parenting and custody, staff perceptions and stigma, modifications of pain and labor management further add to the complexity of the needs of this population.

Psychiatric Comorbidity

In the general population, mood disorders, anxiety disorders, PTSD, and eating disorders are more prevalent in women than men. Amongst women with SUD, the relative prevalence of these psychiatric comorbidities is even higher (compared to women without SUD and to men). Also psychiatric comorbidities are associated with more severe substance use and higher rates of relapse [10–12].

In a study of women with comorbid non SUD psychiatric conditions and SUD, women with comorbid Postraumatic

Table 2 Summary of pharmacologic treatments available for substance use disorders

Alcohol use disorder
Disulfiram, naltrexone, acamprosate
Opioid use disorder
Methadone, buprenorphine, naltrexone (PO and depot IM)
Nicotine use disorder
Nicotine Replacement Therapy (NRT) consisting of lozenges, gum, patch, inhaler, nasal spray
Bupropion, varenicline

Stress Disorder and SUD have more suicidality aggression and psychosocial impairment [13].

Treatment Considerations

Men comprise the majority of patients in SUD treatment, and many programs are not designed to consider the unique needs of women including trauma-informed care, pregnancy specific approaches, and childcare. Data about gender-specific treatments, such as single sex treatment are mixed. However evidence is starting to accumulate that women are more likely to respond to treatment interventions specifically designed to target the unique challenges they might face such as prenatal care, child care, trauma informed care, and need for integrated mental health services [5] (Table 2).

Part II: Specific Substances

Nicotine/Tobacco

Epidemiology and Course

In 2016, 25.4% of Americans over the age of 18 reported current (past month) tobacco use, with higher rates of reported tobacco use in men than women (31.7% vs. 19.5%) [1]. On average women smoke fewer cigarettes per day, tend to use cigarettes with lower nicotine content, and do not inhale as deeply as men [14].

Like other substance use disorders, the development of tobacco use disorder is multifactorial and may be driven by different factors in men and women. Studies have shown that cigarette nicotine dose is more reinforcing and more likely to influence subjective reports of enjoyment in men, whereas women are less likely to be influenced by nicotine dose [15] and more likely to use tobacco in an attempt to regulate negative emotions or with the expectation to manage weight [16].

Treatment Considerations

In a qualitative review of studies, Smith et al. found that women are less likely to be able to quit smoking and sustain abstinence than men [17]. There are also data suggesting that women tend to be driven to smoke more by non-nicotine related factors, such as the smell of the smoke or people they see when smoking or motivation related to weight as compared to men. Additionally there are data that suggest that nicotine replacement therapy is more effective for men than women [15, 18]. Varenicline and bupropion are equally effective between sexes, though varenicline was more effective than nicotine replacement in women [18].

Although the exact mechanisms remain unclear, one hypothesis is that women are less responsive to nicotine replacement therapy than men because they tend to use tobacco to alleviate negative emotions while men use tobacco to experience subjective reward. In earlier studies, women were found to worry twice as much about weight [19] and cite this as a common reason for relapse [20].

Several studies suggest that hormonal factors mediate women's response to nicotine and likelihood for quitting, though findings are conflicting. Perkins and colleagues found that tobacco withdrawal symptoms were worse when women quit during the luteal phase of their menstrual cycle [21]. However, Franklin et al. noted that smoking abstinence was best when quit dates were set during the follicular phase of the menstrual cycle [22]. In another study, quitting outcomes were more favorable during the luteal phase than the follicular phase [23].

Pregnancy

In 2016, rates of past month cigarette use amongst women of childbearing age (15–44 years old) were significantly higher in non-pregnant compared to pregnant women (19.9% vs. 10.0%) [1]. Smoking in pregnancy has been associated with spontaneous abortion, intrauterine growth retardation, premature rupture of membranes, low birth weight, perinatal mortality and placental abruption. Smoking is also associated with poor outcomes for children exposed in utero including sudden infant death syndrome (SIDS), asthma, and obesity [24].

According to United States Preventive Services Task Force recommendations, effective and evidence-based behavioral interventions in pregnant women who smoke include counseling, feedback, health education, incentives, and social support. Compared with usual care or controls, behavioral interventions can increase rates of smoking abstinence from approximately 11% to 15% in pregnant women [25].

In a secondary analysis of a larger metaanalysis, nicotine replacement therapy was associated with a small improvement in abstinence of smoking at the time of delivery. However, the positive effect on smoking abstinence did not remain significant in the postpartum period [26]. More than half of women who quit smoking during pregnancy will resume within 4 months postpartum [27].

Alcohol

Epidemiology and Course

Data from the 2016 National Survey on Drug Use and Health show that adult men of all ages drink more than women on all measures of alcohol use, including past month use, binge drinking (>5 drinks at least 1× in past month), and heavy alcohol use (binge drinking at least 5× in past month). The gender gap becomes more pronounced over time. Whereas male and female youths aged 12–17 report past month alcohol use at similar rates (11.2% male vs. 11.9% female), adult men are more likely to be current users compared to women aged 18–25 (62.3% vs. 56.9%) and older than 26 (62.2% vs. 50.1%). Differences in rates of binge drinking also become more pronounced over time. Amongst adults aged 18–25, 44.4% of males vs. 33.2% of females binge drink, and amongst adults aged 26 and older men are nearly twice as likely to report binge drinking (30.7% vs. 14.7%) [1].

Biologically, women may be predisposed to more rapid progression of alcohol use disorder, including the development of medical sequelae, related to sex differences in body size, water content and alcohol metabolism. The NIAAA defines at-risk drinking for women as more than seven standard drinks per week or more than three standard drinks in a drinking day. (One standard equals 12 oz of beer, 5 oz of wine, and 1.5 oz of 80-proof liquor.) At-risk drinking for men is defined as more than 14 standard drinks per week or more than four standard drinks in a day, reflecting sex differences in body size, water content, and alcohol metabolism [28].

Treatment

Patients with risk for physiologic dependence to alcohol may require medication assisted management of withdrawal symptoms (sometimes referred to colloquially as detox) as well as pharmacologic treatment to decrease use such as disulfiram, naltrexone or acamprosate. Additionally psychosocial treatments are an important component of treatment and can include individual therapy, group therapy and mutual/peer help as in Alcoholics Anonymous. Results from Project MATCH show that women engage in AA more frequently and for longer periods of time than men and some studies suggest that the benefit of mutual help groups does not differ by gender [29].

Pregnancy

Epidemiologic survey data show rates of alcohol use were lower amongst pregnant compared to non-pregnant women aged 15–44, including past month alcohol use (8.3% vs. 53.5%) binge drinking (4.3% vs. 28.6%) and heavy alcohol use (0.9% vs. 5.8%) [1].

A number of organizations, including the American College of Obstetrics and Gynecology (ACOG), The American Academy of Pediatrics (AAP) and the Centers for

Disease Control (CDC) all recommend that women abstain from alcohol during pregnancy [30–32].

Alcohol consumed during pregnancy is rapidly absorbed into fetal blood, resulting in alcohol toxicity and known teratogenicity. Alcohol use during pregnancy is associated with miscarriage and stillbirth, preterm delivery, fetal alcohol spectrum disorders and increased risk for Sudden Infant Death Syndrome (SIDS) [33] May and colleagues describe fetal alcohol spectrum disorders, with associated physical, cognitive, behavioral and emotional features, as affecting between 1% and 5% of births in US communities, making it a prevalent and important outcome of maternal alcohol use as it is a cause of developmental delay and increased risk for mental health and behavioral consequences for affected children [34].

All pregnant and preconception women should be advised that there is no safe amount of alcohol defined in pregnancy. Alcohol use should be assessed in all women during preconception and prenatal visits. The T-ACE and the TWEAK are validated tools for screening for alcohol use disorders in this population [35, 36].

For patients who are physiologically dependent on alcohol, there is a risk for withdrawal that would need to be managed medically to safely achieve abstinence. There is limited data available regarding presentation, assessment and management of alcohol withdrawal in pregnancy. Bhat and colleagues conclude that the risks of alcohol withdrawal, which include autonomic instability and seizures, warrant treatment in the pregnant woman, and they recommend treatment of withdrawal with benzodiazepines (chlordiazepoxide and lorazepam) and monitoring of symptoms with the CIWA-Ar – the revised Clinical Institute withdrawal scale for alcohol [37]. Outside of the treatment for alcohol withdrawal, there is little evidence to support the safety of maintenance medications to decrease the use of alcohol in alcohol use disorders [38].

In lactation, it is important for women to be counseled that alcohol can pass into breastmilk rapidly with more transferring at the time of peak serum level. Alcohol can impact lactogenesis and is associated with alterations in infant sleep-wake cycle [39].

Cannabis

Epidemiology and Course

Marijuana is the most commonly used drug in the United States with 13.9% of the general population age 12 or older reporting use in the past 1 year [1]. The proportion of males meeting criteria for Cannabis Use disorder in the past 12 months is 3.5% as compared to 1.7% in females [40]. Additionally, a growing number of women report cannabis use for medical purposes, which may narrow the gender gap over time [41, 42]. Amongst subjects seeking treatment for cannabis use withdrawal severity is greater in women relative to men despite similar patterns and levels of cannabis use, which may make it more difficult for women to quit [43–45]. The legalization of medical marijuana has increased access to marijuana and to more potent strains of marijuana with higher concentrations of THC [46, 47]. Moreover, young adults tend to view marijuana as less harmful than other illicit drugs [48]. Additionally, the cannabis products available now are more potent and available in more formulations and modes of administration than available when much of the early literature on safety and effect took place.

There is evidence that women may be especially sensitive to the psychoactive and adverse effects of cannabis related to underlying neurobiological mechanisms. For example, healthy non-cannabis using women have been found to have greater cannabinoid receptor availability compared to men [49, 50]. Using positron emission tomography (PET), another study found that cannabis using women exhibited decreased brain glucose metabolism in response to both placebo and methylphenidate administration compared to healthy controls, a finding not observed in men [51]. Hormonally, evidence that endocannabinoid tone fluctuates across the menstrual cycle suggests the behavioral effects of cannabis may be related to variations in gonadal hormones [52].

Treatment

Cannabis Use disorder is primarily treated with behavioral interventions such as Cognitive Behavioral Therapy, Motivational Interviewing and Contingency Management, though results are modest. There is not a well defined pharmacologic treatment approach for cannabis use disorder [53].

Pregnancy

Pregnant women are less likely to report cannabis use in the past month compared to women who are not pregnant (3.9% vs. 7.6%) [54]. However, past-month cannabis use has increased amongst pregnant women overall (from 2.4% in 2002 to 3.9% in 2014) [55]. Tetrahydrocannabinol (THC), the main psychoactive component in cannabis, crosses the placenta readily and is thought to play a major role in fetal neurodevelopment [56, 57]. Although there is not yet enough evidence to fully understand the effects cannabis has on the developing fetus in pregnancy, rising rates of prenatal cannabis use, especially in the context of legalization of recreational and medical use, are a significant cause for concern given findings that such use may adversely effect perinatal outcomes and neurodevelopment.

In the neonate, prenatal cannabis use has been associated with various negative outcomes although it should be noted that studies have yielded mixed results and are often difficult to interpret given the presence of confounding variables (e.g. comorbid tobacco use). Results have been largely mixed regarding prenatal cannabis exposure and the risk of preterm birth, stillbirth, and low birth weight thus there is not enough evidence to draw firm conclusions [46, 57–59]. Other risks include higher rates of neonatal intensive care unit admissions and transient effects in infants at 24–72 h, such as exaggerated startle reflex, tremors, increased irritability, and poor sleep [59–61]. In children, longitudinal studies evaluating the effects of prenatal cannabis exposure over time have found patterns of impaired executive functioning, including deficits in attention, impulsivity and visuospatial integration [60, 62]. In addition to its risks when used prenatally, cannabis also carries significant risks in the postpartum period. For one, cannabis may impact a caregiver's ability to provide safe care to a child. It has also been associated with increased rates of sudden infant death syndrome (SIDS) [63]. Finally, THC is transmitted in breastmilk and has been associated with negative neurodevelopmental effects, such as lethargy, slowed motor development, and poor feeding at 1 year when used during lactation [64]. In chronic users, THC concentrations in breastmilk are eight times those of maternal serum concentration [65].

The American College of Obstetricians and Gynecologists advises against marijuana use during preconception, pregnancy, and lactation, and obstetricians are discouraged from prescribing medical marijuana [66]. Given, the prevalence of marijuana use and the lack of a clear consensus regarding its safety, it is important to educate women of reproductive age and their partners about the potential risks of marijuana use during the perinatal period and to screen for and treat cannabis use disorders effectively in this population [66].

Opioids

Epidemiology and Course

Opioid use disorder is increasing at alarming rates in the United States and the prevalence in women is substantial. While the number of opioid-dependent men in the US remains larger than the number of opioid-dependent women, there are some disturbing trends. Between 1999 and 2016, overdose deaths from prescription pain drugs increased 596% [or sevenfold] in women compared to an increase of 312% [or fourfold] in men [67]. Although nonmedical use of prescription opioids among women has generally been decreasing since 2010 heroin use among women has been increasing faster among women than men. Between 2002 and 2013, heroin use among women increased 100% compared to an increase of 50% among men [68–70]. Disturbingly, there has been an enormous increase in the rates of synthetic opioid-related deaths; with an 850% increase in deaths for women between 1999 and 2015 [67].

Approximately 30–40% of women of reproductive age were prescribed at least one opioid medication per year from 2008 to 2012 [71]. There is some evidence to suggest that women are more sensitive to pain and more likely to have a chronic pain condition, in comparison to men, which may contribute to the high rates of opioid prescriptions among women of reproductive age [72, 73]. Further, women are more likely to report misuse of prescription opioid medications to self-treat pain or anxiety symptoms and may suggest that untreated pain conditions or anxiety disorders are contributing to the increased use of opioids among women [74]. Women who use heroin, in comparison to men who use heroin, tend to be younger, are more likely to use smaller amount of heroin for a shorter period of time, are less likely to inject drugs and drug use is more likely to be influenced by drug-using sexual partners [75–78].

As previously mentioned, there are biological and psychosocial differences between men and women that appear to influence the prevalence, presentation, comorbidity and treatment of SUDs such as telescoping. In support of this in Opioid Use Disorders, an analysis of data from a multisite clinical trial demonstrated that women progressed to opioid dependence more quickly and experienced more craving as compared to men [79]. Women with opioid use disorders are also more likely to have comorbid depression and anxiety disorders and are more likely to attribute use and relapse to negative emotional states and interpersonal conflict [79, 80]. In particular, Back and colleagues found psychological and emotional distress identified as risk factors for hazardous prescription opioid use among women, but not men [79].

Treatment Considerations

The standard of care for the treatment of Opioid Use Disorder is pharmacological treatment including Methadone, Buprenorphine or Naltrexone combined with individual counseling including relapse prevention therapy. There is limited data evaluating gender differences in response to pharmacological treatments for Opioid Use Disorders. In one randomized, controlled trial evaluating gender differences in treatment response to Levomethadyl Acetate (LAAM) (75–115 mg), methadone (60–100 mg) or buprenorphine (16–32 mg) in flexible dosing schedules, overall no significant gender disparities in relapse to substance use were identified [81]. This study did find however that women receiving buprenorphine had significantly fewer illicit-opioid positive urine drug screens compared men also receiving buprenorphine. In addition, women receiving buprenorphine had significantly fewer illicit-opioid positive urine drug screens compared to women receiving methadone. These findings are consistent with another study finding less illicit drug use among women receiving buprenorphine in comparison to men receiving buprenorphine [82]. One potential explanation for this gender difference may be due to the unique pharmacology of buprenorphine (a partial mu-agonist/kappa-antagonist) combined with basic pharmacodynamic sex differences. For example, women of reproductive age have higher mu and kappa opioid receptor concentrations and differences in signal transduction that would lend to a greater sensitivity to opioid pharmacotherapy, compared to men [83–85]. Given that levels of estradiol and progesterone influence binding of endogenous opioids, further investigation into factors such as the phase of the menstrual cycle and age (i.e. menopause) may be important in examining sex and gender differences in response to treatment of Opioid Use Disorders [86].

Prior work has consistently demonstrated important demographic and psychiatric gender differences among women seeking treatment for opioid use disorder in comparison to men. In particular, prior work demonstrates that women entering treatment for Opioid Use Disorders are significantly more likely to be unemployed, have a shorter duration of opioid addiction before starting treatment [i.e., telescoping] and have more psychiatric and family problems compared to males with Opioid Use Disorder entering treatment [82, 87, 88]. Over half of women with Opioid Use Disorder will have a major psychiatric disorder such as mood disorders. Further past and present trauma including sexual abuse are commonly seen. Gender-specific treatment programs are greatly needed to address issues that are more common among women entering substance abuse treatment and often complicate recovering including the need for trauma informed care and treatment, employment and work toward independent financial security, family planning, social services, childcare and treatment of psychiatric comorbidities.

Pregnancy

The use of opioids during pregnancy has grown rapidly in the past decade. In the United States, prescription opioids are dispensed by pharmacies to 14–21% of all pregnant women [89, 90]. Approximately 3–5% of pregnant women are dispensed prescription opioids at least twice during pregnancy, suggesting a long-term pattern of use which has increased fourfold over the past decade [89]. In addition, opioid dependence in pregnant women increased from 1.2 per 1000 deliveries in 2000 to 5.6 per 1000 deliveries in 2009 [91].

There are substantial maternal, fetal and newborn risks associated with perinatal OUD. In addition to risk of unintentional overdose and death as seen in the general population, opioid abuse or dependence during pregnancy is associated with considerable maternal, obstetric, fetal and newborn morbidity and mortality [92]. OUD is associated with a 4.6-fold increased risk for maternal death at delivery as well as an increased risk for intrauterine growth restriction, placental abruption, prematurity, blood transfusion, stillbirth, cesarean section, and preeclampsia or eclampsia [93]. A well-known consequence of opioid use in pregnancy is Newborn Opioid Withdrawal Syndrome (NOWS), formally known as Neonatal Abstinence Syndrome (NAS), with 60% of newborns born to pregnant women with OUDs exhibiting withdrawal following delivery [91]. Over the past decade the incidence of NOWS in the United States has increased approximately 400%, from 1.2 per 1000 hospital births in 2000 to 5.8 per 1000 hospital births in 2012 [91, 94].

The standard of care for pregnant women with Opioid Use Disorder is pharmacotherapy with either methadone or buprenorphine, as opposed to medication withdrawal [95]. These recommendations are largely based on several studies demonstrating that pregnant women using opioids are at high risk for relapse if they undergo medication-assisted withdrawal [96–100]. Although there are obstetric and newborn risks associated with opioid agonist therapy, opioid use, particularly intravenous drug use or illicit opioid use places women at risk for infectious disease, violence, legal consequences, incarceration and poor obstetric outcomes [94, 101]. As such, experts conclude that the risk of relapse outweighs the risk of opioid agonist therapy and treatment with agonist therapy is the standard of care for women with Opioid Use Disorder as part of an overall treatment plan including prenatal care, individual counseling with relapse prevention therapy and social services [94].

Cocaine and Stimulants

Epidemiology and Course

In 2016, the rate of past month cocaine use in people over the age of twelve was greater in men (1.0%) compared to women (0.4%) [1]. Though some studies suggest telescoping effects amongst women using cocaine, including shorter time from first use to abuse and fewer years of pretreatment use, others do not [3, 102–104].

Men are more likely than women to abuse methamphetamine than women in general; however recent statistical analyses suggest that the gender gap is narrowing [105]. In an analysis of over 300,000 young adults aged 18–24 years old admitted for substance abuse treatment in 2011, women were more likely to identify methamphetamine as their primary substance of abuse (8.9%) compared to men (3.7%) [106]. Studies also show that women tend to start using methamphetamine at an earlier age, are more dependent compared to their male counterparts, and are less likely to start using a different substance if they lack access to methamphetamine [104, 107–110].

Gender differences in patterns of cocaine and stimulant use are driven by variable motivators for use. Women are significantly more likely to report that they use methamphetamine for weight loss, increased energy or to deal with emotional problems whereas men are significantly more likely to be motivated by curiosity [104, 111]. Although not statistically significant, men are also more likely to cite ability to work more and better sex as motivators for amphetamine use [104].

Evidence suggests that women may be more susceptible to the rewarding effects of cocaine and psychostimulants depending on their hormonal mileu and menstrual cycle status [112–115]. For example, one study found that women felt a greater subjective high after smoking cocaine during the follicular phase of their menstrual cycle, compared to the luteal phase [8]. Another study found that progesterone administration decreased the subjective reward of smoked cocaine during the follicular phase in women but not in men [113]. Similarly, in another study, women given oral d-amphetamine reported feeling more energetic and euphoric during the follicular compared to the luteal phase of their menstrual cycles, and higher levels of estrogen in the follicular phase were correlated with greater feelings of energy and euphoria in response to d-amphetamine [114]. Taken together these findings suggest that estrogen may enhance the rewarding effects of cocaine and amphetamine whereas progesterone may inhibit them.

Studies have found a number of other physiologic differences in how women respond to cocaine and amphetamine in addition to the hormonally driven differences summarized above. Women may be especially vulnerable to the effects of cocaine on the heart and vasculature though studies have been mixed; whereas men abusing cocaine demonstrate more severely disrupted patterns of blood flow to orbitofrontal neural circuitry compared to women [116, 117]. Compared to men, female methamphetamine users are more likely to report skin problems and have dental complications, including tooth loss and caries [104, 118]. Among users who inject methamphetamine intravenously, women are more likely to develop skin and soft tissue infections than men [119, 120].

Treatment

At present, psychotherapeutic interventions, including cognitive behavioral therapy and contingency management are the mainstays of treating cocaine use disorders as no pharmacologic agent has been shown to be effective or approved for treatment. Gender-specific treatment options for women in general remain understudied, making it difficult to draw firm conclusions from the literature; however at least two recent studies have evaluated the effectiveness of treatments for cocaine use disorders specifically in women. One study found that female cocaine users in a therapeutic community had improved retention when they were able to live at the program with their children, as compared to those whose children stayed with another adult away from the treatment program [121]. Another study provides evidence that contingency management is an effective strategy in promoting abstinence amongst pregnant and postpartum women using cocaine [122].

In addition, women tend to be more receptive than men to methamphetamine treatment [104, 107, 110]. In general, females appear to be more receptive and responsive to treatment for methamphetamine abuse, compared to males. Females, compared to males, are more likely to perceive a need for treatment (18.7% vs 14.6%, respectively) and to acknowledge dependence (13.9% vs 7.8%) on methamphetamine [109]. Importantly, women who use methamphetamine also have high rates of co-occurring depression and therefore treatment of comorbid psychiatric illness should be included as part of patients treatment plan [107, 108, 110].

Pregnancy

It is difficult to accurately assess the prevalence of cocaine use disorders in pregnancy given variable methods of reporting, and estimated rates range anywhere from 1% to 30% [123, 124]. As an example, one study found that only 11% of pregnant women endorsed any substance use on self-report but that on meconium and urine toxicology screen 31% of these women tested positive for cocaine [125].

Maternal use of cocaine in pregnancy is associated with a variety of neonatal and obstetric risks, thought to occur secondary to the vasoconstrictive properties of cocaine. Complications include preterm birth, low birth weight, intrauterine growth restriction, placental abruption, premature rupture of membranes, maternal migraines and seizures [122]. Results from studies examining the long term neurodevelopmental effects of prenatal cocaine exposure have been mixed, with some studies reporting minimal to no effect and others reporting altered stress responses, delayed language and motor development, and impaired mother-child bonding [126–133].

Part III: Summary

Substance Use Disorders in women have distinct epidemiology, natural history and presentation. SUD are increasingly prevalent in younger women and the phenomenon of telescoping describes that while onset of substance use may be later for women, the escalation of severity and decline in function are more rapid. These differences can have implications on management and treatment. Pregnancy is a particularly important life stage for which assessment and management can differ.

References

Introduction References

1. Center for Behavioral Health Statistics and Quality. 2016 national survey on drug use and health: detailed tables. Rockville: Substance Abuse and Mental Health Services Administration; 2017.

2. Hasin DS, O'Brien CP, Auriacombe M, Borges G, Bucholz K, Budney A, Compton WM, Crowley T, Ling W, Petry NM, Schuckit M. DSM-5 criteria for substance use disorders: recommendations and rationale. Am J Psychiatr. 2013;170(8):834–51.

3. Hernandez-Avila CA, Rounsaville BJ, Kranzler HR. Opioid-, cannabis-and alcohol-dependent women show more rapid progression to substance abuse treatment. Drug Alcohol Depend. 2004;74(3):265–72.

4. Grella CE, Scott CK, Foss MA, Joshi V, Hser YI. Gender differences in drug treatment outcomes among participants in the Chicago target cities study. Eval Program Plann. 2003;26(3):297–310.

5. Greenfield SF, Back SE, Lawson K, Brady KT. Substance abuse in women. Psychiatr Clin. 2010;33(2):339–55.

6. Substance Abuse and Mental Health Services Administration. Substance abuse treatment: addressing the specific needs of women, Treatment Improvement Protocol (TIP) Series, No. 51. HHS Publication No. (SMA) 13-4426. Rockville: Substance Abuse and Mental Health Services Administration; 2009.

7. Lindblad R, Hu L, Oden N, Wakim P, Rosa C, VanVeldhuisen P. Mortality rates among substance use disorder participants in clinical trials: pooled analysis of twenty-two clinical trials within the national drug abuse treatment clinical trials network. J Subst Abus Treat. 2016;70:73–80.

8. Sofuoglu M, Dudish-Poulsen S, Nelson D, Pentel PR, Hatsukami DK. Sex and menstrual cycle differences in the subjective effects from smoked cocaine in humans. Exp Clin Psychopharmacol. 1999;7(3):274.

9. McCabe JE, Arndt S. Demographic and substance abuse trends among pregnant and non-pregnant women: eleven years of treatment admission data. Matern Child Health J. 2012;16(8):1696–702.

10. Garcia-Guix A, Mestre-Pinto JI, Tirado-Muñoz J, Domingo-Salvany A, Torrens M. Psychiatric co-morbidity among women with substance use disorders. Adv Dual Diagn. 2018;11(1):1–3.

11. Frem Y, Torrens M, Domingo-Salvany A, Gilchrist G. Gender differences in lifetime psychiatric and substance use disorders among people who use substances in Barcelona. Spain Adv Dual Diagn. 2017;10(2):45–56.

12. Krawczyk N, Feder KA, Saloner B, Crum RM, Kealhofer M, Mojtabai R. The association of psychiatric comorbidity with treatment completion among clients admitted to substance use treatment programs in a US national sample. Drug Alcohol Depend. 2017;175:157–63.

13. Eggleston AM, Calhoun PS, Svikis DS, Tuten M, Chisolm MS, Jones HE. Suicidality, aggression, and other treatment considerations among pregnant, substance-dependent women with post-traumatic stress disorder. Compr Psychiatry. 2009;50(5):415–23.

14. Melikian AA, Djordjevic MV, Hosey J, Zhang J, Chen S, Zang E, Muscat J, Stellman SD. Gender differences relative to smoking behavior and emissions of toxins from mainstream cigarette smoke. Nicotine Tob Res. 2007;9(3):377–87.

15. Perkins KA, Scott J. Sex differences in long-term smoking cessation rates due to nicotine patch. Nicotine Tob Res. 2008;10(7):1245–50. https://doi.org/10.1080/14622200802097506.

16. Aguirre CG, Bello MS, Andrabi N, Pang RD, Hendricks PS, Bluthenthal RN, Leventhal AM. Gender, ethnicity, and their intersectionality in the prediction of smoking outcome expectancies in regular cigarette smokers. Behav Modif. 2016;40(1–2):281–302.

17. Smith PH, Bessette AJ, Weinberger AH, Sheffer CE, McKee SA. Sex/gender differences in smoking cessation: a review. Prev Med. 2016;92:135–40.

18. Smith PH, Weinberger AH, Zhang J, Emme E, Mazure CM, McKee SA. Sex differences in smoking cessation pharmacotherapy comparative efficacy: a network meta-analysis. Nicotine Tob Res. 2017;19(3):273–81.

19. Pirie PL, Murray DM, Luepker RV. Gender differences in cigarette smoking and quitting in a cohort of young adults. Am J Public Health. 1991;81:324–7. [PubMed: 1994740]

20. Swan GE, Ward MM, Carmelli D, et al. Differential rates of relapse in subgroups of male and female smokers. J Clin Epidemiol. 1993;46:1041–53. [PubMed: 8263577]

21. Perkins KA, Levine M, Marcus M, Shiffman S, D'amico D, Miller A, Keins A, Ashcom J, Broge M. Tobacco withdrawal in women and menstrual cycle phase. J Consult Clin Psychol. 2000;68(1):176.

22. Franklin TR, Ehrman R, Lynch KG, Harper D, Sciortino N, O'Brien CP, Childress AR. Menstrual cycle phase at quit date predicts smoking status in an NRT treatment trial: a retrospective analysis. J Women's Health. 2008;17(2):287–92.

23. Allen SS, Bade T, Center B, Finstad D, Hatsukami D. Menstrual phase effects on smoking relapse. Addiction. 2008;103(5):809–21.

24. Committee on Obstetric Practice. Committee opinion no. 721: smoking cessation during pregnancy. Obstet Gynecol. 2017;130(4):e200.

25. Siu AL. Behavioral and pharmacotherapy interventions for tobacco smoking cessation in adults, including pregnant women: US Preventive Services Task Force recommendation statement. Ann Intern Med. 2015;163(8):622–34.

26. Hartmann-Boyce J, Chepkin SC, Ye W, Bullen C, Lancaster T. Nicotine replacement therapy versus control for smoking cessation. Cochrane Database Syst Rev. 2018;5:CD000146.

27. Tong VT, Dietz PM, Morrow B, et al. Trends in smoking before, during, and after pregnancy-pregnancy risk assessment monitoring system, United States, 40 sites, 2000–2010. MMWR Surveill Summ. 2013;62:1–19.

28. National Institute on Alcohol Abuse and Alcoholism. Helping patients who drink too much: a clinician's guide. 2005. NIH publication: 07-3769.

29. Kelly JF, Stout R, Zywiak W, Schneider R. A 3-year study of addiction mutual-help group participation following intensive outpatient treatment. Alcohol Clin Exp Res. 2006;30(8):1381–92.

30. American College of Obstetricians and Gynecologists, Committee on Health Care for Underserved Women. Committee opinion no. 496: at-risk drinking and alcohol dependence: obstetric and gynecologic implications. Obstet Gynecol. 2011;118(2 Pt 1):383.

31. Williams JF, Smith VC, Committee on Substance Abuse. Fetal alcohol spectrum disorders. Pediatrics. 2015;136:e1395. Oct 19:peds-2015.

32. Tan CH, Denny CH, Cheal NE, Sniezek JE, Kanny D. Alcohol use and binge drinking among women of childbearing age—United States, 2011–2013. MMWR Morb Mortal Wkly Rep. 2015;64(37):1042–6.

33. McLafferty LP, Becker M, Dresner N, Meltzer-Brody S, Gopalan P, Glance J, Victor GS, Mittal L, Marshalek P, Lander L, Worley LL. Guidelines for the management of pregnant women with substance use disorders. Psychosomatics. 2016;57(2):115–30.

34. May PA, Chambers CD, Kalberg WO, Zellner J, Feldman H, Buckley D, Kopald D, Hasken JM, Xu R, Honerkamp-Smith G, Taras H. Prevalence of fetal alcohol spectrum disorders in 4 US communities. JAMA. 2018;319(5):474–82.

35. Sokol RJ, Martier SS, Ager JW. The T-ACE questions: practical prenatal detection of risk-drinking. Am J Obstet Gynecol. 1989;160(4):863–70.

36. Chang G, Wilkins-Haug L, Berman S, Goetz MA. The TWEAK: application in a prenatal setting. J Stud Alcohol. 1999;60(3):306–9.

37. Bhat A, Hadley A. The management of alcohol withdrawal in pregnancy—case report, literature review and preliminary recommendations. Gen Hosp Psychiatry. 2015;37(3):273–e1.

38. Rolland B, Paille F, Gillet C, Rigaud A, Moirand R, Dano C, Dematteis M, Mann K, Aubin HJ. Pharmacotherapy for alcohol dependence: the 2015 recommendations of the French Alcohol Society, issued in partnership with the European Federation of Addiction Societies. CNS Neurosci Ther. 2016;22(1):25–37.

39. Giglia R, Binns C. Alcohol and lactation: a systematic review. Nutr Diet. 2006;63(2):103–16.

40. Hasin DS, Kerridge BT, Saha TD, Huang B, Pickering R, Smith SM, Jung J, Zhang H, Grant BF. Prevalence and correlates of DSM-5 cannabis use disorder, 2012-2013: findings from the National Epidemiologic Survey on alcohol and related conditions–III. Am J Psychiatr. 2016;173(6):588–99.

41. Ryan-Ibarra S, Induni M, Ewing D. Prevalence of medical marijuana use in California, 2012. Drug Alcohol Rev. 2015;34(2):141–6.

42. Cooper ZD, Craft RM. Sex-dependent effects of cannabis and cannabinoids: a translational perspective. Neuropsychopharmacology. 2018;43(1):34.

43. Copeland J, Swift W, Rees V. Clinical profile of participants in a brief intervention program for cannabis use disorder. J Subst Abus Treat. 2001;20(1):45–52.

44. Herrmann ES, Weerts EM, Vandrey R. Sex differences in cannabis withdrawal symptoms among treatment-seeking cannabis users. Exp Clin Psychopharmacol. 2015;23(6):415.

45. Sherman BJ, McRae-Clark AL, Baker NL, Sonne SC, Killeen TK, Cloud K, Gray KM. Gender differences among treatment-seeking adults with cannabis use disorder: clinical profiles of women and men enrolled in the achieving cannabis cessation—evaluating N-acetylcysteine treatment (ACCENT) study. Am J Addict. 2017;26(2):136–44.

46. Metz TD, Stickrath EH. Marijuana use in pregnancy and lactation: a review of the evidence. Am J Obstet Gynecol. 2015;213(6):761–78.

47. Volkow ND, Compton WM, Wargo EM. The risks of marijuana use during pregnancy. JAMA. 2017;317(2):129–30.

48. Pearson G, Shiner M. Rethinking the generation gap: attitudes to illicit drugs among young people and adults. Crim Justice. 2002;2(1):71–86.

49. Onaivi ES, Chaudhuri G, Abaci AS, Parker M, Manier DH, Martin PR, Hubbard JR. Expression of cannabinoid receptors and their gene transcripts in human blood cells. Prog Neuro-Psychopharmacol Biol Psychiatry. 1999;23(6):1063–77.

50. Normandin MD, Zheng MQ, Lin KS, Mason NS, Lin SF, Ropchan J, Labaree D, Henry S, Williams WA, Carson RE, Neumeister A. Imaging the cannabinoid CB1 receptor in humans with [11C] OMAR: assessment of kinetic analysis methods, test–retest reproducibility, and gender differences. J Cereb Blood Flow Metab. 2015;35(8):1313–22.

51. Wiers CE, Shokri-Kojori E, Wong CT, Abi-Dargham A, Demiral ŞB, Tomasi D, Wang GJ, Volkow ND. Cannabis abusers show hypofrontality and blunted brain responses to a stimulant challenge in females but not in males. Neuropsychopharmacology. 2016;41(10):2596.

52. El-Talatini MR, Taylor AH, Konje JC. The relationship between plasma levels of the endocannabinoid, anandamide, sex steroids, and gonadotrophins during the menstrual cycle. Fertil Steril. 2010;93(6):1989–96.

53. Sherman BJ, McRae-Clark AL. Treatment of cannabis use disorder: current science and future outlook. Pharmacother: J Hum Pharmacol Drug Ther. 2016;36(5):511–35.

54. Ko JY, Farr SL, Tong VT, Creanga AA, Callaghan WM. Prevalence and patterns of marijuana use among pregnant and non-pregnant women of reproductive age. Am J Obstet Gynecol. 2015;213(2):201–e1.

55. Brown QL, Sarvet AL, Shmulewitz D, Martins SS, Wall MM, Hasin DS. Trends in marijuana use among pregnant and non-pregnant reproductive-aged women, 2002–2014. JAMA. 2017;317(2):207–9.

56. Fantasia HC. Pharmacologic implications of marijuana use during pregnancy. Nurs Womens Health. 2017;21(3):217–23.

57. Varner MW, Silver RM, Hogue CJ, Willinger M, Parker CB, Thorsten VR, Goldenberg RL, Saade GR, Dudley DJ, Coustan D, Stoll B. Association between stillbirth and illicit drug use and smoking during pregnancy. Obstet Gynecol. 2014;123(1):113.

58. El Marroun H, Tiemeier H, Steegers EA, Jaddoe VW, Hofman A, Verhulst FC, Van Den Brink W, Huizink AC. Intrauterine cannabis exposure affects fetal growth trajectories: the Generation R Study. J Am Acad Child Adolesc Psychiatry. 2009;48(12):1173–81.

59. Gunn JK, Rosales CB, Center KE, Nuñez A, Gibson SJ, Christ C, Ehiri JE. Prenatal exposure to cannabis and maternal and child health outcomes: a systematic review and meta-analysis. BMJ Open. 2016;6(4):e009986.

60. Fried PA, Makin JE. Neonatal behavioural correlates of prenatal exposure to marihuana, cigarettes and alcohol in a low risk population. Neurotoxicol Teratol. 1987;9(1):1–7.

61. de Moraes Barros MC, Guinsburg R, de Araújo Peres C, Mitsuhiro S, Chalem E, Laranjeira RR. Exposure to marijuana during pregnancy alters neurobehavior in the early neonatal period. J Pediatr. 2006;149(6):781–7.

62. Richardson GA, Ryan C, Willford J, Day NL, Goldschmidt L. Prenatal alcohol and marijuana exposure: effects on neuropsychological outcomes at 10 years. Neurotoxicol Teratol. 2002;24(3):309–20.

63. Klonoff-Cohen H, Lam-Kruglick P. Maternal and paternal recreational drug use and sudden infant death syndrome. Arch Pediatr Adolesc Med. 2001;155(7):765–70.

64. Astley SJ, Little RE. Maternal marijuana use during lactation and infant development at one year. Neurotoxicol Teratol. 1990;12(2):161–8.

65. Perez-Reyes M, Wall ME. Presence of delta-9-tetrahydrocannabinol in human milk. N Engl J Med. 1982;307:819–20.

66. American College of Obstetricians and Gynecologists. Marijuana use during pregnancy and lactation. Committee opinion no. 722. Obstet Gynecol. 2017;130(4):e205–9.

Opioid References

67. Centers for Disease Control and Prevention (CDC), National Center for Health Statistics. Multiple Cause of Death, 1999–2016 on CDC WONDER Online Database, released 2017. Data are from the Multiple Cause of Death Files, 1999–2016, as compiled from data provided by the 57 vital statistics jurisdictions through the Vital Statistics Cooperative Program. https://wonder.cdc.gov/mcd-icd10.html. Published 2017. Accessed 8 Aug 2018.

68. Jones CM, Logan J, Gladden RM, Bohm MK. Vital signs: demographic and substance use trends among heroin users—United States, 2002–2013. MMWR. Morb Mortal Wkly Rep. 2015;64(26):719.

69. Han B, Compton WM, Jones CM, Cai R. Nonmedical prescription opioid use and use disorders among adults aged 18 through 64 years in the United States, 2003–2013. JAMA. 2015;314(14):1468–78.

70. Cicero TJ, Kasper Z, Ellis MS. Increased use of heroin as an initiating opioid of abuse: further considerations and policy implications. Addict Behav. 2018;87:267–71.

71. Ailes EC, Dawson AL, Lind JN, Gilboa SM, Frey MT, Broussard CS, Honein MA. Opioid prescription claims among women of reproductive age – United States, 2008–2012. MMWR Morb Mortal Wkly Rep. 2015;64(2):37–41.

72. Riley IIIJL, Robinson ME, Wise EA, Myers CD, Fillingim RB. Sex differences in the perception of noxious experimental stimuli: a meta-analysis. Pain. 1998;74(2–3):181–7.

73. Gerdle B, Björk J, Cöster L, Henriksson KG, Henriksson C, Bengtsson A. Prevalence of widespread pain and associations with work status: a population study. BMC Musculoskelet Disord. 2008;9(1):102.

74. McHugh RK, DeVito EE, Dodd D, Carroll KM, Potter JS, Greenfield SF, Connery HS, Weiss RD. Gender differences in a clinical trial for prescription opioid dependence. J Subst Abus Treat. 2013;45(1):38–43.

75. Powis B, Griffiths P, Gossop M, Strang J. The differences between male and female drug users: community samples of heroin and cocaine users compared. Subst Use Misuse. 1996;31(5):529–43.

76. Bryant J, Brener L, Hull P, Treloar C. Needle sharing in regular sexual relationships: an examination of serodiscordance, drug using practices, and the gendered character of injecting. Drug Alcohol Depend. 2010;107(2–3):182–7.

77. Lum PJ, Sears C, Guydish J. Injection risk behavior among women syringe exchangers in San Francisco. Subst Use Misuse. 2005;40(11):1681–96.

78. Dwyer R, Richardson D, Ross MW, Wodak A, Miller ME, Gold J. A comparison of HIV risk between women and men who inject drugs. AIDS Educ Prev Off Publ Int Soc AIDS Educ. 1994;6(5):379–89.

79. Back SE, Lawson KM, Singleton LM, Brady KT. Characteristics and correlates of men and women with prescription opioid dependence. Addict Behav. 2011;36(8):829–34.

80. Gros DF, Milanak ME, Brady KT, Back SE. Frequency and severity of comorbid mood and anxiety disorders in prescription opioid dependence. Am J Addict. 2013;22(3):261–5.

81. Jones HE, Fitzgerald H, Johnson RE, Jones HE, Fitzgerald H, Johnson RE. Males and females differ in response to opioid agonist medications. Am J Addict. 2005;14(3):223–33.

82. Schottenfeld RS, Pakes JR, Kosten TR. Prognostic factors in buprenorphine-versus methadone-maintained patients. J Nerv Ment Dis. 1998;186(1):35–43.

83. Zubieta JK, Smith YR, Bueller JA, Xu Y, Kilbourn MR, Jewett DM, Meyer CR, Koeppe RA, Stohler CS. μ-Opioid receptor-mediated antinociceptive responses differ in men and women. J Neurosci. 2002;22(12):5100–7.

84. Gear RW, Miaskowski C, Gordon NC, Paul SM, Heller PH, Levine JD. Kappa–opioids produce significantly greater analgesia in women than in men. Nat Med. 1996;2(11):1248.

85. Kreek MJ, Schluger J, Borg L, Gunduz M, Ho A. Dynorphin A1–13 causes elevation of serum levels of prolactin through an opioid receptor mechanism in humans: gender differences and implications for modulation of dopaminergic tone in the treatment of addictions. J Pharmacol Exp Ther. 1999;288(1):260–9.

86. Unger A, Jung E, Winklbaur B, Fischer G. Gender issues in the pharmacotherapy of opioid-addicted women: buprenorphine. J Addict Dis. 2010;29(2):217–30.

87. Karuntzos GT, Caddell JM, Dennis ML. Gender differences in vocational needs and outcomes for methadone treatment clients. J Psychoactive Drugs. 1994;26(2):173–80.

88. Zhang Z, Friedmann PD, Gerstein DR. Does retention matter? Treatment duration and improvement in drug use. Addiction. 2003;98(5):673–84.

89. Bateman BT, Hernandez-Diaz S, Rathmell JP, Seeger JD, Doherty M, Fischer MA, Huybrechts KF. Patterns of opioid utilization in pregnancy in a large cohort of commercial insurance beneficiaries in the United States. Anesthesiol: J Am Soc Anesthesiologists. 2014;120(5):1216–24.

90. Desai RJ, Hernandez-Diaz S, Bateman BT, Huybrechts KF. Increase in prescription opioid use during pregnancy among Medicaid-enrolled women. Obstet Gynecol. 2014;123(5):997.

91. Patrick SW, Schumacher RE, Benneyworth BD, Krans EE, McAllister JM, Davis MM. Neonatal abstinence syndrome and associated health care expenditures: United States, 2000–2009. JAMA. 2012;307(18):1934–40.

92. Epstein RA, Bobo WV, Martin PR, Morrow JA, Wang W, Chandrasekhar R, Cooper WO. Increasing pregnancy-related use of prescribed opioid analgesics. Ann Epidemiol. 2013;23(8):498–503.

93. Maeda A, Bateman BT, Clancy CR, Creanga AA, Leffert LR. Opioid abuse and dependence during pregnancy temporal trends and obstetrical outcomes. J Am Soc Anesthesiologists. 2014;121(6):1158–65.

94. Patrick SW, Davis MM, Lehmann CU, Cooper WO. Increasing incidence and geographic distribution of neonatal abstinence syndrome: United States 2009 to 2012. J Perinatol. 2015;35(8):650.

95. ACOG Committee on Health Care for Underserved Women. ACOG committee opinion no. 524: opioid abuse, dependence, and addiction in pregnancy. Obstet Gynecol. 2012;119(5):1070.

96. Luty J, Nikolaou V. Bearn J. Is opiate detoxification unsafe in pregnancy? J Subst Abus Treat. 2003;24(4):363–7.

97. Blinick G, Wallach RC, Jerez E, Ackerman BD. Drug addiction in pregnancy and the neonate. Am J Obstetr Gynecol. 1976;125(2):135–42.

98. Dashe JS, Jackson GL, Olscher DA, Zane EH, Wendel GD Jr. Opioid detoxification in pregnancy. Obstet Gynecol. 1998;92(5):854–8.

99. Jones HE, O'grady KE, Malfi D, Tuten M. Methadone maintenance vs. methadone taper during pregnancy: maternal and neonatal outcomes. Am J Addict. 2008;17(5):372–86.

100. Maas U, Kattner E, Weingart-Jesse B, Schäfer A, Obladen M. Infrequent neonatal opiate withdrawal following maternal methadone detoxification during pregnancy. J Perinat Med-Off J WAPM. 1990;18(2):111–8.

101. McCarthy JJ, Leamon MH, Parr MS, Anania B. High-dose methadone maintenance in pregnancy: maternal and neonatal outcomes. Am J Obstet Gynecol. 2005;193(3):606–10.

102. Haas AL, Peters RH. Development of substance abuse problems among drug-involved offenders: evidence for the telescoping effect. J Subst Abus. 2000;12(3):241–53.

103. White KA, Brady KT, Sonne S. Gender differences in patterns of cocaine use. Am J Addict. 1996;5(3):259–61.

104. Brecht ML, O'Brien A, Von Mayrhauser C, Anglin MD. Methamphetamine use behaviors and gender differences. Addict Behav. 2004;29(1):89–106.

105. Durell TM, Kroutil LA, Crits-Christoph P, Barchha N, Van Brunt DL. Prevalence of nonmedical methamphetamine use in the United States. Subst Abuse Treat Prev Policy. 2008;3(1):19.

106. Substance Abuse and Mental Health Services Administration, Center for Behavioral Health Statistics and Quality. The TEDS report: gender differences in primary substance of abuse across age groups. 2014. Rockville.

107. Hser YI, Evans E, Huang YC. Treatment outcomes among women and men methamphetamine abusers in California. J Subst Abus Treat. 2005;28(1):77–85.

108. Rawson RA, Gonzales R, Obert JL, McCann MJ, Brethen P. Methamphetamine use among treatment-seeking adolescents in Southern California: participant characteristics and treatment response. J Subst Abus Treat. 2005;29(2):67–74.

109. Kim JY, Fendrich M. Gender differences in juvenile arrestees' drug use, self-reported dependence, and perceived need for treatment. Psychiatr Serv. 2002;53(1):70–5.

110. Dluzen DE, Liu B. Gender differences in methamphetamine use and responses: a review. Gend Med. 2008;5(1):24–35.

111. Cretzmeyer M, Sarrazin MV, Huber DL, Block RI, Hall JA. Treatment of methamphetamine abuse: research findings and clinical directions. J Subst Abus Treat. 2003;24(3):267–77.

112. Sofuoglu M, Mitchell E, Kosten TR. Effects of progesterone treatment on cocaine responses in male and female cocaine users. Pharmacol Biochem Behav. 2004;78(4):699–705.

113. Evans SM, Foltin RW. Exogenous progesterone attenuates the subjective effects of smoked cocaine in women, but not in men. Neuropsychopharmacology. 2006;31(3):659.

114. Justice AJ, de Wit H. Acute effects of d-amphetamine during the follicular and luteal phases of the menstrual cycle in women. Psychopharmacology. 1999;145(1):67–75.

115. Justice AJ, De Wit H. Acute effects of d-amphetamine during the early and late follicular phases of the menstrual cycle in women. Pharmacol Biochem Behav. 2000;66(3):509–15.

116. Agabio R, Campesi I, Pisanu C, Gessa GL, Franconi F. Sex differences in substance use disorders: focus on side effects. Addict Biol. 2016;21(5):1030–42.

117. Adinoff B, Williams MJ, Best SE, Harris TS, Chandler P, Devous MD Sr. Sex differences in medial and lateral orbitofrontal cortex hypoperfusion in cocaine-dependent men and women. Gend Med. 2006;3(3):206–22.

118. Shetty V, Harrell L, Murphy DA, Vitero S, Gutierrez A, Belin TR, Dye BA, Spolsky VW. Dental disease patterns in methamphetamine users: Findings in a large urban sample. J Am Dent Assoc. 2015;146(12):875–85.

119. Kittirattanapaiboon P, Srikosai S, Wittayanookulluk A. Methamphetamine use and dependence in vulnerable female populations. Curr Opin Psychiatry. 2017;30(4):247–52.

120. Dahlman D, Håkansson A, Björkman P, Blomé MA, Kral AH. Correlates of skin and soft tissue infections in injection drug users in a syringe-exchange program in Malmö, Sweden. Subst Use Misuse. 2015;50(12):1529–35.

121. Hughes PH, Coletti SD, Neri RL, Urmann CF, Stahl S, Sicilian DM, Anthony JC. Retaining cocaine-abusing women in a therapeutic community: the effect of a child live-in program. Am J Public Health. 1995;85(8_Pt_1):1149–52.

122. Schottenfeld RS, Moore B, Pantalon MV. Contingency management with community reinforcement approach or twelve-step facilitation drug counseling for cocaine dependent pregnant women or women with young children. Drug Alcohol Depend. 2011;118(1):48–55.

123. Bhuvaneswar CG, Chang G, Epstein LA, Stern TA. Cocaine and opioid use during pregnancy: prevalence and management. Prim Care Companion J Clin Psychiatry. 2008;10(1):59.

124. Wendell AD. Overview and epidemiology of substance abuse in pregnancy. Clin Obstet Gynecol. 2013;56(1):91–6.

125. Ostrea EM, Brady M, Gause S, Raymundo AL, Stevens M. Drug screening of newborns by meconium analysis: a large-scale, prospective, epidemiologic study. Pediatrics. 1992;89(1):107–13.

126. Fallone MD, LaGasse LL, Lester BM, Shankaran S, Bada HS, Bauer CR. Reactivity and regulation of motor responses in cocaine-exposed infants. Neurotoxicol Teratol. 2014;43:25–32.

127. Zuckerman B, Frank DA, Mayes L. Cocaine-exposed infants and developmental outcomes: crack kids revisited. JAMA. 2002;287(15):1990–1.

128. Frank DA, Augustyn M, Knight WG, Pell T, Zuckerman B. Growth, development, and behavior in early childhood following prenatal cocaine exposure: a systematic review. JAMA. 2001;285(12):1613–25.

129. Chaplin TM, Freiburger MB, Mayes LC, Sinha R. Prenatal cocaine exposure, gender, and adolescent stress response: a prospective longitudinal study. Neurotoxicol Teratol. 2010;32(6):595–604.

130. Bandstra ES, Vogel AL, Morrow CE, Xue L, Anthony JC. Severity of prenatal cocaine exposure and child language functioning through age seven years: a longitudinal latent growth curve analysis. Subst Use Misuse. 2004;39(1):25–59.

131. Singer LT, Arendt R, Minnes S, Farkas K, Salvator A, Kirchner HL, Kliegman R. Cognitive and motor outcomes of cocaine-exposed infants. JAMA. 2002;287(15):1952–60.

132. Mansoor E, Morrow CE, Accornero VH, Xue L, Johnson AL, Anthony JC, Bandstra ES. Longitudinal effects of prenatal cocaine use on mother-child interactions at ages 3 and 5. J Dev Behav Pediatr: JDBP. 2012;33(1):32.

133. Strathearn L, Mayes LC. Cocaine addiction in mothers. Ann N Y Acad Sci. 2010;1187(1):172–83.

Neurologic Imaging in Pregnancy

Jesse M. Thon, Robert Regenhardt, and Joshua P. Klein

Clinical Case 1

A 26 year-old healthy pregnant woman in her third trimester presents to the emergency department following an acute-onset severe headache. Upon arrival, she is noted to be hypertensive, increasingly lethargic and plegic on the left side of her body. What brain imaging modality should be used in this emergent clinical situation?

Computed Tomography

The choice of imaging modality during pregnancy to evaluate a neurologic disorder should aim to provide the standard of care for diagnosis and treatment while minimizing risks to the fetus [1]. Three governing bodies provide evidence-based guidelines that can offer suggestions, including the American College of Obstetricians and Gynecologists [2], the American College of Radiology [3], and the European Society of Urogenital Radiology [4].

Computed Tomography (CT) involves exposure to ionizing radiation, the effects of which are either stochastic or deterministic [1]. Stochastic effects may theoretically occur after any amount of radiation. Examples include mutagenesis and malignancy, and inform the recommendation to keep exposure "as low as reasonably achievable" [1, 2]. Deterministic effects, however, are dose dependent and associated with specific exposure thresholds. Examples include cataract formation and infertility [1].

Evidence regarding the risk of ionizing radiation during pregnancy has been gathered in a variety of settings. Observational studies of human survivors of atomic warfare in Hiroshima and Nagasaki, observational studies of pregnant patients exposed to radiation before its detrimental effects were understood, and experimental animal model studies have all contributed to our understanding of its pathophysiology [1]. Furthermore, the effects of radiation depend on the dose of absorption, the rate dose absorption, and the gestational age of the fetus [3, 5, 6].

Dose units are often in rad, which is equivalent to 0.01 Gy or 0.01 J/kg. Even low dose radiation to the fetus is associated with an increased risk of childhood cancer [7]. After in utero exposure to 1–2 rad, the rate of leukemia increases from 3.6 to 5 per 10,000 children. A meta-analysis showed that for every 100 rad exposure, there is a 6% increase in risk of childhood cancer [7]. That stated, even with repeated imaging these exposure levels are not reached [1].

The rate of absorption is also important, and varies depending on several factors. Fetal exposure to background environmental radiation over the course of pregnancy is approximately 0.23 rad [6]. When exposed to CT, maternal size, exam parameters, and direct vs indirect exposure all factor into the absorption. Direct exposure occurs with lumbar spine or pelvis imaging. Lumbar spine imaging can cause an exposure of 0.28–2.4 rad, and pelvis imaging can cause up to 3 rad. In contrast, indirect exposure is secondary to attenuated scattered radiation, often from imaging the maternal head or cervical spine. These indirect exposures are estimated to be less than 0.01 rad [6].

Lastly, gestational age of the fetus plays a role in the effects. Days 0–15 (conception to implantation) is a very high risk period, though the risk is all or nothing. In animal models, there is either death or no effect. In atomic bomb

J. M. Thon (✉)
Department of Neurology, Massachusetts General Hospital, Boston, MA, USA

R. Regenhardt
Partners Neurology Residency Program, Brigham and Women's Hospital, Massachusetts General Hospital, Boston, MA, USA
e-mail: rregenhardt@partners.org

J. P. Klein
Department of Neurology, Brigham and Women's Hospital, Boston, MA, USA
e-mail: jpklein@partners.org

© Springer Nature Switzerland AG 2019
M. A. O'Neal (ed.), *Neurology and Psychiatry of Women*, https://doi.org/10.1007/978-3-030-04245-5_12

survivors, there were no effects noted if exposed during this period and the pregnancy was completed. The American College of Radiology cites an increased risk of miscarriages through week 4 [3]. Exposure during weeks 3–8 (organogenesis) is associated with an increased risk of malformations, transient growth retardation, and neonatal death in animal models. Human fetuses exposed before the harmful effects of radiation were recognized suffered malformations, and atomic bomb survivors were noted to have microcephaly [8]. Weeks 6 to birth are also not without risk. While malformations have not been noted, there are associations with mental retardation. The highest risk is from weeks 8 to 15, where a 12–20 rad threshold is associated with mental retardation. The risk is fourfold lower from weeks 15 to 25, and negligible thereafter [3].

Attempts to limit exposure should be made whenever possible, through patient positioning, considerations of body habitus, and advanced image reconstruction techniques. Doses and techniques should be reported in radiology reports, and radiation dosimetry experts can be used to aid in calculations [2]. Counseling is important to help pregnant patients understand the risks and also to reassure them when risks are clearly outweighed by benefits. It is standard to counsel patients that no definitive association of exposure less than 5 rad has been made with spontaneous abortion, developmental malformations, or mental retardation. There is a small association with childhood malignancies. For exposure of 5–15 rad, there is a small increased risk of congenital defects, 10% vs 5% of all births [3]. Although it is optimal to avoid maternal CT imaging completely if possible, it may be required in emergent clinical situations, such as in the evaluation of subarachnoid hemorrhage (as presented in *clinical case 1*), in which the minimal radiation exposure to the fetus is outweighed by the benefits of prompt diagnosis.

CT Angiography and Iodinated Contrast

The contrast used for CT angiography (CTA) and CT with contrast is intravenous iodinated contrast. It is classified by the US Food and Drug Administration as class B and should be avoided if possible during pregnancy. Administration of iodinated contrast in animal models has not shown any teratogenic or mutagenic properties [9]. No controlled human studies with intravenous contrast have been conducted, but contrast injection into the fetal cavity has been associated with hypothyroidism. Recommendations are made to the clinician to obtain informed consent before administration [3], take standard precautions to prevent contrast-induced nephropathy, and send thyroid function testing in the 1st week of life [10].

Digital Subtraction Angiography

Many of the same risks for CT, CTA and CT with contrast exist for digital subtraction angiography (DSA) . It also uses ionizing radiation, which has the same aforementioned properties. Furthermore, the contrast is also iodinated and has the same properties. A study compared 64 slice CTA to DSA, and found that CTA provided near equivalent visualization of the cerebral vessels, with the exception of distal vessels beyond A3/P3 and ICA segments at the skull base, and radiation doses were equivalent [11]. A newer study using more modern CT scanners showed that the CTA uses about 25% of the DSA dose for intracranial vessels, but about 135% of the DSA dose if neck vessels are also included [12]. In some cases, DSA allows the use of a smaller overall volume of contrast. In addition, contrast is injected directly into the relevant arteries, bypassing the fetus at least in first pass.

However, there are also additional risks to the fetus [13]. The procedure often involves sedation, which is not without risk. Groin puncture is associated with a small risk of maternal hemorrhage, including into the retroperitoneal space causing significant blood loss. While there are some advantages to this technique, in most cases this imaging modality should be reserved for emergencies where a direct life-saving intervention can be performed such as aneurysm rupture or stroke from large vessel occlusion [14].

Clinical Case 2

A 31 year-old pregnant woman in her second trimester presents to the neurology clinic for evaluation of right hand weakness that has been persistent for the last 2 days. She has a known history of multiple sclerosis and has been off of beta-interferon treatment since the start of her pregnancy. She has noted that her right hand has lost dexterity, and she has been dropping objects and is unable to write. On neurologic exam, she has significant weakness in all tested muscles of the right hand, without sensory loss or abnormal findings elsewhere. If brain imaging is ordered, which modality should be used in this case?

Magnetic Resonance Imaging

In contrast to computed tomography, magnetic resonance imaging (MRI) does not expose the pregnant patient or her fetus to ionizing radiation. Instead, images are created via radiofrequency pulses applied within a magnetic field. The magnetic field aligns proton spins and the radiofrequency pulses momentarily deflect the spins. The detection of electrical current produced by return to alignment, which occurs at different rates for molecules in different tissues, allows for the construction of a detailed image. Although this technique changes the position of atoms, it does not alter their structure or composition, as opposed to ionizing radiation, and is thus considered a safe imaging modality [15].

However, theoretical risks to the fetus have been raised since the development of MRI, including effects of static magnetic fields, alterations in field gradients, noise exposure, heat transfer to the pregnant mother, and potential teratogenicity [16]. To date, studies have not shown evidence to support these concerns, as heat exposure to the uterus has been found to be negligible, no acoustic damage to infants exposed to MRI has been demonstrated, and animal studies have largely shown no increased teratogenic risk [17, 18]. Based on these findings, the American College of Obstetricians and Gynecologists recommends that with regard to MRI, there are no precautions or contraindications specific to the pregnant woman [19]. In non-emergent clinical situations, such as the one presented in *clinical case 2*, brain MRI is the preferred imaging modality.

Recently, a large retrospective cohort study evaluated the outcomes of MRI exposure during the first trimester, given particular concern for potential risks during this period. In 1737 such pregnancies, there were no statistically significant differences in rates of stillbirths or neonatal deaths, congenital anomalies, neoplasm development, or vision or hearing loss compared to controls over a median post-birth follow up period of 3.6 years. In subgroup analysis, even infants whose mothers underwent abdominal, pelvic, or spine MRI had no elevated risks of the above outcomes. The only potential adverse effect was seen in patients imaged between 5 and 10 weeks' gestation, with infant vision loss rates slightly higher than controls (adjusted risk difference 2.7 per 1000 person-years, 95% CI, 0.2–7.9) but with no increased rates of other adverse outcomes [20].

Gadolinium

Contrast-enhanced MR imaging with gadolinium can provide increased diagnostic clarity in certain clinical situations, such as when evaluating for infection, neoplasm, or active inflammation. However, gadolinium has also been linked to adverse effects, in particular the development of nephrogenic systemic fibrosis in patients with renal failure, which has led to concern regarding its impact on the fetus.

Animal studies have demonstrated the passage of gadolinium into the placenta and subsequent circulation into the fetal kidneys and amniotic fluid. In one primate study, gadolinium was detected in the amniotic fluid 50 days after injection into the mother during the second trimester, and tissue levels were detected in very small amounts in the newborn monkeys [21]. Placental imaging studies have shown similar results in humans of gadolinium passage into the placenta [22, 23].

Outcome studies in animals following maternal gadolinium administration have shown mixed results. Early trials showed an association with growth retardation and congenital anomalies at doses equivalent to two to seven times higher than those used in humans. However, subsequent studies in rodents, rabbits, and primates showed no deleterious effects [24, 25].

Until recently, human studies evaluating the impact of maternal gadolinium exposure have been limited to small case series. One such prospective cohort study of 26 pregnant women who received gadolinium during the first trimester showed no adverse effects on the pregnancies or neonatal outcomes [26]. However, the large retrospective study cited above that evaluated outcomes following noncontrast enhanced MRI during the first trimester also evaluated outcomes following gadolinium administration at any time during pregnancy. This study showed that rates of stillbirth or neonatal death were higher in the 397 gadolinium-exposed pregnancies compared to controls. It also showed that in pregnancies exposed to gadolinium during the first trimester, there were increased rates of infant rheumatologic, inflammatory, or infiltrative skin conditions compared to unexposed pregnancies [20]. At this time, gadolinium-enhanced MR imaging should be avoided in pregnancy unless absolutely clinically necessary.

Take Home Points
1. CT should be avoided in pregnancy if possible due to potential fetal harm from radiation exposure, but it may be required in an emergent setting when benefits of rapid diagnosis outweigh risks, as fetal harm is unlikely if exposure is kept to a minimum.
2. Iodinated contrast with CT and DSA should be avoided in pregnancy unless there is a high pretest probability of a serious neurologic condition and rapid diagnosis could lead to an emergent intervention. One should obtain informed consent, prevent contrast nephropathy, and test thyroid function in the 1st week of life.
3. MRI is considered safe in pregnancy and is the modality of choice in non-emergent clinical situations where neurologic imaging is indicated.
4. There is evidence that gadolinium may increase rates of fetal death and the development of systemic disease in infancy, and thus its use should be avoided unless absolutely clinically indicated to aid diagnosis.

References

1. Bove RM, Klein JP. Neuroradiology in women of childbearing age. Continuum (Minneap Minn). 2014;20(1 Neurology of Pregnancy):23–41.
2. ACOG Committee on Obstetric Practice. ACOG Committee Opinion. Number 299, September 2004 (replaces No. 158, September 1995). Guidelines for diagnostic imaging during pregnancy. Obstet Gynecol. 2004;104(3):647–51.
3. Manual on Contrast Media v10.3 – American College of Radiology [Internet]. [cited 2017 Oct 25]. Available from: https://www.acr.org/Quality-Safety/Resources/Contrast-Manual.
4. Webb JAW, Thomsen HS, Morcos SK. Members of contrast media safety committee of european society of urogenital radiology (ESUR). The use of iodinated and gadolinium contrast media during pregnancy and lactation. Eur Radiol. 2005;15(6):1234–40.
5. Hall EJ, Giaccia AJ. Radiobiology for the radiologist. Philadelphia: Lippincott Williams & Wilkins; 2006. p. 546.
6. Osei EK, Faulkner K. Fetal doses from radiological examinations. Br J Radiol. 1999;72(860):773–80.
7. Wakeford R, Little MP. Risk coefficients for childhood cancer after intrauterine irradiation: a review. Int J Radiat Biol. 2003;79(5):293–309.
8. Yamazaki JN, Schull WJ. Perinatal loss and neurological abnormalities among children of the atomic bomb. Nagasaki and Hiroshima revisited, 1949 to 1989. JAMA. 1990;264(5):605–9.
9. Nelson JA, Livingston GK, Moon RG. Mutagenic evaluation of radiographic contrast media. Investig Radiol. 1982;17(2):183–5.
10. Grüters A, Krude H. Detection and treatment of congenital hypothyroidism. Nat Rev Endocrinol. 2011;8(2):104–13.
11. Klingebiel R, Kentenich M, Bauknecht H-C, Masuhr F, Siebert E, Busch M, et al. Comparative evaluation of 64-slice CT angiography and digital subtraction angiography in assessing the cervicocranial vasculature. Vasc Health Risk Manag. Dove Press. 2008;4(4):901–7.
12. Manninen A-L, Isokangas J-M, Karttunen A, Siniluoto T, Nieminen MTA. Comparison of radiation exposure between diagnostic CTA and DSA examinations of cerebral and cervicocerebral vessels. Am J Neuroradiol. 2012;33(11):2038–42.
13. Moon EK, Wang W, Newman JS, Bayona-Molano MDP. Challenges in interventional radiology: the pregnant patient. Semin Interv Radiol. Thieme Medical Publishers. 2013;30(4):394–402.
14. Grzyska U, Freitag J, Zeumer H. Selective cerebral intraarterial DSA. Complication rate and control of risk factors. Neuroradiology. 1990;32(4):296–9.
15. Hartwig V, Giovannetti G, Vanello N, Lombardi M, Landini L, Simi S. Biological effects and safety in magnetic resonance imaging: a review. Int J Environ Res Public Health. Multidisciplinary Digital Publishing Institute (MDPI). 2009;6(6):1778–98.
16. Kanal E, Shellock FG, Talagala L. Safety considerations in MR imaging. Radiology. 1990;176(3):593–606.
17. Chen MM, Coakley FV, Kaimal A, Laros RK. Guidelines for computed tomography and magnetic resonance imaging use during pregnancy and lactation. Obstet Gynecol. 2008;112(2 Pt 1):333–40.
18. Kanal E, Barkovich AJ, Bell C, Borgstede JP, Bradley WG, Froelich JW, et al. ACR guidance document on MR safe practices: 2013. J Magn Reson Imaging. 2013;37(3):501–30.
19. Committee on Obstetric Practice. Committee opinion No. 723: guidelines for diagnostic imaging during pregnancy and lactation. Obstet Gynecol. 2017;130(4):e210–6.
20. Ray JG, Vermeulen MJ, Bharatha A, Montanera WJ, Park AL. Association between MRI exposure during pregnancy and fetal and childhood outcomes. JAMA. 2016;316(9):952–61.
21. Prola-Netto J, Woods M, Roberts VHJ, Sullivan EL, Miller CA, Frias AE, et al. Gadolinium chelate safety in pregnancy: barely detectable gadolinium levels in the juvenile nonhuman primate after in utero exposure. Radiology. 2017;286:162534.
22. Marcos HB, Semelka RC, Worawattanakul S. Normal placenta: gadolinium-enhanced dynamic MR imaging. Radiology. 1997;205(2):493–6.
23. Tanaka YO, Sohda S, Shigemitsu S, Niitsu M, Itai Y. High temporal resolution dynamic contrast MRI in a high risk group for placenta accreta. Magn Reson Imaging. 2001;19(5):635–42.
24. Sundgren PC, Leander P. Is administration of gadolinium-based contrast media to pregnant women and small children justified? J Magn Reson Imaging. 2011;34(4):750–7.
25. Fraum TJ, Ludwig DR, Bashir MR, Fowler KJ. Gadolinium-based contrast agents: a comprehensive risk assessment. J Magn Reson Imaging. 2017;46(2):338–53.
26. De Santis M, Straface G, Cavaliere AF, Carducci B, Caruso A. Gadolinium periconceptional exposure: pregnancy and neonatal outcome. Acta Obstet Gynecol Scand. 2007;86(1):99–101.

The Normal Physiology of Pregnancy: Neurological Implications

Cesar R. Padilla and Nicole A. Smith

Cardiovascular and Hemodynamic Changes in Pregnancy

Maternal hemodynamic changes are marked in pregnancy, starting as early as 5 weeks gestation. These changes are characterized overall by a decline in systemic vascular resistance, and increase in plasma volume and cardiac output.

Systemic vascular resistance (SVR) begins to decline early, around 5 weeks gestation, with a nadir in the second trimester. Decline in SVR is thought to mediate the drop in systolic and diastolic blood pressures, which starts early and continues into the second trimester. Blood pressures rise in the third trimester, often back to pre-pregnancy values. Systolic pressures of 140 or diastolic pressures of 90 are abnormal in pregnancy and warrant evaluation. Elevated blood pressures in pregnancy may be related to gestational hypertension or preeclampsia, both of which carry risks to mother and fetus.

Perhaps one of the most dramatic maternal physiologic accommodations is the rapid increase in maternal blood volume, hypothesized to provide nutrients to the growing fetus, and protect mothers from excessive blood loss at birth, due to the state of physiologic anemia caused by an increase in plasma volume [1]. Maternal plasma blood volume increases early in the first trimester, by 6 weeks, and expands rapidly, peaking at 30–34 weeks with an average total increase of approximately 50% [1–3]. Change in plasma volume is largely hormone related, causing adaptive changes in renal absorption of sodium through the renin-angiotensin aldosterone system [4].

Decreased afterload from decreased systemic vascular resistance, and increased preload due to plasma volume expansion contribute significantly to the average 30–50% increase in cardiac output. Heart rate is another contributor to increased cardiac output. Rates begin to rise early in the first trimester, and increase progressively throughout pregnancy. While heart rates may increase up to 20% above baseline, peaking in the third trimester, most will remain below 100 beats per minute [4]. The rise in cardiac output is seen from the first trimester onward, with a peak in the second stage of labor (pushing) [5].

Renal Physiology

An increase in plasma volume and cardiac output leads to an increase in blood flow to the kidneys, leading to increased GFR (glomerular filtration rate) and creatinine clearance seen early in the first trimester [6, 7]. Renal sodium retention contributes to an increase in plasma volume expansion which promotes an overall increase in flow and perfusion to the developing fetus and utero-placental circulation [7]. Sodium retention in the renal system is driven largely by an up-regulation in the renin–angiotensin–aldosterone system (RAAS) system [8, 9].

In pregnancy, there is renal-mediated inhibition of natriuretic hormones, which in otherwise non-pregnant patients would permit diuresis of excess plasma volume [10]. This is accomplished by the production of atrial natriuretic peptide (ANP), leading to further volume retention and plasma volume expansion. Hence, two physiologic systems, which normally work to counter one another (RAAS/ANP), work in unison to promote increases in plasma volume while inhibiting diuresis.

These changes in renal physiology have pharmacokinetic implications. Increases in renal blood flow and an increase in hepatic induction promotes clearance and drug elimination of many anti-epileptic medications, leading to a decrease in serum concentrations of many, including: phenobarbital (25–50% decrease), carbamezapine (10–25%), phenytoin (25–50%) and levetiracetam (>50% decrease) [11]. Drug levels typically normalize to pre-pregnancy values by 2 weeks post partum [12].

C. R. Padilla
Brigham and Women's Hospital, Boston, MA, USA
e-mail: Cpadilla3@bwh.harvard.edu

N. A. Smith (✉)
Maternal Fetal Medicine, Brigham and Women's Hospital, Boston, MA, USA

Department of ob/gyn, Brigham and Women's Hospital, Boston, MA, USA
e-mail: NASMITH@PARTNERS.ORG; nasmith@bwh.harvard.edu

© Springer Nature Switzerland AG 2019
M. A. O'Neal (ed.), *Neurology and Psychiatry of Women*, https://doi.org/10.1007/978-3-030-04245-5_13

Hematologic Changes in Pregnancy

Normal pregnancy is a prothrombotic state, characterized by increased procoagulant factors II, VII, VIII, X, XII, and XIII, and von Willbrand's factor, reduced anticoagulant factors including protein S and antithrombin, and reduced fibrinolysis. Coagulation parameters typically normalize by 6–8 weeks postpartum, with earlier resolution of some values. This state of hypercoagulation is somewhat compensated by a state of fibrinolysis, as evidenced by an increase in fibrin degradation products in parturients [4]. Should coagulation testing be indicated, the prothrombin time and activated partial thromboplastin time typically remain normal. D-dimer can be elevated in pregnancy, resulting in low sensitivity and specificity for clot. Negative predictive value is likely unchanged. Evidence of hypercoagulability has been well documented with novel assays, such as thromboelestography, which can give pertinent findings of coagulation activity in the clinical setting [13].

As plasma volume increases, red blood cell mass increases as well, starting in the first trimester. Increase in red blood cell mass will peak at 20–30% in the third trimester, in women taking iron supplementation. Total iron requirements are close to 1000 mg over the entirety of pregnancy. Even in women taking iron supplementation, iron deficiency anemia is relatively common, defined by the Centers for Disease Control and prevention as a hemoglobin value of <11 in g/dL in the first and third trimesters, and 10.5 g/dL in the second trimester [14]. Intravascular volume increases at a rate greater than that of red blood cell volume, however, resulting in physiologic, or dilutional, anemia.

Platelet counts typically remain in the non-pregnant normal range above 150,000. Mild thrombocytopenia (80,000–149,000) may be the result of a physiologic process (gestational thrombocytopenia), or in response to a pregnancy related disease state (pre-eclampsia/eclampsia) [15, 16]. Most cases (70%) of thrombocytopenia occur due to gestational thrombocytopenia, which occurs in up to 10% of all pregnancies. This may represent a state of receptor activated platelet activation, destruction and hemodilution due to an increase in plasma volume [15, 17].

Impact of Pregnancy Physiology on Specific Neurologic Conditions

Intracranial Hemorrhage and Cerebral Infarctions

Intracranial hemorrhage in pregnancy is a result of two major causes- arteriovenous malformation (AVM) and cerebral aneurysms [18]. Although other causes, such as venous bleeding can also occur, AVM and aneurysms have been identified as leading causes of hemorrhagic strokes in pregnancy. A recent retrospective review examining over 11 million deliveries in the U.S. identified a higher increase in subarachnoid hemorrhages (SAH's) with an increase in maternal age and the postpartum period [18]. For example, when comparing women under the age of 25 to women over 35 years of age, the incidence of SAH rises from 2.0 per 100,000 to 5.0 per 100,000. The incidence of SAH rises rapidly in the postpartum period, with incidence in women over 35 at a rate of 66 per 100,000 [18].

AVM is a more likely cause of hemorrhage than is aneurysmal rupture in pregnant patients [19]. The increase in AVM and aneurysmal- related hemorrhage has been attributed to the increase in blood volume, cardiac output and overall hemodynamic stress. Risk is increased at later gestational age and in the postpartum period [20].

Another type of stroke pathology exacerbated by pregnancy is thrombosis of the cerebral venous and sinus vasculature, which may present as headache, seizure, or with vague symptoms such as lethargy, nausea and dizziness, In obstetric patients, the incidence of cerebral vein and sinus thrombosis is 12 per 100,000 deliveries. In contrast, the incidence in the general population is three to four per one million people [21].

Pregnancy may precipitate the development of cerebral venous thrombosis, as it is more likely to occur in late pregnancy (third trimester) and in the postpartum period [22] Possible reasons for this increase in risk include a prothrombotic hematological state in pregnancy and vasculature injury from vaginal delivery [23].

The vague presentation of cerebral venous and sinus thrombosis makes this pathology difficult to diagnose. More severe symptoms, such as focal neurological deficits and seizures have also been reported and should prompt providers to involve neurological specialists. MRI imaging is the most sensitive modality for diagnosing cerebral venous and sinus thrombosis, often revealing characteristic signs such as hyperintense signals [24]. Vigilance by the provider, and a multidisciplinary approach to these patients, prompting timely imaging and diagnosis, is instrumental as severe cases can lead to cerebral herniation and hemorrhage [25].

Epilepsy

Estrogen has been shown in previous studies to be associated with higher rates of seizure frequency [26]. However, a recent systematic review found no differences in the rate of seizure activity in pregnant patients with epilepsy. Hormonal fluctuations in pregnancy, therefore, may not present a clear risk for seizure development as previously believed. Optimal pharmacologic therapy may present the best prevention for seizure free activity in pregnancy, as an important predictor of seizure free activity during the peripartum period is seizure free activity at least 9 months before pregnancy [27].

However, maternal mortality rates are increased in women with epilepsy [28]. Pharmacokinetic changes including increases in renal clearance and hepatic metabolism, and decreases in serum binding protein, can lead to a decrease in serum levels of many anti- seizure medications during pregnancy, often necessitating escalating doses. Given the pharmacokinetic variability between individuals, serum monitoring of anticonvulsants as possible during pregnancy is recommended [29].

Older anticonvulsants, such as valproic acid, have been associated with congenital malformations and long term neurobehavioral conditions [30]. Although large trials assessing the safety of new anticonvulsant medications are lacking, more recently developed medications, such as lamotrigine and levetiracetam, have been shown to have a greater safety profile in pregnancy [30, 31]. Optimal planning with an epileptic patient wishing to become pregnant is recommended to avoid teratogenic anticonvulsants, developing an optimal pharmacologic regimen with seizure free activity prior to conception and serum monitoring during pregnancy.

References

1. Gaiser R. Chestnut's obstetric anesthesia: principles and practice, fifth edition: physiologic changes in pregnancy fifth edition ed. Philadelphia; Elsevier. 2014.
2. Bernstein IM, Ziegler W, Badger GJ. Plasma volume expansion in early pregnancy. Obstet Gynecol. 2001;97(5 Pt 1):669–72.
3. de Haas S, Ghossein-Doha C, van Kuijk SM, van Drongelen J, Spaanderman ME. Physiological adaptation of maternal plasma volume during pregnancy: a systematic review and meta-analysis. Ultrasound Obstet Gynecol. 2017;49(2):177–87.
4. Gerbasi FR, Bottoms S, Farag A, Mammen E. Increased intravascular coagulation associated with pregnancy. Obstet Gynecol. 1990;75(3 Pt 1):385–9.
5. Robson SC, Hunter S, Moore M, Dunlop W. Haemodynamic changes during the puerperium: a Doppler and M-mode echocardiographic study. Br J Obstet Gynaecol. 1987;94(11):1028–39.
6. Dunlop W. Serial changes in renal haemodynamics during normal human pregnancy. Br J Obstet Gynaecol. 1981;88(1):1–9.
7. Sims EA, Krantz KE. Serial studies of renal function during pregnancy and the puerperium in normal women. J Clin Invest. 1958;37(12):1764–74.
8. West CA, Sasser JM, Baylis C. The enigma of continual plasma volume expansion in pregnancy: critical role of the renin-angiotensin-aldosterone system. Am J Physiol Ren Physiol. 2016;311(6):F1125–34.
9. Barron WM, Durr JA, Schrier RW, Lindheimer MD. Role of hemodynamic factors in osmoregulatory alterations of rat pregnancy. Am J Phys. 1989;257(4 Pt 2):R909–16.
10. Irons DW, Baylis PH, Davison JM. Effect of atrial natriuretic peptide on renal hemodynamics and sodium excretion during human pregnancy. Am J Phys. 1996;271(1 Pt 2):F239–42.
11. Sabers A, Tomson T. Managing antiepileptic drugs during pregnancy and lactation. Curr Opin Neurol. 2009;22(2):157–61.
12. Tomson T, Palm R, Kallen K, et al. Pharmacokinetics of levetiracetam during pregnancy, delivery, in the neonatal period, and lactation. Epilepsia. 2007;48(6):1111–6.
13. Karlsson O, Sporrong T, Hillarp A, Jeppsson A, Hellgren M. Prospective longitudinal study of thromboelastography and standard hemostatic laboratory tests in healthy women during normal pregnancy. Anesth Analg. 2012;115(4):890–8.
14. Institute of Medicine. Iron deficiency anemia: Recommended guidelines for the prevention, detection, and management among US children and women of childbearing age. https://www.nap.edu/catalog/2251/iron-deficiency-anemia-recommended-guidelines-for-the-prevention-detection-and. Accessed on 22 Nov 2017.
15. American College of O, Gynecologists' Committee on Practice B-O. Practice bulletin no. 166: thrombocytopenia in pregnancy. Obstet Gynecol. 2016;128(3):e43–53.
16. Samuels P, Bussel JB, Braitman LE, et al. Estimation of the risk of thrombocytopenia in the offspring of pregnant women with presumed immune thrombocytopenic purpura. N Engl J Med. 1990;323(4):229–35.
17. Thornton P, Douglas J. Coagulation in pregnancy. Best Pract Res Clin Obstet Gynaecol. 2010;24(3):339–52.
18. Bateman BT, Olbrecht VA, Berman MF, Minehart RD, Schwamm LH, Leffert LR. Peripartum subarachnoid hemorrhage: nationwide data and institutional experience. Anesthesiology. 2012;116(2):324–33.
19. Bader A. Chestnut's obstetric anesthesia: principles and practice, 5th edition: neurologic and neuromuscular disease. Philadelphia; Elsevier. 2014.
20. Ng J, Kitchen N. Neurosurgery and pregnancy. J Neurol Neurosurg Psychiatry. 2008;79(7):745–52.
21. Stam J. Thrombosis of the cerebral veins and sinuses. N Engl J Med. 2005;352(17):1791–8.
22. Saposnik G, Barinagarrementeria F, Brown RD Jr, et al. Diagnosis and management of cerebral venous thrombosis: a statement for healthcare professionals from the American Heart Association/American Stroke Association. Stroke. 2011;42(4):1158–92.
23. Suresh M. Shnider and Levinson's anesthesia for obstetrics. Lippincott Williams &Wilkins; 2013.
24. Lafitte F, Boukobza M, Guichard JP, et al. MRI and MRA for diagnosis and follow-up of cerebral venous thrombosis (CVT). Clin Radiol. 1997;52(9):672–9.
25. Ferro JM, Canhao P, Stam J, Bousser MG, Barinagarrementeria F, Investigators I. Prognosis of cerebral vein and dural sinus thrombosis: results of the International Study on Cerebral Vein and Dural Sinus Thrombosis (ISCVT). Stroke. 2004;35(3):664–70.
26. Kaplan PW, Norwitz ER, Ben-Menachem E, et al. Obstetric risks for women with epilepsy during pregnancy. Epilepsy Behav. 2007;11(3):283–91.
27. Harden CL, Hopp J, Ting TY, et al. Practice parameter update: management issues for women with epilepsy – focus on pregnancy (an evidence-based review): obstetrical complications and change in seizure frequency: report of the quality standards subcommittee and therapeutics and technology assessment subcommittee of the american academy of neurology and american epilepsy society. Neurology. 2009;73(2):126–32.
28. Edey S, Moran N, Nashef L. SUDEP and epilepsy-related mortality in pregnancy. Epilepsia. 2014;55(7):e72–4.
29. Nau H, Kuhnz W, Egger HJ, Rating D, Helge H. Anticonvulsants during pregnancy and lactation. Transplacental, maternal and neonatal pharmacokinetics. Clin Pharmacokinet. 1982;7(6):508–43.
30. Tomson T, Battino D. Teratogenic effects of antiepileptic drugs. Lancet Neurol. 2012;11(9):803–13.
31. Hernandez-Diaz S, Smith CR, Shen A, Mittendorf R, Hauser WA, Yerby M, Holmes LB, North American AED Pregnancy Registry; North American AED Pregnancy Registry. Comparative safety of antiepileptic drugs during pregnancy. Neurology. 2012;78(21):1692–9.

Epilepsy and Pregnancy

Mariel Velez and Kimford J. Meador

Prepregnancy Planning

It is very important to achieve seizure control prior to pregnancy. The most salient predictor of seizures during pregnancy is the presence of seizures before pregnancy [1]. If a WWE is seizure free for at least 9 months prior to pregnancy, they have a 84–92% chance of remaining seizure-free during pregnancy [2]. In addition to the risks that seizures pose to the mother (injury, risks related to convulsions, sudden unexpected death in epilepsy), seizures can also pose a risk to the fetus. When compared to WWE without seizures during pregnancy, pregnant WWE who have seizures have an increased risk of having infants that are small for gestational age [3]. The occurrence of one or more convulsions during pregnancy is associated with having a shorter gestational age, a five times higher preterm risk and reduced birth weight in boys [4]. According to a large, multi-country pregnancy registry (EURAP), for most WWE (63.6%), seizure frequency remains the same throughout their pregnancy, with 92.7% of those women remaining seizure free [5]. However seizure frequency in many women can go up or down over the course of their pregnancy, without any consistent pattern across studies [2].

A family planning discussion should occur in any WWE of childbearing age during the initial clinic visit, especially if an AED prescribed. This should include: (1) a discussion about if/when the patient is planning for pregnancy, (2) whether the patient is on the most efficacious contraception if they are not planning a pregnancy, (3) which AEDs are most appropriate for the patient with the lowest teratogenic risk, (4) whether the patient's seizures are well controlled on the lowest possible AED dose, and (5) the need for ongoing folic acid supplementation. A 2017 study by Herzog et al. has reemphasized the need to have these discussions even when the patient is not planning for a pregnancy: almost 80% of WWE in their study who became pregnant after their seizure diagnosis reported having at least one unintended pregnancy [6]. Most WWE taking a potentially teratogenic AED do not take contraception at all [7]. Not surprisingly, WWE under the age of 18 are the most at risk for having an unintended pregnancy, which underscores the need to have discussions about sexual activity and contraception in teenagers with epilepsy.

What is the best way to achieve seizure control while minimizing the risks of AED related fetal complications? The goal should be seizure freedom at the lowest possible AED dose. If the patient is planning for pregnancy more than a year from conception, physicians should consider any further evaluation prior to pregnancy, such as inpatient monitoring, consideration of epilepsy surgery if appropriate, AED adjustments, and establishing baseline AED therapeutic levels. Preconception counseling during this time should include a discussion about: (1) what AEDs pose the least risk to the fetus while maintaining the best seizure control for the patient, (2) medication changes if the patient is on an AED with higher rates of teratogenesis such as valproic acid (VPA), (3) potentially decreasing the dose of current AEDs if the patient has been well controlled, and (4) possible withdrawal of AEDs if the patient has been seizure free for 2–4 years, depending on risk factors [8]. In addition, it is important to emphasize the need for contraception during this time and to continue folic acid supplementation. If the patient is currently attempting conception, AED changes or adjustments should only be made if the benefits outweigh the risks. As discussed previously, the best predictor of whether a patient will have a seizure during pregnancy is whether they have been seizure-free for 9–12 months prior to pregnancy, thus medication adjustments should be made prior to pregnancy in an attempt to achieve seizure freedom prior to pregnancy.

M. Velez (✉)
California Pacific Medical Center, California Pacific Neurosciences Institute, San Francisco, CA, USA

K. J. Meador
Department of Neurology and Neurological Sciences, Stanford University, Palo Alto, CA, USA
e-mail: kmeador@stanford.edu

© Springer Nature Switzerland AG 2019
M. A. O'Neal (ed.), *Neurology and Psychiatry of Women*, https://doi.org/10.1007/978-3-030-04245-5_14

Best and Worst AED Choices for Childbearing WWE

Fetal AED exposure in the first trimester increases the risk for birth defects. These defects include major congenital malformations (MCMs), defined as abnormalities that interfere with organ structure or function and may require a major intervention such as surgery. These include anomalies such as cleft palates, neural tube defects, skeletal defects, craniosynostosis, hypospadias and cardiovascular malformations. Most of these defects occur between 3 and 10 weeks of pregnancy, often before the patient even realizes she is pregnant. In the general population, MCMs occur at a rate of 1–3%, and WWE who are not taking AEDs have similar rates. In WWE who are taking AEDs, the overall rate of MCMs are approximately two to three fold higher [9]. However, these rates are based primarily on exposure to older generation AEDs, and recent studies suggest considerable variability across specific AEDs. Not only is there an increased risk of major birth defects, but fetal exposure to certain AEDs, especially VPA, also show poor cognitive and behavioral outcomes in children exposed in utero. Unfortunately, these deficiencies are typically only detected when the child has grown beyond infancy. We will review available AED choices and their teratogenic potential from the poorest choices to the best choices in the following discussion.

Based on the present data, VPA is the worst first choice for women of childbearing potential. Data from many large international pregnancy registries have consistently demonstrated that the risk for congenital MCMs with VPA exposure is high; risks from the two largest registries is 9–10% [10, 11]. These MCMs include neural tube defects, hypospadias, cleft palates, craniosynostosis, and cardiac septal defects. According to data analyzed from the European Surveillance of Congenital Anomalies (EUROCAT) registry, the rates of spina bifida in fetuses exposed to VPA were particularly high (12–16%) depending on the control group) [12]. Furthermore, the association between MCMs and VPA is dose dependent [10, 12–14]; however, MCMs were seen at doses below what most clinicians would consider a standard adult dose for epilepsy (as low as 500 mg/day).

In addition to MCMs, VPA exposure has also been associated with poor cognitive, psychomotor and behavioral outcomes. In a large meta-analysis of neurodevelopmental defects in children exposed to AEDs, VPA alone, or in combination with other AEDS, was associated with a significantly increased risk of cognitive and psychomotor developmental delay [15]. Children born to WWE who took VPA during pregnancy have a decrease in mean IQ by 10 points compared to other AEDs and a control group, even after accounting for maternal IQ [16–18]; this effect is dose dependent. Specific cognitive domains also are affected by VPA exposure: children of WWE who took VPA in the first trimester showed an risk of language deficits [16–19]. Although valproate's effect on cognition is dose dependent, a safe dose is unclear. In one study, even fetal exposure below 800 mg/day were associated with impaired verbal IQ, and these children were more likely to require special educational assistance [18]. In addition, there is a significantly increased risk of autism spectrum disorder and childhood autism in children born to mothers who took VPA during their pregnancy. In a population based study of all children born in Denmark between 1996 and 2006, there was an absolute risk of autism spectrum disorder (4.15%) and childhood autism (2.95%), among 432 children of WWE exposed to VPA vs. respective risks of 2.44% and 1.02% for children not exposed to VPA [20].

While there have been multiple studies on various rates of MCMS for AEDs other than VPA, many of these studies have been small, underpowered or poorly designed, often resulting in conflicting data. A large, comparative meta-analysis published in 2017, sought to rectify this as well as examine the comparative safety of different AED exposures in utero. Veroniki et al. performed a network meta-analysis of 96 high quality studies, and demonstrated that phenobarbital (PB), topiramate (TPM), phenytoin (PHT), ethosuximide (ESM), and carbamazepine (CBZ) (as well as VPA) were all associated with increased risk for MCMs [21]. Their study, as well as others, also revealed that certain AEDs may have a higher probability of having particular MCMs associated with them. This is a salient point given that some MCMs, such as cardiac or neural tube defects, are more potentially life threatening than MCMs which only require comparatively minor surgical interventions (such as hypospadias and cleft lip/palates). ESM, primidone (PRM), TPM, PHB, PHT, and VPA were all associated with a higher risk of developing cleft/lip palate than controls. An increased risk of hypospadias was seen in gabapentin (GBP), clonazepam (CLO), PRM, and VPA. Cardiac malformations were seen in GBP exposure, as well as some polytherapy combinations; however, GBP did not have a higher risk of MCMs overall making this result difficult to interpret. Analysis of fetal risks with newer AEDs from multiple studies have shown that an association between TPM and cleft/lip palate and hypospadias is strong [22]. Prior large registry-based studies have shown an association between PB and cardiovascular malformations [11] as well as CBZ and neural tube defects [12, 23].

Lamotrigine (LTG) and levetiracetam (LEV), represent the safest choices for WWE of childbearing potential based on current data. In the large meta-analysis by Veroniki et al., mentioned above, LEV and LTG were not associated with an increased risk of MCMs. Other studies have demonstrated that, if there is an increased risk for MCMs with LTG and LEV, that risk is small (~2 to 3%) [11, 24, 25].

There appears to be a slight dose dependent increase in the rate of MCMs for lamotrigine; according to data from the EURAP registry, there was an increase in MCMs from 2% at doses <=300 mg/day to 4.5% at doses > than 300 mg/day [14], however other studies have not shown a similar dose dependence.

In terms of cognitive outcomes for AEDs other than VPA, a 2014 Cochrane review of 22 prospective cohort and 6 registry studies did not show consistent deficits with *in utero* exposure to non-VPA AEDs. Studies since then have shown no cognitive deficits for LEV or TPM [26]. In a recent study by Baker et al., while carbamazepine did not have a significant effect on IQ, it was associated with reduced verbal abilities and increased frequency of IQ <85 [18]. A recent large meta-analysis of AEDs exposure in utero and neurodevelopmental outcomes, also by Veroniki et al., suggested that LTG and OXC may be associated with a slightly higher risk of autism, a result which needs to be confirmed by future studies [15].

In sum, it is important to note that despite the fact that most AEDs analyzed seem to carry at least a small increased risk for MCMs, analysis of four class III studies has shown that VPA exposure carries a higher risk to the fetus than all other AEDs combined [27]. There have been quite a few studies looking at risks of MCM and cognitive risks in polypharmacy with various AED combinations potentially causing fetal harm; a 2009 practice parameter states that polypharmacy should be avoided if possible given that it probably contributes to the development of MCMs in the offspring of WWE as compared to monotherapy [9]. However, newer data suggests that most of the risks seen with polypharmacy are driven by combinations that contain VPA [10, 28], but detailed data for multiple polypharmacy combinations are lacking. Furthermore, IQ deficits from VPA exposure are the most consistent cognitive deficit seen in AED exposure *in utero*. Thus, VPA is the main medication to avoid in a WWE of childbearing age. PB and TPM, likely pose intermediate risks for MCMs, CBZ and PHT have somewhat less risks, while LEV and LTG pose the least risk. This is summarized in Table 1.

There is a paucity of data regarding newer AEDs such as oxcarbazepine (OXC), pregabalin, (PGB) zonisamide (ZNS),

Table 1 Stratified risk for major congenital malformations in fetuses exposed to AEDs *in utero*

Risk	Antiepileptic drugs
High risk	Valproic acid
Intermediate risk	Phenobarbital, Topiramate
Low-intermediate risk	Carbamazepine, Phenytoin
Low risk	Levetiracetam, Lamotrigine
Unknown risk (needs more data)	Oxcarbazepine, Pregabalin, Zonisamide, Eslicarbazepine, Perampenal, Brivateracetam, Lacosamide, Clobazam

and no data to date on eslicarbazepine, perampenal, brivateracetam, clobazam and lacosamide in terms of their effect on the developing fetus. A 2016 Cochrane review of 50 studies (31 contributing to the meta-analysis) found no increased risk for MCMs with OXC or ZNS (as well as no increased risk for LEV, PRM, LTG and GBP); however, the authors did caution that there was far less data for these AEDs than for the older medications [29]. A similar result also found in a 2017 metananalysis for OXC; it did not find statistically significant risk to physical development with OXC compared to control; however, the authors cautioned that risks to the fetus could not be ruled out (given the low sample size) [21]. As mentioned above, this group found an increase in the rates of autism in OXC exposed children [15]. There is conflicting data regarding PGB and the risk for MCMs: a 2016 multicenter observational prospective study of 164 pregnancies exposed to PGB in the first trimester showed an increased risk for major birth defects as compared to controls (6% in the PGB group compared with 2.1% in the controls [30]. However, a larger cohort study, published in 2017 with 477 PGB exposed pregnancies showed no increased risks for MCMs [31]. Other than LEV, LTG and OXC, there is no neurocognitive data for any of the newer AEDs. Clearly, elucidating the possible risks for MCMs and/or neurocognitive deficits with these AEDs is an area ripe for further exploration.

Folic Acid Use in WWE

There are suggestions that taking folic acid during preconception and pregnancy may reduce the risk of miscarriage in WWE [32], and may be associated with higher IQs in children of WWE [16]. It makes at least theoretical sense that folic acid supplementation would prevent MCMs in fetuses exposed to AEDs that lower serum levels of folic acid (such as PB, CBZ, PHT and VPA). However, studies have yet to find a direct association between lowering of MCMs with folic acid supplementation in WWE [33, 34]. A 2009 practice parameter by the American Academy of Neurology and American Epilepsy Society examined the effects of folic acid on MCMs in WWE and concluded that there was level C evidence that preconceptional folic acid supplementation may reduce the risk of MCMs [27]. Based on the clear evidence for reduced MCMs in the general population, and the absence of adverse effects of folic acid supplementation, the practice parameter reasonably advised that WWE take folic acid supplementation at the current recommended dose for women of childbearing potential (0.4 mg/day). There is currently no data on the proper dose of folic acid in WWE, and it may be that higher doses would be more appropriate for WWE taking AEDs that interfere with folic acid. Further research is needed to determine the optimal dose of folic acid in WWE.

Epilepsy Management During Pregnancy

As discussed above, it is essential that seizures are controlled both prior and during pregnancy given that seizures can pose a significant risk both to the mother and the fetus. There is some data to suggest that seizure control during pregnancy may depend on the particular AED regimen. The largest study looking into this issue reported a higher risk of seizures in patients taking LTG or OXC [5, 10]. This may be related to the fact that both LTG and OXC rely heavily on glucuronidation for their metabolism; a system that is induced by estrogen. According to one study, in the majority of women, lamotrigine clearance increases by 200% over the course of pregnancy [35]. Several other AEDs have been shown to have marked and variable clearance changes during pregnancy including PHT, LEV and TPM [36, 37].

It is for this reason that careful monitoring of all AEDs is very important in order to maintain seizure control during pregnancy. In addition to the known changes that occur due to liver metabolism of AEDs, there is also significant individual variation in metabolism [35]. Prior to pregnancy, baseline levels of AED should be checked when the patient's seizures are well controlled. Once pregnant, we recommend checking AED levels monthly and adjusting AED doses accordingly. After birth AED metabolism can return quickly back to post partum levels; in the case of LTG this can occur within 1–3 weeks. A common strategy to avoid toxicity is to taper gradually over 1–3 weeks to the near prepregnancy dosages. Given that the patient is likely to be sleep deprived after birth, one may consider leaving the patient on a slightly higher dose than baseline for the first 1–3 months.

Breastfeeding in Pregnancy

Several studies have demonstrated that breastfeeding is safe for children of mothers who are taking an AED. In the general population, the benefits of breastfeeding are widely documented and include nutritional benefits, protection against common childhood infections, and improved survival during the 1st year, including a lower risk of Sudden Infant Death Syndrome [38]. Two studies in WWE showed no increased risk for poor cognitive outcomes at 3 years old [39, 40] and one study showed improved verbal outcomes at age 6 years old in infants that were breastfed [41]. It is important to counsel postpartum women that the benefits of breastfeeding outweigh the risks; however, certain precautions should be kept in mind. Awakening several times at night in order to feed the baby will cause sleep disruption that could lead to increased seizure frequency. We encourage family and friends to help with nighttime feedings so that the mother can get an uninterrupted 6–8 h of sleep.

References

1. Thomas SV, Syam U, Devi JS. Predictors of seizures during pregnancy in women with epilepsy. Epilepsia. 2012;53(5):2010–3.
2. Harden CL, Hopp J, Ting TY, Pennell PB, Jacqueline A, Hauser WA, et al. Management issues for women with epilepsy – focus on pregnancy (an evidence-based review): I. Obstetrical complications and change in seizure frequency neurology and the American Epilepsy. Society. 2009;50(5):1229–36.
3. Chen Y-H, Chiou H-Y, Lin H-C, Lin H-L. Affect of seizures during gestation on pregnancy outcomes in women with epilepsy. Arch Neurol. 2009;66(8):979–84.
4. Rauchenzauner M, Ehrensberger M, Prieschl M, Kapelari K, Bergmann M, Walser G, Neururer S, Unterberger I, Luef G. Generalized tonic–clonic seizures and antiepileptic drugs during pregnancy—a matter of importance for the baby? J Neurol. 2013;260(2):484–8.
5. Battino D, Tomson T, Bonizzoni E, Craig J, Lindhout D, Sabers A, et al. Seizure control and treatment changes in pregnancy: observations from the EURAP epilepsy pregnancy registry. Epilepsia. 2013;54(9):1621–7.
6. Herzog AG, Mandle HB, Cahill KE, Fowler KM, Hauser WA. Predictors of unintended pregnancy in women with epilepsy. Neurology. 2017;88:1–7.
7. Bhakta J, Bainbridge J, Borgelt L. Teratogenic medications and concurrent contraceptive use in women of childbearing ability with epilepsy. Epilepsy Behav [Internet]. 2015 [cited 2017 Sep 6];52:212–217. Available from: http://linkinghub.elsevier.com/retrieve/pii/S152550501500462X.
8. Gerard EE, Meador KJ. Managing epilepsy in women. Continuum (Minneap Minn). 2016;22:204–26.
9. Harden CL, Meador KJ, Pennell PB, Hauser WA, Gronseth GS, French JA, et al. Practice parameter update: management issues for women with epilepsy – focus on pregnancy (an evidence-based review): teratogenesis and perinatal outcomes. Neurology [Internet]. 2009;73(2):133–41.. Available from: http://www.neurology.org/content/73/2/133.abstract
10. Tomson T, Battino D, Bonizzoni E, Craig J, Lindhout D, Perucca E, et al. Dose-dependent teratogenicity of valproate in mono- and polytherapy: an observational study. Neurology. 2015;85(10):866–72.
11. Hernandez S, Shen A, Holmes LB. Comparative safety of antiepileptic drugs during pregnancy. Neurology. 2012;78:1692–9.
12. Janneke J, Loane M, Dolk H, Barisic I, Ester G, Garne E, Morris JK, de Jong-van den Berg L. Valproic acid monotherapy in pregnancy and major congenital malformations. N Engl J Med [Internet]. 2010;362(23):2185–93. https://doi.org/10.1056/NEJMoa0907328.
13. Campbell E, Kennedy F, Russell A, Smithson WH, Parsons L, Morrison PJ, et al. Malformation risks of antiepileptic drug monotherapies in pregnancy: updated results from the UK and Ireland Epilepsy and Pregnancy Registers. J Neurol Neurosurg Psychiatry [Internet]. 2014;85(9):1029 LP–1034.. Available from: http://jnnp.bmj.com/content/85/9/1029.abstract
14. Tomson T, Battino D, Bonizzoni E, Craig J, Lindhout D, Sabers A, et al. Dose-dependent risk of malformations with antiepileptic drugs: an analysis of data from the EURAP epilepsy and pregnancy registry. Lancet Neurol [Internet]. 2011;10(7):609–17. https://doi.org/10.1016/S1474-4422(11)70107-7.
15. Veroniki AA, Rios P, Cogo E, Straus SE, Finkelstein Y, Kealey R, et al. Comparative safety of antiepileptic drugs for neurological development in children exposed during pregnancy and breast feeding: a systematic review and network meta-analysis. BMJ Open [Internet]. 2017;7(7):e017248. https://doi.org/10.1136/bmjopen-2017-017248.
16. Meador KJ, Baker GA, Browning N, Cohen MJ, Bromley RL, Clayton-Smith J, et al. Fetal antiepileptic drug exposure and cogni-

tive outcomes at age 6 years (NEAD study): a prospective observational study. Lancet Neurol [Internet]. 2013;12(3):244–52. https://doi.org/10.1016/S1474-4422(12)70323-X.

17. Meador KJ, Baker GA, Browning N, Cohen MJ, Bromley RL, Clayton-Smith J, et al. Effects of fetal antiepileptic drug exposure: outcomes at age 4.5 years. Neurology. 2012;78(16):1207–14.

18. Baker GA, Bromley RL, Briggs M, Cheyne CP, Cohen MJ, García-Fiñana M, et al. IQ at 6 years after in utero exposure to antiepileptic drugs: a controlled cohort study. Neurology. 2015;84(4):382–90.

19. Nadebaum C, Anderson V, Vajda F, Reutens D, Barton S, Wood A. Language skills of school-aged children prenatally exposed to antiepileptic drugs. Neurology. 2011;76(8):719–26.

20. Christensen J, Grønborg TK, Sørensen MJ, Schendel D, Parner ET, Pedersen LH, et al. Prenatal valproate exposure and risk of autism spectrum disorders and childhood autism. JAMA [Internet]. 2013;309(16):1696. https://doi.org/10.1001/jama.2013.2270.

21. Veroniki AA, Cogo E, Rios P, Straus SE, Finkelstein Y, Kealey R, et al. Comparative safety of anti-epileptic drugs during pregnancy: a systematic review and network meta-analysis of congenital malformations and prenatal outcomes. BMC Med [Internet]. 2017;15(1):95. https://doi.org/10.1186/s12916-017-0845-1.

22. de Jong J, Garne E, de Jong-Van den Berg LTW, Wang H. The risk of specific congenital anomalies in relation to newer antiepileptic drugs: a literature review. Drugs Real World Outcome [Internet]. 2016;3(2):131–43.. Available from: http://www.ncbi.nlm.nih.gov/pmc/articles/PMC4914544/

23. Werler MM, Ahrens KA, Bosco JLF, Mitchell AA, Anderka MT, Gilboa SM, et al. Use of antiepileptic medications in pregnancy in relation to risks of birth defects. Ann Epidemiol [Internet]. 2017;21(11):842–50. https://doi.org/10.1016/j.annepidem.2011.08.002.

24. Meador K, Reynolds MW, Crean S, Fahrbach K, Probst C. Pregnancy outcomes in women with epilepsy: a systematic review and meta-analysis of published pregnancy registries and cohorts. Epilepsy Res [Internet]. 2008;81(1):1–13.. Available from: http://www.ncbi.nlm.nih.gov/pmc/articles/PMC2660205/

25. Tomson T, Battino D. Teratogenic effects of antiepileptic drugs. Lancet Neurol. 2012;11(9):803–13.

26. Bromley RL, Calderbank R, Cheyne CP, Rooney C, Trayner P, Clayton-Smith J, et al. Cognition in school-age children exposed to levetiracetam, topiramate, or sodium valproate. Neurology. 2016;87(18):1943–53.

27. Harden CL, Pennell PB, Koppel BS, Hovinga CA, Gidal B, Meador KJ, et al. Management issues for women with epilepsy-focus on pregnancy (an evidence-based review): III. Vitamin K, folic acid, blood levels, and breast-feeding. Epilepsia [Internet]. 2009;50(5):1247–55. https://doi.org/10.1111/j.1528-1167.2009.02130.x.

28. Holmes LB, Mittendorf R, Shen A, Smith CR, Hernandez-Diaz S. Fetal effects of anticonvulsant polytherapies: different risks from different drug combinations. Arch Neurol [Internet]. 2011;68(10):1275–81. https://doi.org/10.1001/archneurol.2011.133.

29. Weston J, Bromley R, Jackson CF, Adab N, Clayton-Smith J, Greenhalgh J, et al. Monotherapy treatment of epilepsy in pregnancy: congenital malformation outcomes in the child. In: Bromley R, editor. Cochrane Database of Systematic Reviews [Internet]. Chichester: Wiley; 2016. https://doi.org/10.1002/14651858.CD010224.pub2.

30. Winterfeld U. Pregnancy outcome following maternal exposure to pregabalin may call for concern. Neurology. 2016;86(24):2251–7.

31. Patorno E, Bateman BT, Huybrechts KF, Macdonald SC, Cohen JM, Panchaud A, et al. Pregabalin use early in pregnancy and the risk of major congenital malformations. 2017;88(21):2020–5.

32. Pittschieler S, Brezinka C, Jahn B, Trinka E, Unterberger I, Dobesberger J, et al. Spontaneous abortion and the prophylactic effect of folic acid supplementation in epileptic women undergoing antiepileptic therapy. J Neurol [Internet]. 2008;255(12):1926–31. https://doi.org/10.1007/s00415-008-0029-1.

33. Morrow JI, Hunt SJ, Russell AJ, Smithson WH, Parsons L, Robertson I, et al. Folic acid use and major congenital malformations in offspring of women with epilepsy: a prospective study from the UK Epilepsy and Pregnancy Register. J Neurol Neurosurg Psychiatry [Internet]. 2009;80(5):506 LP–511.. Available from: http://jnnp.bmj.com/content/80/5/506.abstract

34. Jentink J, Bakker MK, Nijenhuis CM, Wilffert B, de Jong-van den Berg LTW. Does folic acid use decrease the risk for spina bifida after in utero exposure to valproic acid? Pharmacoepidemiol Drug Saf [Internet]. 2010. [cited 2017 Oct 27];19(8):803–7. https://doi.org/10.1002/pds.1975.

35. Polepally AR, Pennell PB, Brundage RC, Stowe ZN, Newport DJ, Viguera AC, et al. Model-based lamotrigine clearance changes during pregnancy: clinical implication. Ann Clin Transl Neurol. 2014;1(2):99–106.

36. Vajda FJE, O'Brien T, Lander C, Graham J, Eadie M. The efficacy of the newer antiepileptic drugs in controlling seizures in pregnancy. Epilepsia. 2014;55(8):1229–34.

37. Reisinger TL, Newman M, Loring DW, Pennell PB, Meador KJ. Antiepileptic drug clearance and seizure frequency during pregnancy in women with epilepsy. Epilepsy Behav [Internet]. 2013;29(1):13–8.. Available from: http://www.ncbi.nlm.nih.gov/pmc/articles/PMC3775962/

38. Breastfeeding and the use of human milk. Pediatrics [Internet]. 2012;129(3):e827 LP–e841. Available from: http://pediatrics.aappublications.org/content/129/3/e827.abstract.

39. Meador KJ, Baker GA, Browning N, Clayton-Smith J, Combs-Cantrell DT, Cohen M, et al. Effects of breastfeeding in children of women taking antiepileptic drugs. Neurology. 2010;75(22):1954–60.

40. Veiby G, Engelsen BA, Gilhus NE. Early child development and exposure to antiepileptic drugs prenatally and through breastfeeding. JAMA Neurol [Internet]. 2013;70(11):1367. Available from: https://doi.org/10.1001/jamaneurol.2013.4290.

41. Meador KJ, Baker GA, Browning N, Cohen MJ, Bromley RL, Clayton-Smith J, et al. Breastfeeding in children of women taking antiepileptic drugs. JAMA Pediatr [Internet]. 2014;168(8):729. https://doi.org/10.1001/jamapediatrics.2014.118.

Headaches in Pregnancy and Postpartum

Mary Angela O'Neal

Introduction

Headache during pregnancy and the postpartum period is one of the most common reasons for neurologic consultation. Over 90% of these headaches are primary and benign [1]. However there are a number of secondary causes of headache for which the neurologist must be vigilant and aware of concerning features in the history and exam that warrant further investigation. In addition, how to manage headaches in pregnancy and postpartum raises special issues around medication safety both as regards potential teratogenicity and safety during breast feeding. This chapter will review the most common primary headache, migraine, as well as some of the secondary headaches which occur during pregnancy and postpartum. A practical approach to diagnosis and management will be emphasized.

General Considerations

There are a number of features on the history and exam which should raise concern that the headache may not be benign. These are listed in Fig. 1. The time of onset of the headache is another helpful feature in predicting the likely etiology. For example, PEE would be rare prior to 20 weeks of gestation, so would be an unlikely cause for a first trimester headache. The hypercoaguable changes in pregnancy are most pronounced in the last trimester and the first 6 weeks postpartum [2]. Thus, this is the time that CVT is most often encountered. See Fig. 2.

Medications are classified as to their safety during pregnancy. See Table 1 I have a couple of salient points about this classification. First, a medication's classification may change by trimester. An example of this are the nonsteroidal anti-inflammatory medications which are class B in the second trimester, but class D in the third trimester due to their association with premature closure of the patent ductus arteriosis. Next, a medication's risk is disease specific. So if the medication is being used for a more serious disorder such as epilepsy it could be classified differently than when being used for a more benign disorder such as migraine. Valproate is class D when used for epilepsy, but a class X when used for migraine. Last, the drug classification is based on currently available knowledge such that the classification may not be so reliable for newer medications.

Imaging

In the case where the history or physical exam raises a concern appropriate imaging should be obtained. The imaging should adequately exclude the concerning diagnoses and be aligned with the situation acuity. In an emergency situation, such as stroke or intracranial hemorrhage, a computerized axial tomography (CT) scan or CT angiography should be obtained. The radiation dose from such imaging is orders of magnitude less than that known to cause fetal harm, so called deterministic effects, and maternal well being takes precedent [3]. However, there still can be stochastic effects-

- New onset headaches without prior history
- Change in headache character or pattern
- Wake up headaches
- Cough headache
- Associated with elevated blood pressure
- Thunderclap onset
- Exertional/valsalva component
- Abnormal neurologic exam
- Headaches associated with systemic disorders

Fig. 1 Concerning headache features

M. A. O'Neal (✉)
Department of Neurology, Brigham and Women's Hospital, Boston, MA, USA
e-mail: maoneal@bwh.harvard.edu

© Springer Nature Switzerland AG 2019
M. A. O'Neal (ed.), *Neurology and Psychiatry of Women*, https://doi.org/10.1007/978-3-030-04245-5_15

Fig. 2 Frequency of headache type by trimester

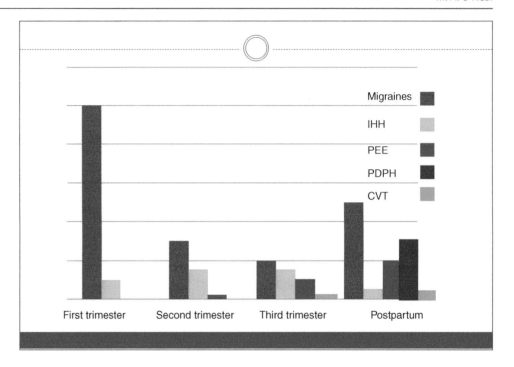

defined as an effect for which there is no threshold for it to occur like cancer- you either have it or not.

When imaging is not an emergency, magnetic resonance imaging (MRI) is preferred over CT. Vessel imaging can be obtained with time of flight technology and gadolinium is avoided. There have been no documented deleterious effects from MRI. Gadolinium is avoided due to concerns over fetal kidney injury [4]. Table 2 summarizes historical features and radiographic imaging that can be helpful to distinguish different headache types.

Migraine

Definitions

The International Classification of Headache Disorders, ICHD, defines migraine without aura (common migraine) as at least five headaches lasting four or up to 72 h which have at least two of the following characteristics: are unilateral, pulsating in quality, of moderate to severe intensity and aggravated by physical activity. In addition, they have one of the following: nausea, vomiting, photophobia or phonophobia. Last, the headaches cannot be attributable to another disorder.

Migraine with aura (classic migraine) is defined by the ICHD as headaches which fulfill the same criteria as migraine without aura and have two attacks which fulfill criteria of classic aura. The aura symptoms can be visual, sensory, speech or language, motor or related to brainstem symptoms.

Further the aura has to have at least two of the following four characteristics:

1. At least one aura symptom spreads gradually over 5 min, and/or two or more symptoms occur in succession
2. Each individual aura symptom lasts 5–60 min
3. At least one aura symptom is unilateral
4. The aura is accompanied, or followed within 1 h, by headache

Epidemiology in Pregnancy and Postpartum

Prospective studies have shown migraine improvement generally by the second trimester with a decrease in frequency migraines ranging from 77% to 83% [5–7]. Menstrually triggered migraines are more frequent in migraneurs without aura. Although pregnancy has a beneficial effect on both forms of migraine, studies show that a higher percent of migraineurs without aura improve as compared to women who had migraine with aura, 77% versus 44% [8].

Migraine is associated with both an increased risk of pre-eclampsia and gestational hypertension. In one report of primiparous women with migraine compared with those without migraine, the association with migraine before pregnancy was reported by 16% of pre-eclamptic women compared to only 8% of controls [9]. Other studies have corroborated the finding that women with a history of migraines had a 1.8-fold increased risk of preeclampsia [10].

Table 1 Medications are classified as to their safety during pregnancy

FDA pharmaceutical pregnancy categories

A Adequate and well controlled human studies have failed to demonstrate a risk to the fetus in the first trimester of pregnancy (and there is no risk in later trimesters).

B Animal reproduction studies have failed to demonstrate a risk to the fetus and there are no adequate and well controlled studies in pregnant women OR Animal studies have shown an adverse effect, but adequate and well-controlled studies in pregnant women have failed to demonstrate a risk to the fetus in any trimester.

C Animal reproduction studies have shown an adverse effect on the fetus and there are no adequate and well-controlled studies in humans, but potential benefits may warrant use of the drug in pregnant women despite potential risks.

D There is positive evidence of human fetal risk based on adverse reaction data from investigational or marketing experience or studies in humans, but potential benefits may warrant use of the drug in pregnant women despite potential risks

X Studies in animals or humans have demonstrated fetal abnormalities and/or there is positive evidence of human fetal risk based on adverse reaction data from investigational or marketing experience, and the risks involved in use of the drug in pregnant women clearly outweigh potential benefits.

Table 2 Summarizes historical features and radiographic imaging that can be helpful to distinguish different headache types

Historical features	Headache type	Helpful radiographic studies
Thunderclap onset	SAH, RCVS, CVT	MRI, MRV, MRA
Postural	PDPH	MRI with gadolinium
First trimester	Likely migraine or tension type	None
Prior similar headache	Benign	Not needed
Hypertension, proteinuria	PEE	MRI

SAH subarachnoid hemorrhage, *MRV* magnetic resonance venogram, *MRA* magnetic resonance angiogram

Treatment

Given that migraine is a benign condition which often improves as pregnancy progresses, the general strategy is to start with behavioral treatments. Biofeedback, relaxation training and physical therapy can be beneficial in managing headaches.

Pharmacologic therapy is generally restricted to symptomatic rather than preventative medication. The logic behind this strategy is the following: it may take months to assess the effectiveness of a preventative therapy, the teratogenic risk of prophylactic medication does not warrant their use for a benign condition and migraines generally improve during pregnancy. Table 3 lists the pregnancy risk category and breast feeding safety of many of the commonly used symptomatic medications for migraine.

Table 3 Lists the pregnancy risk category and breast feeding safety of many of the commonly used symptomatic medications for migraine

Symptomatic therapies		
Generic name	Level of risk in pregnancy	Breastfeeding-hale lactation rating
Metoclopramide	B	L2
Nonsteroidal anti-inflammatory drugs	B (D in 3rd trimester)	L1-L2
Acetaminophen	B	L1
Triptans	C	L3
Prochlorperazine	C	L3
Magnesium	A (D when used in high doses over 3–5 days)	L1
Dihydroergotamine	X	L4
Butalbital	C	L3

Hale lactation ratings:

L1 SAFEST – Drug has been taken by many breastfeeding women without evidence of adverse effects in nursing infants OR controlled studies have failed to show evidence of risk.

L2 SAFER – Drug has been studied in a limited number of breastfeeding women without evidence of adverse effects in nursing infants.

L3 MODERATELY SAFE – Studies in breastfeeding have shown evidence for mild non-threatening adverse effects OR there are no studies in breastfeeding for a drug with possible adverse effects.

L4 POSSIBLY HAZARDOUS – Studies have shown evidence for risk to a nursing infant, but in some circumstances the drug may be used during breastfeeding.

L5 CONTRAINDICATED – Studies have shown significant risk to nursing infants. The drug should NOT be used during breastfeeding

Idiopathic Intracranial Hypertension (IIH)

Definition

IIH is defined by the ICHD as a headache caused by elevated cerebrospinal fluid pressure, CSF, >250 mm CSF as measured by a lumbar puncture. Causation is linked to the elevated CSF pressure by at least two of the following:

1. Headache has developed in temporal relation to IIH
2. Headache is relieved by reducing intracranial hypertension
3. Headache is aggravated in temporal relation to increase in intracranial pressure
4. The headache is not better accounted for by another diagnosis

Usually IIH is usually associated with papilledema, but not always. The character and location of the headache is quite variable. Typically, there are other associated symptoms including visual dimming or obscurations, postural tinnitus and sixth nerve palsies. IIH is strongly associated with obesity.

Epidemiology

IIH is increasing in incidence in parallel with the current epidemic of obesity [11]. The prevalence of obesity in pregnancy has increased from around 10% in the 1990s to 16–19% in 2006. IIH has a female to male ratio of 8:1. The incidence of IIH in women of childbearing age is 19.3/100000 in obese women [12]. The usual onset of IIH is in the first half of pregnancy and relapse of IIH usually happens before week 20 which corresponds to the time of maximal weight gain [13]. Loss of vision is the most devastating complication of IIH. In pregnancy the visual outcomes are the same as in the non-pregnant state [14].

Making the Diagnosis

Confirming the diagnosis of IIH in pregnancy is the same as in the non-pregnant state. Both the brain and venous sinuses need to be imaged to exclude mimics. MRI of the brain and cerebral veins without gadolinium is preferred over CT. If these studies are normal, a lumbar puncture should be performed to measure opening pressure. An ophthalmology referral should also be made to carefully follow the patient's visual fields [15].

Treatment

Treatment is focused on lowering the intracranial pressure. In pregnancy, controlled weight gain rather than weight loss is appropriate. A nutrition consult is helpful in managing these women. Acetazolamide is used in these women to control their intracranial pressure. No major congenital malformations have been reported associated with its use [13].

Preeclampsia/Eclampsia (PEE) Causing Headache

Definition

Pre-eclampsia (PE) is a multisystem organ disorder unique to human pregnancy and refers to the new onset of hypertension and either proteinuria or end-organ dysfunction or both after 20 weeks of gestation in a woman without a history of hypertension. Severe PE is marked by any of the following features: two blood pressures separated by 4 h above 160/110 mmHg, hepatic dysfunction, acute renal insufficiency, thrombocytopenia (platelet count <100,000/ μL), pulmonary edema, and cerebral or visual symptoms. One particularly severe form of PE is that associated with hemolytic anemia, elevated liver enzymes, and low platelets – the HELLP syndrome. Eclampsia is defined by the onset of seizures in a woman with PE. PE usually presents after 20 weeks of gestation and is typically improved after delivery of the placenta. However, PEE may occur postpartum.

Morbidity and Mortality

PEE is a significant cause of both maternal and fetal morbidity and mortality. It complicates 2–8% of pregnancies and accounts for 50,000–60,000 maternal deaths annually worldwide [16, 17]. The maternal risks include abruption placentae, disseminated coagulopathy, acute renal failure, stroke, hemorrhage, death and long term cardiovascular consequences. For the infant, the risks are premature birth, intrauterine growth restriction, hypoxic injury, and death, as well as long-term cardiovascular morbidity [18].

Pathophysiology

PEE is a placentally mediated multiorgan system disease. It is felt that abnormal placental implantation interfers with the development of a low capacitance placental unit. This results in ischemia, cytokine production, hypertension and endothelial injury. The manifestation depends on the end organ. For example, in the kidney endothelial dysfunction causes proteinuria, in the liver, coagulopathy and in the brain white matter edema. The posterior circulation has less ability to autoregulate so the endothelial dysfunction typically affects the posterior parietal occipital regions leading rise to the radiographic entity known as posterior reversible encephalopathy syndrome (PRES). See Fig. 3.

Treatment

Treatment of PEE includes rapid control of hypertension usually with intravenous labetolol, hydralazine or nicardipine and prevention and control of seizures. Magnesium is the agent which has been shown to be to be superior to antiepileptic medications for seizure prevention and control. In a landmark trial, women randomized to receive magnesium had a 67% lower risk of recurrent seizures compared to women who received phenytoin [19].

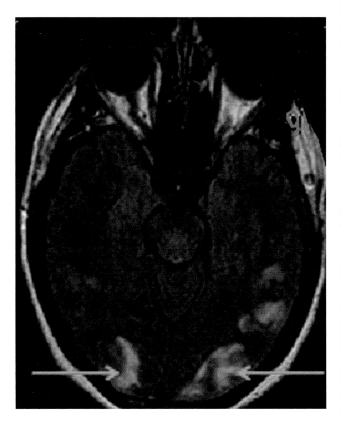

Fig. 3 Axial flair MRI showing typical white matter changes seen in posterior reversible encephalopathy syndrome in a woman with PEE

Reversible Cerebral Vasocontriction Syndrome (RCVS)

Definition

RCVS is characterized by thunderclap headaches, usually maximal in seconds. Other neurologic manifestations can include ischemic stroke, often in a border zone (end territory) distribution, hemorrhages both parenchymal as well as convexity subarachnoid bleeds. Vascular imaging shows diffuse segmental narrowing which usually spontaneously resolves by 3 months. RCVS is a monophasic illness usually lasting 1–2 weeks [20].

Epidemiology

The true incidence of RCVS is unknown as it has until recently likely been under reported. Two thirds of the cases occur in the 1st week postpartum [21]. This is likely due to the overlap of RCVS and PRES. In addition, RCVS can be precipitated by a number of vasoactive medications. Common culprits in the postpartum setting include bromocriptine which is used to inhibit lactation and ergometrine for postpartum hemorrhage.

Pathophysiology

It is known that there is a strong association between PEE and RCVS. The hypothesis is that the endothelial injury initiated by PEE makes the vessels more vulnerable to changes in vascular tone [21]. This can result in breakdown of vascular autoregulation causing PRES, vessel expansion and rupture causing subarachnoid or intracranial hemorrhage or vasospasm leading to ischemic stroke. See Fig. 4.

Treatment

Treatment for RCVS includes controlling blood pressure, symptomatic treatment of headaches and seizures as well as removal of any precipitating medications. Given the association of RCVS with endothelial injury, use of antihypertensive medications and magnesium even in the absence of PEE is often advocated [22]. The associated headaches have been shown to respond to calcium channel blockers, although they do not seem to be effective in treatment of vasospasm [23].

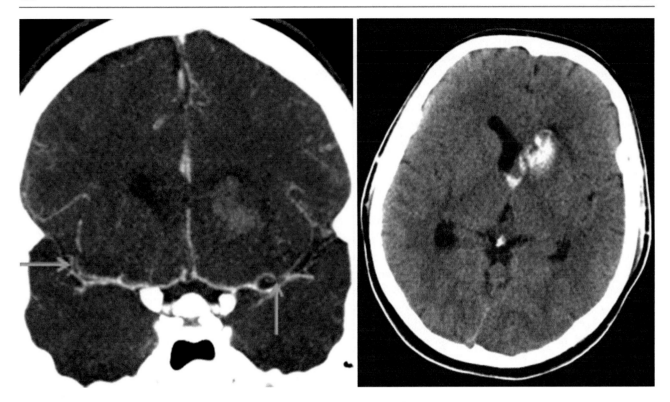

Fig. 4 Imaging findings seen in RCVS. Coronal MR angiogram on the left with arrows depicting areas of vasospasm in the middle cerebral arteries. On the right is the Head CT showing a left caudate hemorrhage with intraventricular extension

Cerebral Venous Thrombosis (CVT)

Epidemiology

In a study in a large tertiary care hospital, CVT occurred in 9 of approximately 1,000,000 pregnancies. Risk factors include dehydration, C- section, and older age. In eight of our nine cases, the women had some predisposing factor in addition to pregnancy, most commonly an underlying hypercoagulable state [24].

Pathophysiology and Clinical Manifestations

Pregnancy is a hypercoaguable state. Fibrin generation is increased and fibrinolytic activity is decreased. Levels of factors II, VII, VIII and X are all increased. Protein S and acquired resistance to activated protein C is common. The hypercoaguable condition is a normal response in preparation for birth to limit bleeding. It is maximal in the last trimester and persists to 6 weeks postpartum [2]. CVT causes venous congestion leading to increased intracranial pressure.

Common clinical manifestations include headache, seizures and focal deficits from hemorrhagic or ischemic stroke. The deficits are often multifocal/bilateral due to involvement of multiple veins, deep veins or the superior sagittal sinus. The headache may be thunderclap in onset or more insidious in onset related to the elevated intracranial pressure associated with visual obscurations and papilledema mimicking IIH.

Treatment

The treatment for CVT is anticoagulation even in the presence of hemorrhage [25, 26]. Warfarin is avoided in pregnancy due to teratogenic side effects. The length of anticoagulation depends on if any additional underlying hypercoagulable state is identified. If there is no other hypercoagulable condition discovered, anticoagulation is typically continued for about 6 months following CVT [27].

Postdural Puncture Headache (PDPH)

Definition

PDPH results following epidural anesthesia when there is a dural puncture. This results in a low pressure headache. Typically the headache is relieved when lying flat after 1–2 min and returns once the patient is upright. The postural nature of the headache is a characteristic feature, but this can decrease over time. The International Headache Society defines headache after lumbar puncture as a headache which worsens within 15 min of resuming the upright position and disappears or improves within 30 min of resuming the recumbent position and occurring within 1 week of a dural puncture [28]. Other clinical features besides the headache can include: dizziness, nausea, diplopia, tinnitus and hearing changes.

Epidemiology

There is a 1.5% risk of an accidental dural puncture in parturients. Of these, about half will result in PDPH. Nonmodifiable risk factors for PDPH include female sex, younger age, prior history of a headache disorder and a history of a prior PDPH. The modifiable risks which increase the incidence of PDPH include larger needle size, use of a cutting needle, orientation of needle bevel perpendicular rather than parallel to the long axis of the spine and difficulty in placing the epidural [29–31].

Pathophysiology

The leakage of cerebrospinal fluid causes the brain to sag resulting in stretching of the pain sensitive structures. In order to maintain the total volume of brain constituent's constant there is associated vasodilatation [32]. This pathophysiology explains the MRI findings in this condition which include: leptomeningeal enhancement, "pseudo- Chiari malformation" and apparent enlargement of the pituitary gland, (due to brain sagging) and subdural hematoma (from stretching of the bridging veins).

Treatment

Conservative management with bed rest and use of caffeine containing analgesics is the first line. In a review of over 10,000 patients with PDPH, 72% improved by 1 week [33]. For those who do not improve an epidural blood patch is the treatment of choice. Ninety percent of patients following a single epidural blood patch report dramatically improved headache [34].

Summary

- Headaches in pregnancy and the postpartum period are common.
- The majority of headache in pregnancy are benign.
- Secondary headaches are more commonly encountered in the third trimester and postpartum.

- A headache presenting with any red flags requires further evaluation.

References

1. Klein A, Loder E. Postpartum headache. Int J Obstet Anesth. 2010;19:422–30.
2. Kamel H, Babak N, Sriram N, et al. Risk of a thrombotic event after the 6-week postpartum period. N Engl J Med. 2014;370:1307–15.
3. McCollough CH, Schueler BA, Atwell TD, et al. Radiation exposure and pregnancy: when should we be concerned? Radiographics. 2007;27:909–17.
4. Patel SJ, Reede DL, Katz DS, et al. Imaging the pregnant patient for nonobstretric conditions: algorithms and radiation dose consideration. Radiographics. 2007;27:1705–22.
5. Somerville BW. A study of migraine in pregnancy. Neurology. 1972;22:824–8.
6. Sances G, Granella F, Nappi RE, et al. Course of migraine during pregnancy and postpartum: a prospective study. Cephalalgia. 2003;23(3):197–205.
7. Kvisvik EV, Stovner LJ, Helde G, et al. Headache and migraine during pregnancy and puerperium: the MIGRA-study. J Headache Pain. 2011;12(4):443–51.
8. Granella F, Sances G, Pucci E, et al. Migraine with aura and reproductive life events: a case control study. Cephalalgia. 2000;20(8):701–7.
9. Marcoux S, Bérubé SB, Brisson J, et al. History of migraine and risk of pregnancy-induced hypertension. Epidemiology. 1992;3:53–6.
10. Adeney KL, Williams MA, Miller RS, et al. Risk of preeclampsia in relation to maternal history of migraine headaches. J Matern Fetal Neonatal Med. 2005;18(3):167–72.
11. Durcan FJ, Corbett JJ, Wall M. The incidence of pseudotumor cerebri: population studies in Iowa and Louisiana. Arch Neurol. 1988;45:875–7.
12. Radhakrishnan K, Ahlskog JE, Cross SA, et al. Idiopathic intracranial hypertension (pseudotumor cerebri). Descriptive epidemiology in Rochester, Minn, 1976 to 1990. Arch Neurol. 1993;50(1):78–80.
13. Digre KB, Varner MW, Corbett JJ. Pseudotumor cerebri and pregnancy. Neurology. 1084;34:721–9.
14. Huna-Baron R, Kupersmith MJ. Idiopathic intracranial hypertension in pregnancy. J Neurol. 2002;249(8):1078–81.
15. Mollan SP, Markey KA, Benzimra JD, et al. A practical approach to, diagnosis, assessment and management of idiopathic intracranial hypertension. Pract Neurol. 2014;14(6):380–90.
16. Khan KS, Wojdyla D, Say L, Gulmezoglu AM, Van Look PFA. WHO analysis of causes of maternal death: systematic review. Lancet. 2006;367:1066–74.
17. Task force on hypertension in pregnancy. Hypertension in pregnancy 2013. American College of Obstetricians and Gynecologists.
18. Sibai B, Dekkar G, Kuperminc M. Pre-eclampsia. Lancet. 2005;365:785–99.
19. Lucas MJ, Leveno KJ, Cunningham FG. A comparison of magnesium sulfate with phenytoin for the prevention of eclampsia. NEJM Med. 1995;333:201–5.
20. Singhai AB, Hajj-Ali RA, Topcuoglu MA, et al. Reversible cerebral constriction syndromes: analysis of 130 cases. Arch Neurol. 2011;68(8):1005–12.
21. Ducros A, Bousser MG. Reversible cerebral vasoconstriction syndrome. Pract Neurol. 2009;9:256–67.
22. Singhal AB. Postpartum angiopathy with reversible posteriorleukoencephalopathy. Arch Neurol. 2004;61:411–6.

23. Chen SP, Fuh JL, Lirng JF, Chang FC, Wang SJ. Recurrent primary thunderclap headache and benign CNS angiopathy: spectra of the same disorder? Neurology. 2006;67:2164–9.

24. Feske SK, Klein AM, Ferrante KL. Clinical risk factors predict pregnancy-associated strokes. Stroke. 2009;40(4):e18.

25. Einhaupl KM, Villringer A, Meister W, et al. Heparin treatment in sinus venous thrombosis. Lancet. 1991;338:597–600.

26. de Bruijn SF, Stam J. Randomized, placebo-controlled trial of anti-coagulation treatment with low-molecular- weight heparin for cerebral sinus thrombosis. Stroke. 1999;30(3):484–8.

27. Saposnik G, Barinagarrementeria F, Brown RD, et al. Diagnosis and management of cerebral venous thrombosis a statement for healthcare professionals from the American Heart Association/ American Stroke Association. Stroke. 2011;42:1158–92.

28. Olsen J, Bousser MG, Diener H-C, et al. The international classification of headache disorders: 2nd edition. Cephalalgia. 2004;33(9):629–808.

29. Lybecker H, Møller JT, Ole M, et al. Incidence and prediction of postdural puncture headache a prospective study of 1021 spinal anesthesias. Anesth Analg. 1990;70:389–94.

30. Vilming ST, Schrader H, Monstad I. The significance of age, sex, and cerebrospinal fluid pressure in post-lumbar-puncture headache. Cephalalgia. 1989;9(2):99–106.

31. Kuntz KM, Kokmen E, Stevens JC, et al. Post-lumbar puncture headaches: experience in 501 consecutive procedures. Neurology. 1992;42(10):1884–7.

32. Bezov D, Lipton RB, Ashina S. Post-dural puncture headache: part I diagnosis, epidemiology, etiology, and pathophysiology. Headache. 2010;50(7):1144–52.

33. Vandam LD, Dripps RD. Long-term follow up of patients who received 10 098 spinal anesthetics. JAMA. 1956;161:586–91.

34. Bezov D, Ashina S, Lipton R. Post-dural puncture headache: part II – prevention, management, and prognosis. Headache. 2010;50(9):1482–98.

Stroke in Pregnancy

Steven K. Feske

Introduction: Importance and Magnitude of the Problem

Pregnancy has historically been a dangerous event, having taken many women in their youth and young adulthood. By lowering the risk dramatically, modern obstetrics has earned the right to be counted among the miracles of modern medicine. Although, stroke is a very uncommon complication of pregnancy, the risk to life and long-term function without disability that stroke confers makes this a serious medical concern.

Pathophysiology

Many physiologic changes of pregnancy prepare the mother to carry the developing fetus and to deliver a healthy baby. Several of these adaptive changes confer some increased risk of stroke. In addition, several pathologic conditions, some unique to pregnancy, also confer stroke risk [1, 2].

Hemodynamic Changes

Pregnancy represents a state of high metabolic, and so circulatory, demand. Increased aldosterone and renin lead to retention of water and sodium resulting in increased plasma volume. Increased prostaglandins and nitric oxide and refractoriness to angiotensin II promote vasodilation as flow distribution to the low-resistance uteroplacental, breast, and renal circulations lowers systemic vascular resistance (SVR). These changes lead to lower BP with increased stroke volume (SV), heart rate (HR), and cardiac output (CO) to meet the increase demand and plasma volume. Plasma volume remains elevated throughout pregnancy until about 6–12 weeks postpartum. Low SVR and the changes in BP, SV, and CO begin to develop in the middle of the first trimester and reach a stable plateau in the late second or early third trimester. BP may rise then toward normal until delivery. HR tends to increase until term. HR and SV and CO all increase with the stress of labor and delivery. Susceptible women may not be refractory to angiotensin II and may develop hypertension in the setting of these cardiovascular changes.

Hypercoagulability

Three pathways converge on hypercoagulability during pregnancy, peaking in effect in the days after delivery. Compression of the gravid uterus on the inferior vena cava and aorta and uterine veins and arteries causes vascular injury and stasis of flow; venous stasis is augmented in the lower extremities by an increase in venous compliance. Levels of pro- and anticoagulant proteins are altered, promoting coagulation [3]. The procoagulants factors I, VII, VIII, IX, X, XII, and XII increase, as do fibrinogen, fibrin, and von Willebrand factor. The anticoagulant proteins antithrombin III and protein S decrease [4]. Although the level of protein C remains stable, a large minority of women develop functional activated protein C resistance. These effects are greatest at the end of pregnancy. Their effects persist after pregnancy, gradually waning and approaching normal around 6–12 weeks postpartum [5]. Finally, pregnancy is a state of low-grade intravascular thrombosis, platelet activation, and decreased fibrinolysis mediated by an increase in levels of plasminogen activator inhibitor and the tissue factor pathway inhibitor. These changes are accompanied by elevation of the erythrocyte sedimentation rate, fibrinogen, and fibrin degradation products and a slight fall in platelets [6]. All of these processes and the effects of the acute hemorrhagic trauma of delivery converge to create the greatest degree of hypercoagulability in the days just after delivery.

S. K. Feske (✉)
Harvard Medical School, Division of Stroke and Cerebrovascular Disease, Neurology Department, Brigham and Women's Hospital, Boston, MA, USA
e-mail: sfeske@bwh.harvard.edu

© Springer Nature Switzerland AG 2019
M. A. O'Neal (ed.), *Neurology and Psychiatry of Women*, https://doi.org/10.1007/978-3-030-04245-5_16

Immune-Mediated Changes

Local and systemic immune modifications allow the fetus to develop within the immunologically foreign mother. The syncytiotrophoblasts that make up the placenta closest to the mother lack identifying major histocompatibility complex class I molecules making the mother immunologically blind to the fetus. Humoral factors inhibit cytotoxic T cells and natural killer cells and T lymphocytes.

Alterations in Connective Tissues/Remodeling

Hormonally-mediated remodeling of connective tissues, including vascular structures, may confer some added risk of stroke. The arterial wall contents of collagen and elastin are decreased during pregnancy. These changes might weaken vascular lesions, such as aneurysms and arteriovenous malformations, and render them more vulnerable to rupture under the increased hemodynamic stress of pregnancy. If so, this effect might be expected to peak during the stress of labor and delivery.

Preeclampsia-Eclampsia

Preeclampsia-eclampsia is a systemic disorder of mid to late pregnancy characterized by hypertension and proteinuria. Systemic hypertension and endothelial dysfunction play major roles in the pathogenesis of preeclampsia-eclampsia. The resulting hypertension, activation of thrombogenesis, decreased fibrinolysis, and enhanced vascular permeability may contribute to both ischemic and hemorrhagic strokes.

Rare Causes of Stroke in Pregnancy

Very rarely, stroke can be caused by embolism of material other than thrombus. During labor and delivery, amniotic fluid or air that enters the venous system can embolize to the lungs and, via a patent foramen ovale or the capillaries of the lungs, into the arterial circulation. Tumor cells of metastatic choriocarcinoma may also enter the circulation to cause pulmonary involvement and cerebral infarction, often with hemorrhage.

Epidemiology

Stroke is uncommon in women during the reproductive years. In large epidemiologic studies, incident rates of stroke in pregnancy range from approximately 10 per 100,000, to 25 per 100,000 [7–9]. The latter higher figure was obtained in a population of women up to age 49, so it likely captured some patients with risk factors that tend to emerge with aging. Pregnancy confers an increased risk of both ischemic and hemorrhagic stroke which is greatest in late pregnancy and especially during the early puerperium. Several studies have failed to show an increased incidence of ischemic stroke *during* pregnancy itself [7, 9, 10], however there is a many-fold increased incidence postpartum (relative risk 8.7 in the Kittner study following women for 6 weeks postpartum) [7, 9]. Studies have shown an increased risk of hemorrhagic stroke, including subarachnoid hemorrhage (SAH), during pregnancy (Kittner RR = 2.5) and, especially, during the puerperium (Kittner RR = 28.3). The increase during pregnancy, especially for SAH, occurs mainly during the third trimester. The relative influence of race has been hard to determine, however, increased risks have been found in studies of Caucasian, African-American, and Asian women [7, 10, 11]. Although, observer bias may influence comparisons across time, it appears that the risk of pregnancy-related stroke increased in comparisons from 1994–1995 to 2006–2007, paralleling increases in obesity, hypertension, and heart disease [12]. Although the incidence of stroke remains low, the toll of chronic disability is relatively high in this, otherwise, young and healthy population.

Pregnancy-associated ischemic strokes are most commonly due to cardioembolism, preeclampsia-eclampsia, or venous sinus thrombosis. The interactions of physiologic and pathologic hypercoagulability in pregnancy with and without preeclamptic-eclampsia are complex. Many women with pregnancy-associated strokes have additional personal or family risk factors. Cardiomyopathy induced by pregnancy is a rare but important cause. Most hemorrhagic strokes are due to preeclampsia-eclampsia followed by various vascular malformations: aneurysm, arteriovenous malformations, and cavernous malformations [2].

Diagnosis

It may seem facile to say that diagnosis depends first on attention to risk factors in a disorder that is so uncommon. However, as we have noted, strokes typically occur in women with suggestions of increased risk based on personal or family histories. Therefore, it is important to be alert for strokes, if symptoms might suggest it. For any woman with severe unexplained headache during late pregnancy and the puerperium, cerebral venous thrombosis and preeclampsia-eclampsia with associated posterior reversible encephalopathy syndrome (PRES) or reversible cerebral vasoconstriction syndrome (RCVS) and cerebral hemorrhage from other causes should be considered and sought by proper diagnostic studies. All patients with sudden onset of focal deficits should undergo urgent evaluations to diagnosis stroke or distinguish it from stroke mimickers, such as migraine and seizure.

It is important that physicians pursue proper neuroimaging studies whenever acute stroke is considered. During pregnancy, unenhanced MRI is the preferred modality, because it confers very little risk to the mother or developing fetus. However, non-contrast CT and contrast CT angiography and catheter angiography can all be performed safely and should be pursued with proper shielding when it is felt that urgent diagnosis is important to direct potential urgent therapies. To allow for prompt decision making for available therapies discussed below, it is important to proceed rapidly to perform brain imaging to define the extent of infarction and vessel imaging to identify sites of vascular occlusion for acute ischemic strokes. For hemorrhagic strokes, it is important to pursue imaging adequate to establish the presence of urgent complications, the stability of the hemorrhage, and the nature of the bleeding lesion. A detailed discussion of imaging in pregnant and breast-feeding women is beyond the scope of his chapter, so I refer interested readers to the excellent review by Chansakul and Young [13].

Acute Treatment

For ischemic stroke, it is most important to emphasize the gravity of major strokes and the principle that pregnant women should be offered the same therapies as nonpregnant patients to minimize stroke size and ultimate disability. In 2018 the American Heart Association/American Stroke Association published revised guidelines for the early management and treatment of acute ischemic stroke [14]. The guidelines continue to support rapid evaluation and triage of patients with acute stroke symptoms and the earliest possible use of intravenous tPA (alteplase) in eligible patients with potentially disabling strokes who can receive this therapy within 4.5 h of symptom onset [15, 16]. These guidelines offer a weak (Class IIb) permissive recommendation concerning the application to pregnant and early postpartum women. This recommendation is based on limited data (Level C-LD) and not on evidence of harm. Although high quality data do not exist to support its use during pregnancy and the early puerperium strongly, the many cases reported suggest that thrombolytic agents can be given with good safety for the mother and the fetus (Table 1). Therefore, acknowledging the limits of knowledge, I would recommend use in such women, unless specific issues, beyond the pregnancy itself, are judged to be contraindications. The current guidelines also recognize the proven benefit of mechanical thrombectomy in otherwise eligible patients with moderate-to-large strokes and established large vessel occlusion and small established infarcts on presentation. These recommendations are based on multiple studies showing major benefit in selected patients within about 6 h, and in more strictly selected patients up to 24 h after onset [17–24]. It is important that these therapies be made available to pregnant and postpartum women who might benefit.

Table 1 Outcomes of intravenous tPA use for stroke during pregnancy

Study	Maternal outcome	Fetal outcome
Dapprich [38]	Minor ICH	NC
Wiese [39]	NC	NC
Leonhardt [40]	NC	NC
Murugappan [41]	Minor uterine bleeding	Medical termination
Murugappan [41]	NC	Medical termination
Murugappan [41]	Died	Died
Yamaguchi [42]	NC	NC
Hori [43]	NC	NC
Tassi [44]	NC	NC
Ritter [45]	NC	NC

ICH intracerebral hemorrhage, *NC* no complications

Stroke associated with preeclampsia-eclampsia should be treated with magnesium sulfate, close monitoring of hemodynamic status, strict control of hypertension, and early delivery, when feasible [25–27].

For all hemorrhagic and ischemic strokes, urgent neurosurgical issues should be addressed based on neurosurgical principles guided by imaging acquired as needed with proper shielding. For hemorrhages due to aneurysms and arteriovenous malformations, issues of timing are important. In general, for subarachnoid hemorrhage due to aneurysmal rupture, both maternal and fetal mortality appear to be markedly decreased by early surgery to secure the aneurysm [28]. Similarly, women and their fetuses probably have lower mortality if ruptured arteriovenous malformations are treated surgically, when otherwise indicated [28]. Unruptured aneurysms that are considered for surgical clipping or coiling can usually be observed and managed surgically after delivery.

Patients with cerebral venous sinus thrombosis may benefit from anticoagulation with heparins during pregnancy, with therapy extended on warfarin postpartum. The duration of therapy will depend on the presence or absence of ongoing underlying risks [29, 30].

Secondary Prevention

Issues of secondary prevention after pregnancy-related stroke have not been studied systematically. All women with known stroke risk factors should be optimally treated for these. The answers to many questions concerning pregnancy-specific issues are left to expert opinion based on limited evidence:

Should women avoid pregnancy after a pregnancy-associated stroke?

In a study of the risk of recurrent stroke in 441 young (age 15–40 years) women who had had a prior stroke, the risk of recurrent stroke was about 2.3% within 5 years. Pregnancy and the puerperium did appear to increase the risk of recurrent stroke. However, only one stroke occurred during pregnancy and one during the puerperium, and both of these occurred in women with uncommon disorders that were definite causes of their strokes (essential thrombocythemia in one and antiphospholipid antibody syndrome in another). Of 37 women who had had a first stroke during pregnancy, none had recurrent stroke during pregnancy. This study is limited by the low numbers of subjects and events, however, I would conclude with the authors that, for women without an identified ongoing disorder that confers increased risk, and especially in younger women, it is reasonable to consider pregnancy after stroke, taking proper precautions to minimize risk [31].

Should antiplatelet agents be given for secondary prevention during a subsequent pregnancy?

There are no studies that address the question of antithrombotic therapy for stroke prevention during pregnancy. However, because antiplatelet agents have been proven to confer benefits for secondary stroke prevention for strokes of many types, it is reasonable to extrapolate to this population as well. There is good evidence that low-dose aspirin can be given during pregnancy with minimal risk to the mother and fetus [32, 33]. Therefore, low-dose aspirin seems to be a reasonable approach to stroke prevention during pregnancy in women deemed to have elevated stroke risk.

Should anticoagulation be given for secondary prevention during a subsequent pregnancy?

For women who suffered arterial ischemic strokes during pregnancy, this decision should be based on the presence or absence of ongoing established indications for anticoagulation, such as atrial fibrillation and other heart diseases that warrant anticoagulation and underlying hypercoagulable states. For cerebral venous sinus thrombosis, the overall recurrence rate is relatively low [34]. However, for women who have suffered venous sinus thrombosis, anticoagulation during late pregnancy and the puerperium is more strongly indicated. Low-molecular-weight heparin can be given beginning in the second trimester, held in anticipation of deliver, and resumed (or warfarin can be used) for 6–12 weeks postpartum [35–37].

Should prior stroke influence the mode of delivery?

Although some studies of the timing of hemorrhagic strokes have suggested an increased risk around the time of labor and delivery, there is no evidence that cesarean section leads to better outcomes for pregnancies after a prior stroke, nor for patients with unruptured aneurysms or arteriovenous malformations. Therefore, most such women can safely undergo vaginal delivery. Obstetricians will need to individualize these decisions in consultation with neurologists and neurosurgeons and patients. When vaginal delivery is chosen, they may wish to take measures to minimize the trauma and stress of the second stage of labor.

Conclusions

Though uncommon, because of its severity and potential for major long-term disability, stroke is an important complication of pregnancy. Many of the physiologic changes of pregnancy increase the risk of stroke, especially in the early puerperium, and preeclampsia-eclampsia further increases risk. With new effective therapies for stroke, it is more important than ever to emphasize that the response to stroke must be rapid and that, with simple accommodations, pregnant women should get urgent imaging and should be provided the optimal therapies without delay to minimize the size and long-term sequelae of strokes. This goal is best accomplished with close collaboration in a team effort by obstetricians, emergency physicians, radiologists, neurologists, and neurosurgeons.

References

1. Feske SK, Klein AM. Neurology of pregnancy and the puerperium. In: Schapira A, editor. Neurology and clinical neuroscience. 1st ed. Philadelphia: Mosby Elsevier; 2007. p. 1490–503.
2. Feske SK, Singhal A. Cerebrovascular disorders complicating pregnancy. Continuum. 2014;20:80–99.
3. Clark P, Brennand J, Conkie JA, et al. Activated protein C sensitivity, protein C, protein S, and coagulation in normal pregnancy. Thromb Haemost. 1998;79:1166–70.
4. Wickström K, Edelstam G, Löwber CH, Hansson LO, Sieghahn A. Reference intervals for plasma levels of fibrinogen, von Willebrand factor, free protein S and antithrombin during third-trimester pregnancy. Scand J Clin Lab Invest. 2004;64:31–40.
5. Kamel H, Navi BB, Sriram N, Hovsepian DA, Devereux RB, Elkind MSV. Risk of thrombotic event after the 6-week postpartum period. N Engl J Med. 2014;370:1307–15.
6. Cerneca F, Ricci G, Simeone R, et al. Coagulation and fibrinolysis changes in normal pregnancy. Increased levels of procoagulants and reduced levels of inhibitors during pregnancy induce a hypercoagulable state, combined with a reactive fibrinolysis. Eur J Obstet Gynecokl Reprod Biol. 1997;73:31–6.
7. Kittner SJ, Stern BJ, Feeser BR, et al. Pregnancy and the risk of stroke. N Engl J Med. 1996;335:768–74.
8. Petitti DB, Sidney S, Quesenberry CP Jr, Bernstein A. Incidence of stroke and myocardial infarction in women of reproductive age. Stroke. 1997;28:280–3.
9. Ban L, Sprigg N, Abdul Sultan A, et al. Incidence of first stroke in pregnant and nonpregnant women of childbearing age: a

population-based cohort study from England. J Am Heart Assoc. 2017;6:e004601.

10. Sharshar T, Lamy C, Mas JL, Stroke in Pregnancy Study Group. Incidence and causes of strokes associated with pregnancy and puerperium: a study in public hospitals of Ile de France. Stroke. 1995;26:930–6.

11. Jeng JS, Tang SC, Yip PK. Incidence and etiologies of stroke during pregnancy adn puerperium as evidenced in Taiwanese women. Cerebrovasc Dis. 2004;18:290–5.

12. Kuklina EV, Tong X, Bansil P, George MG, Callaghan WM. Trends in pregnancy hospitalizations that included a stroke in the United States from 1994 to 2007: reasons for concern? Stroke. 2011;42:2564–70.

13. Chansakul T, Young GS. Neuroimaging in pregnant women. Semin Neurol. 2017;37:712–23.

14. Powers WJ, Rabinstein AA, Ackerson T, et al. 2018 guidelines for the early management of patients with acute ischemic stroke: a guideline for healthcare professionals from the American Heart Association/American Stroke Association. Stroke. 2018;49:e46.

15. The National Institute of Neurological Disorders and Stroke rt-PA Stroke Study Group. Tissue plasminogen activator for acute ischemic stroke. N Engl J Med. 1996;333:1581–7.

16. Hacke W, Kaste M, Bluhmki E, ECASS Investigators, et al. Thrombolysis with alteplase 3 to 4.5 hours after acute ischemic stroke. N Engl J Med. 2008;359:1317–29.

17. Berkhemer OA, Fransen PS, Beumer D, et al. A randomized trial of intraarterial treatment for acute ischemic stroke. N Engl J Med. 2015;372:11–20.

18. Goyal M, Demchuk AM, Menon BK, et al. Randomized assessment of rapid endovascular treatment of ischemic stroke. N Engl J Med. 2015;372:1019–30.

19. Campbell BC, Mitchell PJ, Kleinig TJ, et al. Endovascular therapy for ischemic stroke with perfusion-imaging selection. N Engl J Med. 2015;372:1009–18.

20. Saver JL, Goyal M, Bonafe A, et al. Stent-retriever thrombectomy after intravenous t-PA vs. t-PA alone in stroke. N Engl J Med. 2015;372:2285–95.

21. Jovin TG, Chamorro A, Cobo E, et al. Thrombectomy within 8 hours after symptom onset in ischemic stroke. N Engl J Med. 2015;372:2296–306.

22. Bracard S, Ducrocq X, Mas JL, et al. Mechanical thrombectomy after intravenous alteplase versus alteplase alone after stroke (THRACE): a randomised controlled trial. Lancet Neurol. 2016;15:1138–47.

23. Nogueira RG, Jadhav AP, Haussen DC, et al. Thrombectomy 6 to 24 hours after stroke with a mismatch between deficit and infarct. N Engl J Med. 2018;378:11–21.

24. Albers GW, Marks MP, Kemp S, et al. Thrombectomy for stroke at 6 to 16 hours with selection by perfusion imaging. N Engl J Med. 2018;378:708–18.

25. Altman D, Carroli G, Duley L, et al. Do women with pre-eclampsia, and their babies, benefit from magnesium sulphate? The magpie trial: a randomised placebo-controlled trial. Lancet. 2002;359:1877–90.

26. The Eclampsia Trial Collaborative Group. Which anticonvulsant for women with eclampsia? Evidence from the collaborative eclampsia trial. Lancet. 1995;345:1455–63.

27. Lucas MJ, Leveno KJ, Cunningham FG. A comparison of magnesium sulfate with phenytoin for the prevention of eclampsia. N Engl J Med. 1995;333:201–5.

28. Dias MS, Sekhar LN. Intracranial hemorrhage from aneurysms and arteriovenous malformations during pregnancy and the puerperium. Neurosurgery. 1990;27:855–65, discussion 865–856.

29. Einhäupl KM, Villringer A, Meister W, et al. Heparin treatment in sinus venus thrombosis. Lancet. 1991;338:597–600.

30. de Bruijn SFTM, Starn J, for the Cerebral Venous Sinus Thrombosis Study Group. Randomized, placebo-controlled trial of anticoagulant treatment with low-molecular-weight heparin for cerebral sinus thrombosis. Stroke. 1999;30:484–8.

31. Lamy C, Hamon JB, Coste J, Mas JL. Iachemic stroke in young women: risk of recurrence during subsequent pregnancies. Neurology. 2000;55:269–74.

32. CLASP (Collaborative Low-dose Aspirin Study in Pregnancy) Collaborative Group. CLASP: a randomised trial of low-dose aspirin for the prevention and treatment of pre-eclampsia among 9364 pregnant women. Lancet. 1994;343:619–29.

33. Bujold E, Roberge S, Lacasse Y, et al. Prevention of preeclampsia and intrauterine growth retardation with aspirin started in early pregnancy: a meta-analysis. Obstet Gynecol. 2010;116:402–14.

34. Ferro JM, Canhao P, Stam J, Bousser MG, Barinagarrementeria F, Investigators I. Prognosis of cerebral vein and dural sinus thrombosis: results of the International Study on Cerebral Vein and Dural Sinus Thrombosis (ISCVT). Stroke. 2004;35:664–70.

35. Bushnell C, McCullough LD, Awad IA, et al. Guidelines for the prevention of stroke in women: a statement for healthcare professionals from the American Heart Association/American Stroke Association. Stroke. 2014;45:1545–88.

36. Dentali F, Poli D, Sconditti U, CErebral VEin Thrombosis International Study Investigators, et al. Long-term outcomes of patients with cerebral vein thrombosis: a multicenter study [published correction appears in J Thromb Haemost 2013;11:3991]. J Thromb Haemost. 2012;10:1297–302.

37. Saposnik G, Barinagarrementeria F, Brown RD, American Heart Association Stroke Council and the Council on Epidemiology and Prevention, et al. Diagnosis and management of cerebral venous thrombosis: a statement for healthcare professionals from the American Heart Association/American Stroke Association. Stroke. 2011;42:1158–92.

38. Dapprich M, Boessenecker W. Fibrinolysis with alteplase in a pregnant woman with stroke. Cerebrovasc Dis. 2002;13:290.

39. Wiese KM, Talkad A, Mathews M, Wang D. Intravenous recombinant tissue plasminogen activator in a pregnant woman with cardioembolic stroke. Stroke. 2006;37:2168–9.

40. Leonhardt G, Gaul C, Nietsch HH, Buerke M. Thrombolytic therapy in pregnancy. J Thromb Thrombolysis. 2006;21:271–6.

41. Murugappan A, Coplin WM, Al-Sadat AN, et al. Thrombolytic therapy of acute ischemic stroke during pregnancy. Neurology. 2006;66:768–70.

42. Yamaguchi Y, Kondo T, Ihara M, et al. Intravenous recombinant tissue plasminogen activator in an 18-weeks pregnant woman with embolic stroke. Clin Neurol. 2010;50:315–9.

43. Hori H, Yamamoto F, Ito Y, Hashimoto Y, Hirano T, Uchino M. Intravenous recombinant tissue plasminogen activator therapy in a 14-week pregnant woman with embolic stroke due to protein S deficiency. Rinsho Shinkeigaku. 2013;53:212–6.

44. Tassi R, Acampa M, Marotta G, et al. Systemic thrombolysis for stroke in pregnancy. Am J Emerg Med. 2013;31:448e441–3.

45. Ritter LM, Schüler A, Gangopadhyay R, et al. Successful thrombolysis of stroke with intravenous alteplase in the third trimester of pregnancy. J Neurol. 2014;26:632–4.

Demyelinating Disease and Pregnancy

Tamara B. Kaplan and Riley Bove

Introduction

Multiple sclerosis (MS) is a chronic demyelinating disease of the central nervous system (CNS). MS affects two to threefold more women than men, and the disease often first presents in women during their peak childbearing years (20s–30s) [1]. Therefore, conception, pregnancy, delivery and breastfeeding are significant issues for both patients and their treating physicians.

Effects of MS on Fertility, Gestation and Neonatal Outcomes

Fertility, to a large extend, does not appear to be impaired in women with MS [2]. There is a small field of research into hormonal markers, including follicle-stimulating hormone (FSH), luteinizing hormone (LH), estrogen and anti-Müllerian hormone (AMH, a marker of ovarian reserve [3]) levels in women with MS [4, 5], but data remain too patchy to reach any conclusions on whether women with MS do experience reduced fertility [2, 6, 7] beyond therapy-related amenorrhea [6] or even premature ovarian failure [8]. Reproductive decision making could be affected by hormonal levels [6], decreased libido and sexual dysfunction [9], and concerns about parenting given the risk of worsening MS and disabilities.

Additionally, MS does not appear to increase the risk of early pregnancy loss, stillbirth, or fetal malformations in most studies [6]. Some reports suggest that mothers with MS may be more likely to give birth to neonates who are small for gestational age and with reduced birth weight [10], however,

this remains controversial and potential causes are unknown. Other studies have shown no associated between a patient's MS status and either birth weight or gestational age [11].

Women with MS often ask about the risk of transmitting MS to their children. The genetic risk factors for MS are complex and more than 200 risk alleles have been identified [12, 13]. The absolute risk of a child of a child developing MS who is born to a woman with MS is about 3–5% [14]. However, children born to parents who both have MS have about a 20% risk of developing MS later in life [14]. To date, no predictive genetic testing is available for MS.

Low levels of vitamin D are thought to be a risk factor for the development of MS [15], including prenatally. In a cohort study of women with MS from the Finnish Maternity Cohort, low levels of vitamin D (25(OH)D levels <30 nmol/L) during the first trimester were associated with nearly a two times increase in the risk of MS among offspring [16]. However, there was no significant dose-response effect with increasing levels of 25(OH)D. Currently, the American College of Obstetrics and Gynecology suggests that screening for vitamin D deficiency may be performed in women potentially at risk, but does not recommend routine screening in all pregnant women, and notes that 1000–2000 international units per day of vitamin D is safe for those who are deficient [17]. However, the ideal serum levels for women with MS are unknown, and variable doses will likely be required to achieve these effects in different women.

Effects of Pregnancy on the Course of MS

Short-Term Effects

The landmark 1998 Pregnancy in Multiple Sclerosis (PRIMS) study, is the best large-scale prospective study published [18]. PRIMS enrolled 254 women (246 with relapsing MS), following them for a total of 269 pregnancies until at least 12 months postpartum. Compared to pre-pregnancy, annualized relapse rate fell by 70% during the third trimester

T. B. Kaplan (✉)
Department of Neurology, Harvard Medical School, Brigham and Women's Hospital, Boston, MA, USA
e-mail: tbkaplan@bwh.harvard.edu

R. Bove
Department of Neurology, Weill Institute for the Neurosciences, University of California, San Francisco, CA, USA

© Springer Nature Switzerland AG 2019
M. A. O'Neal (ed.), *Neurology and Psychiatry of Women*, https://doi.org/10.1007/978-3-030-04245-5_17

of pregnancy. However, during the first 3 months postpartum, the relapse rate increased to 70% above the pre-pregnancy level, eventually returning to the pre-pregnancy rate after those initial 3 months. The annualized relapse rate from postpartum months 3–12 was not significantly different from that of the pre-pregnancy year [18]. Clinical predictors of a likelihood of postpartum relapse in PRIMS included: an increased relapse rate in the year before pregnancy, an increased relapse rate during pregnancy, and a higher Expanded Disability Status Scale (EDSS) score at the onset of pregnancy [19]. Epidural anesthesia and breastfeeding were not predictive of a postpartum relapse or of disability progression. The findings of the PRIMS study have been replicated by numerous other studies since its initial publication [20, 21], including in countries such as Italy and the Czech Republic.

One important variable that has changed since PRIMS is the availability and now-widespread use of disease-modifying therapies (DMTs) for the care of patients with relapsing MS, most of which are discontinued during pregnancy. Therefore, evaluation of the effect of pregnancies in MS must now consider potential confounding effects of treatment interruption and resumption on the risk of relapse.

Longer-Term Effects

Longer-term, the effects of childbearing on disability progression are unclear, and often confounded by patient choice (women with worse disability may be more likely to choose not to become pregnant).

A population cohort study demonstrated a significantly lower overall risk of conversion to a progressive form of MS in women who became pregnant after the onset of the disease, suggesting a possible beneficial effect of pregnancy on the disease course. For each year of observation, the risk of entering a progressive course was higher in a non-pregnant state compared with the risk after pregnancy (p = 0.0029) [22]. A prospective 5-year study compared the rate of disability progression between childless women, women who had onset of MS after childbirth, and women who had onset before or during their pregnancy. The rates of disability increased most rapidly in nulliparous women [23]. However, another retrospective population-based study of 185 women with MS showed no association between disability and total number of term pregnancies, timing of pregnancy relative to onset of MS, or either onset or worsening of MS in relation to a pregnancy [24]. While awaiting further prospective studies to clarify the long-term effects of childbearing on MS disease course, it is reassuring that pregnancy does not appear to worsen disease and disability in the long-term.

Management of MS In Women Planning A Pregnancy

General Pre-conception Care and Counseling

General Guidelines

Many pregnancies may be unintentional, and thus, it is imperative that clinicians provide a measure of pregnancy counseling with all women of reproductive age to inform them of the potential risks of conception on various DMTs (see below), and to provide anticipatory guidance about the pregnancy and postpartum periods. Women with MS who are of childbearing age may not have regular encounters with other clinicians (internists or obstetricians) prior to a pregnancy, and therefore may need to be informed of general pre-conception recommendations, including smoking cessation, weight management and folate intake [25]). Additionally, low prenatal vitamin D levels appear to be associated with increased risk of MS in offspring [16]. While awaiting definitive evidence from trials that replete these levels, women with MS may be advised to aim for normal or high-normal serum levels of vitamin D before and during conception, to reduce long-term risk of MS in potentially genetically at-risk children.

Optimizing Chances of Conception Off DMT

For women on DMTs who are planning to discontinue these prior to conception, optimizing their chances of conceiving off DMT may include careful planning of the timing of DMT discontinuation, and consideration of fertility evaluation if conception has not occurred after 6 months (while in the general population, it is typical to wait 12 months [26]).

Assisted Reproductive Technology and Relapse Risk

Several small, heterogeneous studies have reported an increase in relapse rate in the 3-month period following use of assisted reproductive technology (ART), possibly increased when ART protocols included GnRH agonists rather than GnRH antagonists, and following unsuccessful cycles [2, 27–32]. While all of these studies suggest some increase in relapse rate in the 3-month period following ART, they could not adequately account for the effects of DMT interruption or other factors (pregnancy loss, maternal stress) on inflammatory activity. Larger prospective studies are clearly needed to better understand this trend. In women with MS pursuing ART, dialogue between fertility and MS clinicians is recommended.

Whether and When to Discontinue Disease Modifying Therapies?

Since 1993, over 15 disease-modifying medications (DMTs) have been approved by regulatory bodies including the U.S. Food and Drug Administration (FDA) for the treatment of relapsing forms of MS; and one has been approved for primary progressive MS. While data are limited in humans, some of these medications have been shown to be teratogenic in animal studies (Table 1). When the clinical objective is complete elimination prior to conception, a period of five maximal half-lives is recommended – except for teriflunomide, which requires a specific wash out protocol. Based on these principles, a short (days) washout period is likely sufficient for interferon β, glatiramer acetate, and dimethyl fumarate [33] but longer wash-out periods are required for the other oral and infusion DMTs.

Per the FDA and the National MS Society consensus statements, DMTs should not be used in patients with MS who are pregnant, trying to become pregnant, or breastfeeding (https://www.nationalmssociety.org/Living-Well-With-MS/Diet-Exercise-Healthy-Behaviors/Womens-Health/Pregnancy). In practice, there is wide variability of practice patterns relating to DMT discontinuation prior to conception [34]. In the absence of definitive evidence, the decision whether and when to discontinue a DMT should be personalized for each patient. The treating clinician and patient should discuss the risks (and risk tolerance) that the patient should experience increased MS activity off DMT before and early during pregnancy, the timing and risks of potential rebound disease activity when stopping certain DMTs [35–37], and the unique safety profile of each drug (Table 2). Careful documentation of communication of risks and benefits is recommended, and referral of patients to a disease-specific MS registry (eg. https://mothertobaby.org/ongoing-study/multiple-sclerosis/) is recommended.

Gestation: Interferon βs are the oldest class of DMTs. There is no animal evidence of teratogenicity and the large macromolecule is unlikely to be able to cross the placenta in any significant dosing. In humans, an initial suspicion of dose-dependent abortive effect observed from non-human primates has not been confirmed [33, 39, 40]. Some reports suggest maternal interferon beta exposure is associated with lower infant birth weights and length, and higher incidence of premature births [41–43]. However, these studies have been faulted for small sample size, a retrospective study design, the lack of confounder analysis, and/or the absence of a control group [40], and more recent studies do not confirm these findings [33, 39]. A prospective cohort study from the German Multiple Sclerosis and Pregnancy Registry,

Table 1 Disease modifying therapies in pregnancy and lactation

Immunomodulating agents	FDA Class	Drug Half Life	Fetal and maternal risks	Secretion in breast milk
Interferon β-1-b and β-1-a	Class C	10 h	Spontaneous abortions in animals. Not seen in humans	Minimal, may be safe in lactation
Glatiramer acetate	Class B	6.76 h	None reported	Minimal, may be safe in lactation
Intravenous immunoglobulin	Class C	25–32 days	Probably safe in pregnancy	Unknown; may be compatible with lactation
Fingolimod	Class C	6–9 days	Teratogenicity seen in animals and humans. No specific pattern observed.	Yes, avoid in lactation
Dimethyl fumarate	Class C	1 h	Increased spontaneous abortion in animals. Not reported in humans	Unknown, but likely. Avoid in lactation due to potential drug side effects.
Teriflunomide	Class X	18–19 days	Teratogenicity seen in animals; precursor leflunomide is a known human teratogen. No malformations in humans observed thus far	Yes, in animals. Avoid in lactation
Daclizumab	Class C	20 days	Embryofetal deaths observed in animals with early exposure. No fetal malformations in humans observed thus far	Yes, in animals, Avoid in lactation
Natalizumab	Class C	7–15 days	Reduced neonatal survival at supratherapeutic doses in primates. Transient hematologic abnormalities in late pregnancy exposure in humans	Yes, and may increase with subsequent infusions. Avoid in lactation
Alemtuzumab	Class C	12 days	In animals, increased rates of fetal loss, decreased B- and T-lymphocytes in offspring. No human malformations seen, but thyroid monitoring necessary for mother throughout pregnancy. No evidence for spontaneous abortion or birth defects	Minimal secretion of IgG in breastmilk. Avoid in lactation due to potential drug side effects
Rituximab/ Ocrelizumab	Class C	22 days/26 days	No human malformations seen; transient B-cell depletion in human neonates and animal following pregnancy exposure	Minimal secretion of IgG in breastmilk Avoid in lactation due to potential drug side effects

Table 2 Perspectives from two patients

A 32-year-old woman with clinically isolated syndrome has experienced no new lesions or relapses after 3 years on glatiramer acetate. Her current EDSS is 1	A 34-year-old woman with aggressive MS has finally experienced 12 months of stable MRIs on natalizumab, after experiencing breakthrough disease activity on injectable therapies for several years. Her current EDSS is 3.5 and her walking has declined
She chooses to discontinue her DMT at the time of ovulation and conception attempt. While she understands that there is no current evidence of adverse pregnancy-related outcomes in women exposed to GA during pregnancy, she is concerned that there could be longer-term effects on her fetus that might not manifest until later childhood or adulthood, and therefore remain currently undetected	She opts to continue treatment into her pregnancy due to her high baseline rate of MS activity, the risk of rebound activity off natalizumab [36], low risk of natalizumab transfer across the placenta during the first trimester, and initial safety reports from observational studies [38]. She is planning close clinical monitoring during her pregnancy, and a neonatologist will be available at delivery to evaluate her newborn for hematologic and other abnormalities

including 251 pregnancies in mothers treated with interferon-β1a, found no association between exposure during early pregnancy and mean birth weight, risk of preterm birth, or other adverse pregnancy outcomes [40]. Additionally, several post-marketing cohort studies have shown that the risk of spontaneous abortion on IFN-β1a is not significantly different from the general population [44]. There is no data-driven argument to support pregnancy terminations, if conceived during active interferon use [45].

Lactation: IFN-β1a is not generally excreted in breast milk due to its large protein size, and because it remains in a bound state with low plasma levels in the mother's body. A small study reported that breast milk contained only 0.006% of the maternal dose of intramuscular interferon beta-1a [46]. Additionally, beta IFNs are not orally bioavailable. In a study of six nursing mothers using IFN-β1a, there were no side effects seen in infants [47].

Glatiramer Acetate (Copaxone)

Gestation: Glatiramer acetate (GA) is the only DMT with a former FDA "category B." It has been safe in animals. GA is not believed to cross the placenta nor does it have measurable blood levels in the mother [48], and thus far in over 500 human pregnancies, has shown no association with low birth weight, congenital anomaly, preterm birth or spontaneous abortion [44, 48–50]. Overall, no major concerns have been raised with using GA, and currently, some neurologists treat women with GA during pregnancy.

Lactation: GA may be considered safe with breastfeeding [51]. No adverse events were reported in nine mothers who breastfed their infants for a mean period of 3.6 months while taking GA [48] It is unlikely that this drug is transmitted in breast milk but there are no definitive studies. Even if some GA does cross over into breast milk, given its large molecular weight, this amino acid polymer is likely degraded in the infant's gastrointestinal tract upon oral ingestion.

Dimethyl Fumarate (Tecfidera)

Evidence from animal studies shows that dimethyl fumarate (DMF) at doses two times higher than the approved human dose is associated with embryo lethality in rats [33]. Additionally, when given at a dose equivalent to 16 times the normal human therapeutic dose, there was an increased spontaneous abortion rate in rabbits [52]. Despite these studies, in a case series of 45 women exposed to DMT in early pregnancy, no significant adverse effects were noted. Overall, post-marketing studies of human pregnancy exposures to date have not detected any signal of elevated fetal abnormalities after first trimester exposure [53]. DMF has a very short half-life (less than 60 min), and therefore a short wash-out or no wash-out is currently recommended.

Lactation: The active drug component in DMF, monomethyl fumarate, has a low molecular weight (129 Daltons) and low protein binding (27–45%), and consequently, a significant amount it thought to enter milk[54]. Until there are further studies, caution is advised when using DMF in breastfeeding mothers.

Fingolimod (Gilenya)

Fingolimod crosses the placenta and is secreted in breast milk. In animal studies, there is evidence for both teratogenicity and embryolethality (including ventricular septal defect, persistent truncus arteriosis, Tetralogy of Fallot, acrania, malformation of the tibia, and fetal death). In a limited number of human pregnancies, there seems to be a slightly higher rate of spontaneous abortion, as well as malformations [55]. In 66 human exposure cases there was a reported 7.6% rate of fetal abnormalities at birth [56]. In the fingolimod clinical trial program, among 34 pregnancies, there were 13 healthy infants, 1 with a tibia malformation (thought to be unrelated to treatment), 5 spontaneous abortions, 9 elective abortions, and 6 ongoing pregnancies at the time of publication [57]. Currently, fingolimod should be discontinued at least 2 months prior to conceiving (half-life about 9 day) [58]. Patients should also be counseled about the possibility of relapses occurring in the period during which they are trying to conceive, including of rebound inflammatory activity after fingolimod discontinuation [35], and bridging therapies considered.

Lactation: Fingolimod is present in breast milk of rodents, and it is orally bioavailable. While there are no human studies, given this drug's high volume of distribution and high protein binding [54], levels in human milk are likely low. However, breastfeeding is not advised at this time, as even small amounts transmitted in breast milk would be orally available to the infant.

Teriflunomide (Aubagio)

Teriflunomide is the active metabolite of leflunomide, which has long been used to treat rheumatoid arthritis. Teriflunomide must be discontinued and eliminated from the body prior to conception [59]. Leflunomide has shown teratogenic an embryo lethal effects in multiple animals species at doses lower than those used for therapies in humans [60]. Specifically, leflunomide has caused fetal abnormalities such as craniofacial, axial and appendicular skeletal malformations in pregnant rats and rabbits. Despite these findings, of the recorded human pregnancies with exposure to teriflunomide, the rate of spontaneous abortion was not different from the general population and no serious malformations were reported [61].

While the mean half-life of teriflunomide is 16–18 days, it may persist in the body for as long as 24 months. Conception should only occur once teriflunomide levels are lower than 0.02 ug/ml. If an unplanned pregnancy occurs, or if the patient desires pregnancy within 1 year of treatment, a rapid elimination protocol with oral cholestyramine or activated charcoal over several days is used to lower the teriflunomide levels to less than 0.02 ug/ml [56]. In addition to its ability to cross the placenta, teriflunomide is also present in the semen of men taking the drug [62].

Lactation: Teriflunomide has been detected in rat milk following a single dose [58], and while rodent studies are not necessarily indicative of human transfer, use of teriflunomide is contraindicated with breastfeeding.

Daclizumab (Zinbryta)

Daclizumab is an anti-CD25 monoclonal antibody administered monthly subcutaneously. Animal reproductive and developmental toxicology studies suggest no effect on fertility, on teratogenicity, or on pre-and post-natal development in experimental animal models. However, administration of daclizumab to monkeys during gestation did result in embryofetal death and reduced fetal growth at maternal exposures greater than 30 times that expected clinically [63].

Among human pregnancies in the daclizumab clinical program with known outcomes (n = 38), 20 were live births, 4 (11%) spontaneous abortions, 8 elective terminations, 2 ectopic pregnancies. Incidence of spontaneous abortions in women exposed to daclizumab was consistent with the early pregnancy loss rate (12–22%) in the general population. Among the 20 live births, one congenital heart defect was noted and was thought not to be related to daclizumab exposure [52, 63, 64]. However, this number of pregnancies is small, and it is difficult to draw broad conclusions. Currently, there is no large-scale post marketing information on pregnancy outcomes with this drug.

Lactation: With a low volume of distribution (2.5 L/kg), daclizumab probably remains in the plasma for a considerable amount of time [54], but this drug has been shown to cross into breast milk of animals [65], and therefore, should be avoided in lactation.

Natalizumab (Tysabri)

Natalizumab is a humanized monoclonal antibody against the cell adhesion molecule α4-integrin. This drug works by preventing lymphocytes from crossing the blood brain barrier and gaining access to the CNS. Natalizumab likely does not cross into fetal circulation until the placenta is established (13–14 weeks gestation) and then, it can do so via an active transport mechanism in the placenta. In animal studies, supratherapeutic doses of natalizumab have been shown to decrease fertility and reduced neonatal survival. This medication has also been shown to cause transient hematologic abnormalities in primates following maternal exposure. According to the Tysabri Pregnancy Exposure Registry, which reported 375 human pregnancies, resulting in 314 live births, the rates of miscarriage and malformation were not increased compared to the general population. However, mild to moderate hematologic alterations such as thrombocytopenia and anemia have been reported in 75% of newborns who were exposed to natalizumab after the 30th gestational week; and natalizumab was detected in the cord blood of 5 out of 5 newborns tested [66].

Rebound disease activity after natalizumab withdrawal is a well described, and there has been concern that this may occur during pregnancy. A recent prospective case series of 40 women receiving natalizumab during pregnancy observed fewer hematologic abnormalities in those newborns who were exposed to natalizumab for less than 24 weeks gestation and less than 30 weeks gestation, but significantly more relapses in the women who discontinued therapy before 24 weeks gestation [66, 67] Based on these findings, in women with highly active disease, natalizumab withdrawal around 30 weeks gestation could represent a reasonable compromise between maternal and child safety, as long as a pediatrician is available at the time of delivery to evaluate for hematologic abnormalities or other complications [66].

Lactation: Natalizumab has been detected in breast milk and should not be used in lactating women. The volume of distribution of this drug is 3.8–7.6 L/kg, the half-life is 7–15 days, but the time to reach steady state is about 28 weeks, so actual concentration in breast milk at steady state is still uncertain [54]. In fact, it may increase: milk samples from a breastfeeding mother on natalizumab collected over a 50-day period after the patient's first infusion, showed a relative infant dose of 1.74% of the weight-adjusted maternal dose after first infusion, but relative infant dose of 5.3% on day 50 [68]. Even if some drug is transmitted in breast milk, as with other monoclonal antibodies, it is unclear how much would be absorbed through the infant's gastrointestinal mucosa. Still, further research is needed to evaluate any potential risk to the breastfed infant.

B-Cell Depleting Therapies: Rituximab (Rituxan)/Ocrelizumab (Ocrevus)

Over the last few years, rituximab has been used more frequently as off-label treatment for MS. [69] Rituximab is a chimeric mouse monoclonal antibody that selectively targets CD20 positive B cells. Ocrelizumab was more recently approved by the FDA in March 2017 for treatment of relapsing and primary progressive forms of MS, and is a humanized anti -CD20 antibody. Most of what we know about anti-CD20 therapy comes from our experience with rituximab.

Rituximab is thought to cross the placenta in both animals and humans [70], however these studies showed no evidence of increased risk of miscarriage or teratogenicity. Transient newborn B-cell depletion has been seen in exposed animal and human pregnancies [71]. The risk of B-cell depletion in the newborn appears to be higher when the mother is exposed to the drug during the second or third trimester. According to the current Ocrelizumab Product Information (PI) the current recommendation is for women to use contraception while on treatment and for 6 months after the last infusion [72].

Lactation: Low levels of rituximab have been detected in the breast milk of cynomolgus monkeys, with concentrations of 0.19% and 0.26% of maternal serum level [73]. Women treated with rituximab and ocrelizumab are typically advised not to breastfeed given a lack of human data. In general, excretion of maternal IgG antibodies into human breast milk is extremely limited and comprise only about 2% of the total immunoglobulin content [74]. Furthermore, much that IgG is degraded in the infant's gastrointestinal system [74].

Recently, the serum and milk samples of a patient with granulomatosis with polyangiitis who had received rituximab during her lactation period were analyzed. The patient received an infusion of 1000 mg of rituximab and serum and milk samples were collected 7 days later for several consecutive days. Results showed that while the mother's serum contained rituximab levels of 130 μg/ml and 110 μg/ml on subsequent days, the levels in mother's milk were 0.5 μg/ml and 0.4 μg/ml respectively, suggesting minimal excretion into the milk [75]. While no case reports have been published regarding levels of ocrelizumab in breast milk, it is reasonable to assume that the results are similar.

Alemtuzumab (Lemtrada)

Alemtuzumab is an anti-CD52 humanized monoclonal antibody that is administered annually, and is typically used in patients with very aggressive or refractory MS. In animal studies, early maternal administration of alemtuzumab resulted in increased rates of fetal loss as well as decreased B- and T-lymphocytes in offspring at birth [33].

As of 2015, pregnancy outcomes were documented in 167 cases from the clinical development program, including 16 ongoing pregnancies and 10 women lost to follow-up. Of the completed pregnancies, 110 resulted in live births with healthy neonates, 37 (22.2%) pregnancies ended in a spontaneous abortion, 19 elective terminations were observed and in one case, a stillbirth occurred. This reflects the expected range of pregnancy outcomes in the general population [76].

While plasma concentration of alemtuzumab approaches zero at 30 days post last treatment dose, it is advised that women avoid conception for at least 4 months after the infusion. [33, 38] given the risk of secondary autoimmune thyroid disease in the child-bearing patient and its potential effects on the pregnancy. Maternal thyroid-stimulating hormone receptor antibodies can pass the placental barrier and cause transient neonatal Graves' disease [76]. All pregnant women with exposure should be checked for hypothyroidism as this is a known complication from this medication [76].

Lactation: Alemtuzumab is present in milk of lactating mice [33]. Due to the large molecular weight (150 kD) of this monoclonal antibody, alemtuzumab is unlikely to enter breast milk in any significant amounts [54]. However, given the lack of human data and the risk of potential side effects, caution should be used in breastfeeding mothers.

Evaluating and Treating a Relapse During Pregnancy

New neurological symptoms suggestive of a relapse during pregnancy warrant careful evaluation, to distinguish a relapse from "pseudoexacerbations" (due to such factors as urinary tract infections) and other neurological phenomena common in pregnancy (e.g. nerve entrapment). New lesionzs suggestive of a relapse can be visualized on MRI without gadolinium, if a baseline pre-pregnancy scan is available for comparison. There are no conclusive data to show that MRI exposure up to 3 Tesla is associated with harm to the fetus, but gadolinium should be avoided in pregnancy unless the benefit clearly outweighs the risk [77]. Gadolinium can enter fetal circulation and in animal studies, high doses of gadolinium were associated with miscarriage and developmental abnormalities [77]. If a relapse is severe enough to warrant therapy, methylprednisolone is preferred to other steroids as it is metabolized before crossing the placenta. For many years it was assumed that the use of steroids in the second and third trimesters was probably safe but there was potentially an increased risk of cleft palate if used during the first trimester [78–80]. Reassuringly two more recent analyses, from a National Birth Defect Prevention Study (NBDPS) [81], and a large Danish prevalence study of over a thousand women who used inhaled or oral corticosteroids from a period of time 30 days before conception through the first trimester [82], observed no associated risk of cleft lip/palate or other congenital malformations in offspring. In addition, intravenous immunoglobulin (IVIG) therapy is safe to use during pregnancy. Studies suggest that IVIG may help prevent relapses both during pregnancy and postpartum when given to a pregnancy MS patient [83].

Postpartum Management

General Postpartum Management and Counseling

A surveillance MRI with gadolinium is recommended within the first few months postpartum, to provide a new baseline for women resuming DMTs immediately, and to monitor for subclinical disease activity in women who are breastfeeding off DMT, where it may help guide whether to resume DMTs earlier than planned. Of note, gadolinium is unlikely to be excreted into breast milk or absorbed into the infant gut and neither the American College of Obstetrics and Gynecologists or the American College of Radiologists recommend a "pump and dump" strategy [84, 85].

In general, women with MS may need to take special precautions to ensure their own health. This may include sleep management, help with feeding (with pumped milk or formula) and potentially physical and pelvic floor therapy. The clinician may help guide seeking concrete help from available friends, family and social services (e.g. gift cards for food home delivery, partner taking night-time bottle feed, etc.).

Additionally, the risk of peripartum depression (before and after delivery), common in the general population [86], is anticipated to be higher in women with MS given the higher baseline risk of depression in persons with MS [87]. As postpartum women with MS may face challenges in fulfilling the competing needs on their limited time (for newborn care and medical appointments, maternal recovery and MS care, and other household, familial and professional responsibilities), the MS clinician may play an important role in screening for depression and encouraging appropriate treatment.

Prevention and Management of Relapses

In general, is it advised to resume immunomodulating therapy as soon as possible. For some women, this means after they finish breastfeeding. Other women defer breastfeeding and resume their therapy immediately.

Breastfeeding

Beyond the general beneficial effects of breastfeeding, several studies have suggested that breastfeeding may influence postpartum relapse rate, but the true effect continues to be debated. While some studies have reported an association between breastfeeding and decreased relapses [88] (A small study of women with MS suggested that exclusive breastfeeding might protect against postpartum relapse, possibly through promoting ongoing anti-inflammatory changes [89]), other studies [90], including the PRIMS cohort [18], showed no association between breastfeeding and postpartum relapses or disability. There is broad variability in breastfeeding practices, both in intensity (on-demand vs. scheduled), frequency, duration, and degree of supplementation (exclusive breastfeeding versus supplementing breastfeeding with formula). A meta-analysis reported that overall, women with MS who breastfeed were almost half as likely to experience a post-partum relapse compared to women who did not. However, limitations to this pooled analysis included confounding by maternal choice (women who chose to breastfeed were less likely to be using a DMT before pregnancy, likely had more benign disease activity during pregnancy and overall and had less severe forms of MS) [91]. It is likely that while women who breastfeed appear to do better, they may be preselected as having milder disease. Further research is needed to assess if breastfeeding may alter post-partum MRI disease activity.

Although there are still many questions, the available evidence suggests that breastfeeding is safe and possibly even beneficial for MS patients. Therefore, while each case should be considered individually, the choice to breast-feed can generally supported. However, breastfeeding mothers are generally advised not to start DMT until the infant is weaned, as there are limited data available on drug transfer into milk and the effects on newborns.

Steroids and IV Immunoglobulin

Both steroids and IVIg can be used to prevent relapses in women who choose to breastfeed but are considered high-risk for postpartum relapses, or to treat postpartum relapses.

Pulses of monthly intravenous methylprednisolone may play a role in prevention relapses. When given for 6 months postpartum, monthly intravenous methylprednisolone was associated with a decreased rate of relapses compared to an untreated group (p = 0.018), suggesting a beneficial effect of this mode of therapy [92]. However, there was no difference in overall neurologic function or progression of disease between those treated and controls. Frequent IV steroids in the postpartum period should be considered on an individual basis.

Historically women were advised to stop breastfeeding and "pump and dump" after receiving IV steroids, due to possible excretion into breast milk. These doses may be very small. In serial sampling of breast milk from a mother with MS who was receiving IV methylprednisolone once a day for 3 days, breast milk concentrations of methylprednisolone were highest 1 h after steroid administration and then quickly tapered off [93]. Another study showed that even with large doses of steroids given to the mother, the amount ingested by the infant was only between 1.1% and 1.5% of maternal dose, i.e. well below the accepted relative infant dose (RID) of 10% for medications excreted into breast milk, and well below the dose of methylprednisolone on an mg/kg/day basis for infants who require steroid treatment [47]. However, if the mother wishes to limit infant exposure even further, she could wait 2–4 h after receiving IV methylprednisolone, which will significantly reduce the amount of drug in her milk.

Other clinicians may use IV immunoglobulin (IVIG), which is safe during pregnancy. IVIg administration has a very low rate of maternal side effects and no known negative influence on the developing fetal immune system. Breastfeeding is not contraindicated during IVIg therapy, and there is no negative effect on the developing immune system of the new baby. A pilot study of 104 patients reported a lower rate of postpartum relapses in patients treated with IVIg. Significant post-partum relapse rate reduction (p < 0.05) was observed in patients who received IVIg continuously through-

out pregnancy and within the first week after delivery until 12 weeks postpartum [94]. Other studies have also suggested that post-partum administration of IVIG could be beneficial in preventing relapses during this period [95].

Exogenous Hormones and MS Course in Women of Childbearing Age

Observational and interventional studies have evaluated the use of exogenous hormones in women with MS, and any effects of common doses of oral contraceptives (OCs) on inflammatory activity may be sub-clinical. For example, in an observational study of 162 women of childbearing age with new-onset MS, OC use, past or current, did not appear to be associated with greater risk of relapses [96]. In an interventional trial of 150 women with relapsing remitting MS were randomized to receive IFN-β-1a alone, IFN-β-1a plus a low dose OC (ethinylstradiol 20 μg and desogestrel 150 μg), or IFN-β-1a plus a high dose OC (ethinylestradiol 40 μg and desogestrel 125 μg). Both groups receiving OC showed reduced cumulative number of unique active lesions on brain MRI at 96 weeks relative to the group not on OC (decreases of 14.1% (p = 0.24) and 26.5% (p = 0.04)), but there was no benefit on relapse rate or disability [97]. Overall, more research is needed in this area to better understand the role of exogenous estrogens in MS on inflammatory markers.

Based on putative associations between the hormonal changes that occur during pregnancy and observed changes in MS inflammatory activity, several trials have sought to harness these hormonal changes for MS management in the non-pregnant state. It has been postulated that progesterone, may have an immunomodulatory effect by inducing a shift in the Th1/Th2 balance towards a Th2 anti-inflammatory response, and this sex steroids may also play a role in remyelination. A multicenter, randomized placebo controlled trial investigated the effect of high dose progestin in combination with protective doses of estradiol on post-partum relapses [98]. The analysis included 202 patients but the study was stopped early due to difficulties with enrollment. Overall, investigators found no effect from these exogenous hormones on postpartum relapse rates [99]. Additionally, other studies have investigated the role of estriol. Estriol, an estrogen made by the fetal placenta, is minimally present in non-pregnant states, but during pregnancy its levels increase progressively and peak in the third trimester. In animal studies, estriol has been associated with an expansion of the T-cell subsets, Treg and Th2 [100], and to ameliorate experimental allergic encephalomyelitis and rheumatoid arthritis when administered at pregnancy levels to non-pregnant female mice [101]. In humans, following an initially promising small crossover Phase I trial in twelve patients [102], a follow up randomized, double blind, placebo controlled

Phase II trial has been conducted [103]. In this study, 164 women with MS, ages 18–50, received 8 mg oral estriol or placebo daily in addition to their glatiramer acetate injections. The primary end point, annualized relapse rate (ARR) at 24 months, was 0.25 in the estriol group versus 0.37 in the placebo group (P = 0.077). There was no significant change in number or volume of T2 or gadolinium enhancing lesions, or in total brain volume [103]. The possible benefits of high-dose estrogen therapy in MS need to be carefully weighed against possible adverse events associated with chronic high-dose estrogen use such as carcinogenesis, thrombogenesis, and dysfunctional uterine bleeding [104].

Neuromyelitis Optica Spectrum Disorders in Pregnancy

Neuromyelitis optica (NMO) is a relapsing inflammatory neurologic disease that primarily effect the optic nerves and spinal cord. Since its discovery, a broader term, neuromyelitis optica spectrum disorders (NMOSD), is now used. Most patients (68–91%) are seropositive for pathogenic antibodies targeting Aquaporin-4 (AQP4–immunoglobulin G [IgG]). AQP4 is a water channel present in many tissues (CNS, kidneys, muscle and others) but most greatly expressed on the foot processes of astrocytes [105–107]. NMOSD is female-predominant (7–9 F:1 M) [108, 109], often affects women during their child-bearing years [110], and seropositivity for AQP4-IgG appears more frequent in women [107], In contrast to MS, NMOSD is more common in non-white populations [109, 111].

Women with NMOSD appear to be at higher risk for relapses not only in the first 3 months postpartum as seen with MS, but also during pregnancy, where they do not seem to benefit from protection by the immunotolerant state of pregnancy. These observations have been borne out in a number of case series [112–115] and appear analogous to gestational exacerbations of systemic lupus erythematosis [116]. Further, women with NMO may also experience higher rates of other pregnancy complications, such as miscarriage and preeclampsia. For example, in one study of 40 AQP4-seropositive women with 85 pregnancies, 11 pregnancies (12.9%) ended in miscarriages. Of those, seven were in the first trimester, one in the second trimester, and three at an unknown time within the first 24 weeks [115]. Further, rates of preeclampsia were higher among NMOSD patients compared to the general population (11.5% vs 3.2% respectively) [115]. Finally, the mean ARR from 9 months preconception to the end of pregnancy was higher in the miscarriage subgroup compared to the viable pregnancy subgroup [115]. Thus, it is postulated that patients with more active disease may have more complications.

While the exact immunologic mechanisms for these pregnancy complications in NMOSD are unknown, they may include an effect of increased estrogen levels during pregnancy on AQP4-IgG antibody type, amount, and glycosylation pattern, on inflammatory mediators, and potentially on survival of self-reactive B cells [117]. Placental expression of AQP4, leading to an AQP4-antibody mediated attack on the placenta, could also be a contributing factor. For example, the placenta of an NMOSD patient was examined after a second trimester miscarriage and was found to contain regions of necrosis as well as deposits of membrane attack complexes [118].

There are several therapeutic options used for relapse prevention in NMOSD including azathioprine, mycophenolate and rituximab [119]. Rituximab has been shown in a retrospective multicenter case series of 25 NMOSD patients to reduce the frequency of relapses, and ultimately offer stabilization or improvement in disability [120]. Given that the half-life of rituximab is 22 days, it would theoretically be safe to begin conception attempts 3.5–4 months post infusion after the drug has cleared maternal circulation, without risk of significant fetal exposure, while conferring some protection against relapses during the pregnancy. Inone case report, treatment with rituximab 1 week prior to unplanned pregnancy was associated with NMO disease stability during pregnancy and no adverse events to mother and child [121]. While no large clinical trials have been performed using rituximab in pregnancy, low B cells in newborns of mothers treated with rituximab before and during pregnancy have been reported, and normalize by 6 months [122] The potential risks and benefits should be weighed with each individual patient according to parental risk tolerance with medication and overall disease course.

Conclusion

Providers caring for women with MS can reassure them that planning a pregnancy is unlikely to lead to long-term adverse outcomes, and to provide a framework to discuss still-limited information about DMT safety in pregnancy and breastfeeding, uncertainty about the course of their MS and the possible effect that pregnancy may have on the disease [123]. Women with NMOSD, however, while also at risk of postpartum relapses, may not experience such a relatively benign course during pregnancy. Specific recommendations regarding whether and when to discontinue DMTs will continue to evolve in light of accumulating clinical experience. Anticipatory guidance at each clinical visit for a woman of childbearing age with MS and NMOSD is recommended to ensure initial selection of appropriate DMT, optimization of chances of conceiving off DMT, reduction of risk to the fetus, and a benign postpartum period.

Table 3 FDA drug risk categories

Category	Description
A	Controlled studies in humans show no risk to fetus
B	No controlled studies have been conducted in humans; animal studies show no risk to fetus
C	No controlled studies have been conducted in animals or humans. Risk to fetus cannot be ruled out
D	Evidence of human risk to the fetus exists; however, benefits may outweigh risks in certain situations
X	Controlled studies in both animals and humans demonstrate fetal abnormalities; the risk in pregnant women outweighs any possible benefit

Interferons (Betaseron, Rebif, Avonex, Extavia, Plegridy)

Disease Modifying Agents During Pregnancy

Until 2015, the FDA used a five-letter system (A, B, C, D and X) to categorize the known risks of taking a drug or biological product during pregnancy (Table 3). The FDA is now utilizing a more narrative approach for any new drug approved after June 30th, 2015. Due to reader familiarity, we will include both approaches for DMTs approved prior to 2015.

References

1. Bove R, Chitnis T. The role of gender and sex hormones in determining the onset and outcome of multiple sclerosis. Mult Scler J. 2014;20(5):520–6.
2. Hellwig K, Correale J. Artificial reproductive techniques in multiple sclerosis. Clin Immunol. 2013;149(2):219–24.
3. Visser JA, Schipper I, Laven JS, Themmen AP. Anti-Müllerian hormone: an ovarian reserve marker in primary ovarian insufficiency. Nat Rev Endocrinol. 2012;8(6):331–41.
4. Thöne J, Kollar S, Nousome D, et al. Serum anti-Müllerian hormone levels in reproductive-age women with relapsing–remitting multiple sclerosis. Mult Scler J. 2015;21(1):41–7.
5. Grinsted L, Heltberg A, Hagen C, Djursing H. Serum sex hormone and gonadotropin concentrations in premenopausal women with multiple sclerosis. J Intern Med. 1989;226(4):241–4.
6. Bove R, Alwan S, Friedman JM, et al. Management of multiple sclerosis during pregnancy and the reproductive years: a systematic review. Obstet Gynecol. 2014;124(6):1157–68.
7. Cavalla P, Rovei V, Masera S, et al. Fertility in patients with multiple sclerosis: current knowledge and future perspectives. Neurol Sci. 2006;27(4):231–9.
8. Harward L, Mitchell K, Pieper C, Copland S, Criscione-Schreiber L, Clowse M. The impact of cyclophosphamide on menstruation and pregnancy in women with rheumatologic disease. Lupus. 2013;22(1):81–6.
9. Demirkiran M, Sarica Y, Uguz S, Yerdelen D, Aslan K. Multiple sclerosis patients with and without sexual dysfunction: are there any differences? Mult Scler J. 2006;12(2):209–11.
10. Dahl J, Myhr K-M, Daltveit A, Hoff J, Gilhus N. Pregnancy, delivery, and birth outcome in women with multiple sclerosis. Neurology. 2005;65(12):1961–3.
11. van der Kop ML, Pearce MS, Dahlgren L, et al. Neonatal and delivery outcomes in women with multiple sclerosis. Ann Neurol. 2011;70(1):41–50.
12. Beecham AH, Patsopoulos NA, Xifara DK, et al. Analysis of immune-related loci identifies 48 new susceptibility variants for multiple sclerosis. Nat Genet. 2013;45(11):1353.
13. Didonna A, Oksenberg JR. Genetic determinants of risk and progression in multiple sclerosis. Clin Chim Acta. 2015;449:16–22.
14. Langagergaard V, Pedersen L, Gislum M, Nørgard B, Sørensen HT. Birth outcome in women treated with azathioprine or mercaptopurine during pregnancy: a Danish nationwide cohort study. Aliment Pharmacol Ther. 2007;25(1):73–81.
15. Ascherio A, Munger KL, Lünemann JD. The initiation and prevention of multiple sclerosis. Nat Rev Neurol. 2012;8(11):602–12.
16. Munger KL, Åivo J, Hongell K, Soilu-Hänninen M, Surcel H-M, Ascherio A. Vitamin D status during pregnancy and risk of multiple sclerosis in offspring of women in the Finnish maternity cohort. JAMA Neurol. 2016;73(5):515–9.
17. ACOG Committee on Obstetric Practice. Vitamin D: screening and supplementation during pregnancy. Committee opinion no. 495. Obstet Gynecol 2011;118:197–198.
18. Confavreux C, Hutchinson M, Hours MM, Cortinovis-Tourniaire P, Moreau T, Group PiMS. Rate of pregnancy-related relapse in multiple sclerosis. N Engl J Med. 1998;339(5):285–91.
19. Vukusic S, Hutchinson M, Hours M, et al. Pregnancy and multiple sclerosis (the PRIMS study): clinical predictors of post-partum relapse. Brain. 2004;127(6):1353–60.
20. Salemi G, Callari G, Gammino M, et al. The relapse rate of multiple sclerosis changes during pregnancy: a cohort study. Acta Neurol Scand. 2004;110(1):23–6.
21. Hanulíková P, Vlk R, Meluzínová E, et al. Pregnancy and multiple sclerosis-outcomes analysis 2003–2011. Ceska Gynekol/Ceska Lekarska Spolecnost J Ev Purkyne. 2013;78(2):142–8.
22. Runmarker B, Andersen O. Pregnancy is associated with a lower risk of onset and a better prognosis in multiple sclerosis. Brain. 1995;118(1):253–61.
23. Stenager E, Stenager E, Jensen K. Effect of pregnancy on the prognosis for multiple sclerosis. A 5-year follow up investigation. Acta Neurol Scand. 1994;90(5):305–8.
24. Mueller BA, Zhang J, Critchlow CW. Birth outcomes and need for hospitalization after delivery among women with multiple sclerosis. Am J Obstet Gynecol. 2002;186(3):446–52.
25. Dwosh E, Guimond C, Sadovnick A. Reproductive counselling for MS: a rationale. Int MS J. 2003;10(2):52–9.
26. Boivin J, Bunting L, Collins JA, Nygren KG. International estimates of infertility prevalence and treatment-seeking: potential need and demand for infertility medical care. Hum Reprod. 2007;22(6):1506–12.
27. Laplaud D-A, Leray E, Barriere P, Wiertlewski S, Moreau T. Increase in multiple sclerosis relapse rate following in vitro fertilization. Neurology. 2006;66(8):1280–1.
28. Michel L, Foucher Y, Vukusic S, et al. Increased risk of multiple sclerosis relapse after in vitro fertilisation. J Neurol Neurosurg Psychiatry. 2012;83(8):796–802.
29. Correale J, Farez MF, Ysrraelit MC. Increase in multiple sclerosis activity after assisted reproduction technology. Ann Neurol. 2012;72(5):682–94.
30. Hellwig K, Beste C, Brune N, et al. Increased MS relapse rate during assisted reproduction technique. J Neurol. 2008;255(4):592–3.
31. Hellwig K, Schimrigk S, Beste C, Müller T, Gold R. Increase in relapse rate during assisted reproduction technique in patients with multiple sclerosis. Eur Neurol. 2009;61(2):65–8.
32. Bove R, Rankin K, Lin C, Zhao C, Correale J, Michel L, Chitnis T. Assisted reproductive technologies and relapse risk: a new case series, and pooled analysis of existing studies. Poster presented at ECTRIMS 2017 Oct 25–28; Paris; 2017.
33. Coyle PK. Management of women with multiple sclerosis through pregnancy and after childbirth. Ther Adv Neurol Disord. 2016;9(3):198–210.

34. Wundes A, Pebdani RN, Amtmann D. What do healthcare providers advise women with multiple sclerosis regarding pregnancy? Mult Scler Int. 2014;819216.

35. Hatcher SE, Waubant E, Nourbakhsh B, Crabtree-Hartman E, Graves JS. Rebound syndrome in patients with multiple sclerosis after cessation of fingolimod treatment. JAMA Neurol. 2016;73(7):790–4.

36. Novi G, Ghezzi A, Pizzorno M, et al. Dramatic rebounds of MS during pregnancy following fingolimod withdrawal. Neurol-Neuroimmunol Neuroinflammation. 2017;4(5):e377.

37. Sempere A, Berenguer-Ruiz L, Feliu-Rey E. Rebound of disease activity during pregnancy after withdrawal of fingolimod. Eur J Neurol. 2013;20(8):e109–10.

38. Thöne J, Thiel S, Gold R, Hellwig K. Treatment of multiple sclerosis during pregnancy–safety considerations. Expert Opin Drug Saf. 2017;16(5):523–34.

39. Coyle PK, Sinclair S, Scheuerle A, Thorp J, Albano J, Rametta M. Final results from the betaseron (interferon β-1b) pregnancy registry: a prospective observational study of birth defects and pregnancy-related adverse events. BMJ Open. 2014;4(5):e004536.

40. Thiel S, Langer-Gould A, Rockhoff M, et al. Interferon-beta exposure during first trimester is safe in women with multiple sclerosis—a prospective cohort study from the German multiple sclerosis and pregnancy registry. Mult Scler J. 2016;22(6):801–9.

41. Amato M, Portaccio E, Ghezzi A, et al. Pregnancy and fetal outcomes after interferon-β exposure in multiple sclerosis. Neurology. 2010;75(20):1794–802.

42. Boskovic R, Wide R, Wolpin J, Bauer D, Koren G. The reproductive effects of beta interferon therapy in pregnancy a longitudinal cohort. Neurology. 2005;65(6):807–11.

43. Patti F, Cavallaro T, Fermo SL, et al. Is in utero early-exposure to interferon beta a risk factor for pregnancy outcomes in multiple sclerosis? J Neurol. 2008;255(8):1250–3.

44. Lu E, Wang BW, Guimond C, Synnes A, Sadovnick D, Tremlett H. Disease-modifying drugs for multiple sclerosis in pregnancy a systematic review. Neurology. 2012;79(11):1130–5.

45. Waubant E, Sadovnick AD. Interferon beta babies. Neurology. 2005;65(6):788–9.

46. Hale TW, Siddiqui AA, Baker TE. Transfer of interferon β-1a into human breastmilk. Breastfeed Med. 2012;7(2):123–5.

47. Voskuhl R, Momtazee C. Pregnancy: effect on multiple sclerosis, treatment considerations, and breastfeeding. Neurotherapeutics. 2017;14:1–11.

48. Fragoso YD, Finkelsztejn A, Kaimen-Maciel DR, et al. Long-term use of glatiramer acetate by 11 pregnant women with multiple sclerosis. CNS Drugs. 2010;24(11):969–76.

49. Herbstritt S, Langer-Gould A, Rockhoff M, et al. Glatiramer acetate during early pregnancy: a prospective cohort study. Mult Scler J. 2016;22(6):810–6.

50. Neudorfer O, Melamed-Gal S, Baruch P. Pregnancy outcomes in patients with multiple sclerosis and exposure to branded glatiramer acetate during all three trimesters. Poster presented at ECTRIMS 2017 Oct 25–28; Paris; 2017.

51. Hellwig K. Pregnancy in multiple sclerosis. Eur Neurol. 2014;72(Suppl. 1):39–42.

52. Gold R, Phillips JT, Havrdova E, et al. Delayed-release dimethyl fumarate and pregnancy: preclinical studies and pregnancy outcomes from clinical trials and postmarketing experience. Neurol Ther. 2015;4(2):93–104.

53. Biogen Idec Inc. Tecfidera, Dimethy; Fumarte package insert. Massachusetts: Biogen Idec; 2014.

54. Almas S, Vance J, Baker T, Hale T. Management of multiple sclerosis in the breastfeeding mother. Mult Scler Int. 2016;2016:6527458.

55. Karlsson G, Francis G, Koren G, et al. Pregnancy outcomes in the clinical development program of fingolimod in multiple sclerosis. Neurology. 2014;82(8):674–80.

56. Houtchens MK, Sadovnick AD. Health issues in women with multiple sclerosis. Springer; 2017.

57. Collins W, Francis G, Koren G, et al. Lack of interaction between fingolimod (FTY720) and oral contraceptives, and pregnancy experience in the clinical program of fingolimod in multiple sclerosis. Paper presented at: Neurology. 2011.

58. Buraga I, Popovici R-E. Multiple sclerosis and pregnancy: current considerations. Sci World J. 2014;513160.

59. Vukusic S, Marignier R. Multiple sclerosis and pregnancy in the 'treatment era'. Nat Rev Neurol. 2015;11(5):280–9.

60. Brent Robert L. Teratogen update—reproductive risks of leflunomide (Arava TM); a pyrimidine synthesis inhibitor: counseling women taking leflunomide before or during pregnancy and men taking leflunomide who are contemplanting fathering a child. Teratology. 2001;63:106–12.

61. Cassina M, Johnson D, Robinson L, et al. Pregnancy outcome in women exposed to leflunomide before or during pregnancy. Arthritis Rheumatol. 2012;64(7):2085–94.

62. AUBAGIO prescribing information. Cambridge: Genzyme Corporation, a Sanofi company; 2012. Available from: http://products.sanofi.us/aubagio/aubagio.pdf. Accessed 18 Jan 2018.

63. Biogen Idec Inc. Daclizumab package insert. Massachusetts: Biogen Idec; 2016.

64. Gold R, Stefoski D, Selmaj K, et al. Pregnancy experience: nonclinical studies and pregnancy outcomes in the daclizumab clinical study program. Neurol Ther. 2016;5(2):169–82.

65. EMA. Zinbryta® (daclizumab) – EPAR summary of product characteristics. Available from: http://www.ema.europa.eu/docs/en_GB/document_library/EPAR_-_Product_Information/human/003862/WC500210598.pdf.

66. Haghikia A, Langer-Gould A, Rellensmann G, et al. Natalizumab use during the third trimester of pregnancy. JAMA Neurol. 2014;71(7):891–5.

67. Kümpfel T, Thiel S, Meinl I, Gold R, Hellwig K. Long-term exposure to natalizumab during pregnancy – a prospective case series from the German multiple sclerosis and pregnancy registry. Poster presented at ECTRIMS 2017 Oct 25–28; Paris; 2017.

68. Baker TE, Cooper SD, Kessler L, Hale TW. Transfer of natalizumab into breast milk in a mother with multiple sclerosis. J Hum Lact. 2015;31(2):233–6.

69. Gelfand JM, Cree BA, Hauser SL. Ocrelizumab and other CD20+ B-cell-depleting therapies in multiple sclerosis. Neurotherapeutics. 2017;14:1–7.

70. Klink D, Van Elburg R, Schreurs M, Van Well G. Rituximab administration in third trimester of pregnancy suppresses neonatal B-cell development. Clin Dev Immunol. 2008;2008(1):1.

71. Chakravarty EF, Murray ER, Kelman A, Farmer P. Pregnancy outcomes after maternal exposure to rituximab. Blood. 2011;117(5):1499–506.

72. Genentech. Ocrelizumab package insert. San Francisco: Genentech; 2017.

73. Vaidyanathan A, McKeever K, Anand B, Eppler S, Weinbauer GF, Beyer JC. Developmental immunotoxicology assessment of rituximab in cynomolgus monkeys. Toxicol Sci. 2010;119(1):116–25.

74. Hurley WL, Theil PK. Perspectives on immunoglobulins in colostrum and milk. Nutrients. 2011;3(4):442–74.

75. Bragnes Y, Boshuizen R, de Vries A, Lexberg Å, Østensen M. Low level of Rituximab in human breast milk in a patient treated during lactation. Rheumatology. 2017;56(6):1047–8.

76. Oh J, Achiron A, Chambers C, et al. Pregnancy outcomes in patients with RRMS who received alemtuzumab in the clinical development program (S24. 008). Neurology. 2016;86(16 Supplement):S24.008.

77. Bove RM, Klein JP. Neuroradiology in women of childbearing age. Continuum Lifelong Learn Neurol. 2014;20(1):23–41.

78. Argyriou AA, Makris N. Multiple sclerosis and reproductive risks in women. Reprod Sci. 2008;15(8):755–64.

79. Fraser F, Sajoo A. Teratogenic potential of corticosteroids in humans. Teratology. 1995;51(1):45–6.

80. Carmichael SL, Shaw GM. Maternal corticosteroid use and risk of selected congenital anomalies. Am J Med Genet A. 1999;86(3):242–4.

81. Skuladottir H, Wilcox AJ, Ma C, et al. Corticosteroid use and risk of orofacial clefts. Birth Defects Res A Clin Mol Teratol. 2014;100(6):499–506.

82. Bjørn A-MB, Ehrenstein V, Hundborg HH, Nohr EA, Sørensen HT, Nørgaard M. Use of corticosteroids in early pregnancy is not associated with risk of oral clefts and other congenital malformations in offspring. Am J Ther. 2014;21(2):73–80.

83. Achiron A, Kishner I, Dolev M, et al. Effect of intravenous immunoglobulin treatment on pregnancy and postpartum-related relapses in multiple sclerosis. J Neurol. 2004;251(9):1133–7.

84. Webb JA, Thomsen HS, Morcos SK, Members of Contrast Media Safety Committee of European Society of Urogenital Radiology (ESUR). The use of iodinated and gadolinium contrast media during pregnancy and lactation. Eur Radiol. 2005;15(6):1234–40.

85. ACOG Committee on Obstetric Practice. ACOG committee opinion. number 299, September 2004 (replaces no. 158, September 1995). Guidelines for diagnostic imaging during pregnancy. Obstet Gynecol. 2004;104(3):647.

86. Milgrom J, Gemmill AW, Bilszta JL, et al. Antenatal risk factors for postnatal depression: a large prospective study. J Affect Disord. 2008;108(1):147–57.

87. Feinstein A. Multiple sclerosis and depression. Mult Scler J. 2011;17(11):1276–81.

88. Langer-Gould A, Beaber BE. Effects of pregnancy and breastfeeding on the multiple sclerosis disease course. Clin Immunol. 2013;149(2):244–50.

89. Hellwig K, Rockhoff M, Herbstritt S, et al. Exclusive breastfeeding and the effect on postpartum multiple sclerosis relapses. JAMA Neurol. 2015;72(10):1132–8.

90. Portaccio E, Ghezzi A, Hakiki B, et al. Breastfeeding is not related to postpartum relapses in multiple sclerosis. Neurology. 2011;77(2):145–50.

91. Pakpoor J, Disanto G, Lacey MV, Hellwig K, Giovannoni G, Ramagopalan SV. Breastfeeding and multiple sclerosis relapses: a meta-analysis. J Neurol. 2012;259(10):2246–8.

92. De Seze J, Chapelotte M, Delalande S, Ferriby D, Stojkovic T, Vermersch P. Intravenous corticosteroids in the postpartum period for reduction of acute exacerbations in multiple sclerosis. Mult Scler J. 2004;10(5):596–7.

93. Cooper SD, Felkins K, Baker TE, Hale TW. Transfer of methylprednisolone into breast milk in a mother with multiple sclerosis. J Hum Lact. 2015;31(2):237–9.

94. Achiron A, Rotstein Z, Noy S, Mashiach S, Dulitzky M, Achiron R. Intravenous immunoglobulin treatment in the prevention of childbirth-associated acute exacerbations in multiple sclerosis: a pilot study. J Neurol. 1996;243(1):25–8.

95. Brandt-Wouters E, Gerlach OH, Hupperts RM. The effect of postpartum intravenous immunoglobulins on the relapse rate among patients with multiple sclerosis. Int J Gynecol Obstet. 2016;134(2):194–6.

96. Bove R, Rankin K, Chua AS, et al. Oral contraceptives and MS disease activity in a contemporary real-world cohort. Mult Scler J. 2017; https://doi.org/10.1177/1352458517692420.

97. Pozzilli C, De Giglio L, Barletta VT, et al. Oral contraceptives combined with interferon β in multiple sclerosis. Neurol-Neuroimmunol Neuroinflammation. 2015;2(4):e120.

98. Vukusic S, Ionescu I, El-Etr M, et al. The prevention of postpartum relapses with progestin and estradiol in multiple sclerosis (POPARTMUS) trial: rationale, objectives and state of advancement. J Neurol Sci. 2009;286(1):114–8.

99. Durand-Dubief F, El-Etr M, Ionescu I, et al. The POPARTMUS French-Italian multicentric trial of postpartum progestin and estradiol in multiple sclerosis: MRI findings. Paper presented at: Multiple Sclerosis Journal 2014.

100. Haghmorad D, Amini AA, Mahmoudi MB, Rastin M, Hosseini M, Mahmoudi M. Pregnancy level of estrogen attenuates experimental autoimmune encephalomyelitis in both ovariectomized and pregnant C57BL/6 mice through expansion of Treg and Th2 cells. J Neuroimmunol. 2014;277(1):85–95.

101. Jansson L, Olsson T, Holmdahl R. Estrogen induces a potent suppression of experimental autoimmune encephalomyelities and collagen-induced arthritis in mice. J Neuroimmunol. 1994;53(2):203–7.

102. Sicotte NL, Liva SM, Klutch R, et al. Treatment of multiple sclerosis with the pregnancy hormone estriol. Ann Neurol. 2002;52(4):421–8.

103. Voskuhl RR, Wang H, Wu TJ, et al. Estriol combined with glatiramer acetate for women with relapsing-remitting multiple sclerosis: a randomised, placebo-controlled, phase 2 trial. Lancet Neurol. 2016;15(1):35–46.

104. Rizvi SA, Bashir K. Other therapy options and future strategies for treating patients with multiple sclerosis. Neurology. 2004;63(12 suppl 6):S47–54.

105. Lennon VA, Kryzer TJ, Pittock SJ, Verkman A, Hinson SR. IgG marker of optic-spinal multiple sclerosis binds to the aquaporin-4 water channel. J Exp Med. 2005;202(4):473–7.

106. Matiello M, Schaefer-Klein J, Sun D, Weinshenker BG. Aquaporin 4 expression and tissue susceptibility to neuromyelitis optica. JAMA Neurol. 2013;70(9):1118–25.

107. Quek AM, McKeon A, Lennon VA, et al. Effects of age and sex on aquaporin-4 autoimmunity. Arch Neurol. 2012;69(8):1039–43.

108. Marrie RA, Gryba C. The incidence and prevalence of neuromyelitis optica: a systematic review. Int J MS Care. 2013;15(3):113–8.

109. Mealy MA, Wingerchuk DM, Greenberg BM, Levy M. Epidemiology of neuromyelitis optica in the United States: a multicenter analysis. Arch Neurol. 2012;69(9):1176–80.

110. Wingerchuk DM, Lennon VA, Lucchinetti CF, Pittock SJ, Weinshenker BG. The spectrum of neuromyelitis optica. Lancet Neurol. 2007;6(9):805–15.

111. Pandit L, Asgari N, Apiwattanakul M, et al. Demographic and clinical features of neuromyelitis optica: a review. Mult Scler J. 2015;21(7):845–53.

112. Klawiter EC, Bove R, Elsone L, et al. High risk of postpartum relapses in neuromyelitis optica spectrum disorder. Neurology. 2017; https://doi.org/10.1212/WNL.0000000000004681.

113. Kim W, Kim S-H, Nakashima I, et al. Influence of pregnancy on neuromyelitis optica spectrum disorder. Neurology. 2012;78(16):1264–7.

114. Fragoso YD, Adoni T, Bichuetti DB, et al. Neuromyelitis optica and pregnancy. J Neurol. 2013;260(10):2614–9.

115. Nour MM, Nakashima I, Coutinho E, et al. Pregnancy outcomes in aquaporin-4–positive neuromyelitis optica spectrum disorder. Neurology. 2016;86(1):79–87.

116. Reichlin M. Systemic lupus erythematosus and pregnancy. J Reprod Med. 1998;43:355–60.

117. Davoudi V, Keyhanian K, Bove RM, Chitnis T. Immunology of neuromyelitis optica during pregnancy. Neurol-Neuroimmunol Neuroinflammation. 2016;3(6):e288.

118. Reuß R, Rommer PS, Brück W, et al. A woman with acute myelopathy in pregnancy: case outcome. London: BMJ Publishing Group; 2009.

119. Kimbrough DJ, Fujihara K, Jacob A, et al. Treatment of neuromyelitis optica: review and recommendations. Mult Scler Relat Disord. 2012;1(4):180–7.

120. Jacob A, Weinshenker BG, Violich I, et al. Treatment of neuromyelitis optica with rituximab. Arch Neurol. 2008;65(11):1443–8.

121. Pellkofer H, Suessmair C, Schulze A, Hohlfeld R, Kuempfel T. Course of neuromyelitis optica during inadvertent pregnancy in a patient treated with rituximab. Mult Scler J. 2009;15(8):1006–8.

122. Azim HA Jr, Azim H, Peccatori FA. Treatment of cancer during pregnancy with monoclonal antibodies: a real challenge. Expert Rev Clin Immunol. 2010;6(6):821–6.

123. Prunty M, Sharpe L, Butow P, Fulcher G. The motherhood choice: themes arising in the decision-making process for women with multiple sclerosis. Mult Scler J. 2008;14(5):701–4.

Mood Disorders in Pregnancy

Kara Brown and Dylan Kathol

Abbreviations

AAP	American Academy of Pediatrics
ACOG	American College of Obstetricians and Gynecologists
CBT	Cognitive behavioral therapy
CRH	Corticotropin-releasing hormone
EPDS	Edinburgh Postnatal Depression Scale
ECT	Electroconvulsive therapy
EEG	Electroencephalography
EPS	Extrapyramidal symptoms
FGAs	First-generation antipsychotics
HPA	Hypothalamic-Pituitary-Adrenal
IPT	Interpersonal psychotherapy
MCMs	Major congenital malformations
MDQ	Mood Disorder Questionnaire
NMDA	N-methyl-D-aspartate
PHQ	Patient Health Questionnaire
PNAS	Postnatal adaptation syndrome
RID	Relative infant dose
SGAs	Second generation antipsychotics
SSRIs	Selective serotonin reuptake inhibitors
SNRIs	Serotonin-norepinephrine reuptake inhibitors
TCAs	Tricyclic antidepressants
WHO	World Health Organization

Baby Blues

Baby blues is a common phenomenon affecting up to 70–85% of women following delivery [1, 2]. Baby blues is time-limited, lasting no more than 2 weeks [3]. It may con-

K. Brown (✉)
Southeast Louisiana Verterans Health Care System,
New Orleans, LA, USA

D. Kathol
Department of Psychiatry, NorthShore University Health System,
Evanston, IL, USA

sist of mood lability, crying spells (not necessarily associated with low mood), irritability, poor concentration, feelings of overwhelmed and be associated with neurovegetative symptoms such as poor appetite and difficulty sleeping [1, 2]. It does not result in impaired functioning and resolves without treatment. Women should receive psychoeducation regarding baby blues and be encouraged to reach out for further care if symptoms persist past 2 weeks [2]. Postpartum blues is not a risk factor for postpartum depression [2].

Perinatal Depression

Epidemiology

The prevalence of both major and minor depression during pregnancy has been found to range from 7.5% to 12.7% with discrete major depressive episodes occurring in 3.1–4.9% of women [4–6]. The prevalence of major and minor depression in the postpartum (defined as the 12 months post-birth) is approximately 10–22% [3, 6–8]. The incidence of perinatal depression is thought to be between 14% and 23%, with nearly one in seven women experiencing a depressive episode in the postpartum period [4, 6, 9, 10]. This makes perinatal depression one of the most common complications of pregnancy.

In a large cohort study, Wisner, et al. identified that 60% of women with postpartum depression were symptomatic while pregnant, with nearly 30% beginning before the pregnancy [11]. Studies determining point prevalence over the course of pregnancy find higher prevalence rates during the first trimester and in the first 3 months postpartum with rates lowest during the second trimester [4].

Risk Factors

The strongest risk factor for a perinatal depressive episode is a history of prior perinatal depression; risk of recurrence in this population has been shown to be as high as 50% [12]. For women who are depressed during pregnancy, their risk of having postpartum depression increases sixfold [13]. Previous history of depression or anxiety, previous history of trauma, previous history of substance use, and previous history of suicidal ideation or self-injurious behaviors are also risk factors [2]. Women with the personal or family history of vulnerability to hormonal fluctuations are also at risk; this includes mood changes during menarche and premenstrually, mood worsening in response to oral contraceptives, and family history of mood changes during perimenopause. Psychosocial stressors are also known to contribute to increased risk: unplanned pregnancy, partner conflict, perceived lack of support, financial strain, limited access to resources, and belonging to a racial or ethnic minority all increase risk [2, 3, 8].

Etiology

Research continues to focus on elucidating the etiology of perinatal depression, although numerous models have been proposed based on humans and other animal data.

Estrogen and progesterone decline in the early postpartum period has been implicated; while many women with postpartum depression note absolute hormone levels equal to non-depressed women, the work of Block et al. suggests that the flux in estrogen levels is responsible for precipitating mood symptoms in a vulnerable population [3, 14–16]. Estrogen has been demonstrated to have prominent antidepressant properties [17]. This has been further supported by examining the role of estrogen on the hypothalamic-pituitary-adrenal (HPA) axis. Data regarding progesterone levels are conflicting [2].

During pregnancy, estrogen stimulates the HPA axis; this is further augmented by the placenta, which also creates and secretes corticotropin-releasing hormone (CRH) which operates in a positive feedback loop, leading to hypercortisolemia [18]. After delivery, progesterone and estrogen levels drop, and placental CRH disappears. A transient blunting of HPA activity is observed with hypothalamic CRH hyposecretion as the system returns to operating as in the prepregnant state with negative feedback resulting from elevated cortisol [3, 17, 18]. During the postpartum, in women without depression, HPA activity is briefly refractory to external CRH challenge as cortisol levels initially remain elevated. On the other hand, in women with postpartum depression, a blunted response to CRH at up to 12 weeks has been found [3, 18].

Clinical Features

Symptoms of perinatal depression are similar to a traditional major depressive episode. However, in the perinatal patient, sleep disturbance, appetite changes, fatigue and poor concentration is often normal and not indicative of mood pathology. This is important for the discerning clinician to consider when assessing a patient. Loss of pleasure, irritability, low mood, thoughts of dying or suicide and impaired functioning are important in making the diagnosis [2]. Women may report low self-efficacy and note difficulty making decisions [19]. Similarly, anxiety is a common feature of perinatal depression with ruminations, ego-dystonic thoughts (often aggressive) and agitation reported [3, 11].

Course

Pregnant women with depression may paradoxically present to prenatal care later and be noncompliant with routine appointments while simultaneously utilizing acute obstetrical services more frequently [20]. With respect to obstetrical outcomes, the literature has inconsistently shown associations with higher rates of Caesarean section, increased epidural requirements, maternal urinary tract infections, pre-eclampsia, anemia and placental abnormalities [20–23]. Untreated depression has been more consistently linked with low birth weight and preterm delivery, with the proposed mechanism related to cortisol levels impacting placental growth and umbilical blood flow [24–27]. Babies born to mothers with depression have associated lower levels of dopamine and serotonin, greater relative right frontal electroencephalography (EEG) activation and lower vagal tone; they also have higher rates of irritability and decreased activity and facial expressions compared to infants of non-depressed mothers [26].

Maternal depression has also been linked with decreased use of safety measures such as car seats and childproof latches, lower rates of compliance with routine vaccination schedules and pediatrician appointments [3]. Rates of breastfeeding initiation are lower in depressed women [28].

Maternal suicide is one of the most serious complications of perinatal depression. While overall, rates of suicide in this population are lower than in the general public, suicide accounts for 20% of all postpartum mortality [29]. Women who attempt suicide during this period are more likely to be young and unmarried, and they use more violent means, which may indicate seriousness of intent or even presence of psychosis [29, 30]. Women who attempt have an increased risk of resulting fetal morbidity, even when the attempt is unsuccessful [29, 31].

Even an initial depressive episode in pregnancy or postpartum increases the risk of recurrent depressive episodes outside of the peripartum [32]. Maternal depression during pregnancy has not been associated with an increased risk of suicide in the offspring although in one study, the presence of illness requiring hospitalization did increase the risk of attempts in female offspring, and presence of a clinical diagnosis increased the risk of completed suicide in male offspring [33].

Perinatal Bipolar Disorder

Bipolar disorder is a common psychiatric disorder characterized by episodes of depression, mania, hypomania, and mixed depressive/manic symptoms. Manic episodes have been associated with increased risk-taking behavior, excessive substance or alcohol use, aggression, and disinhibited behavior that can have life-threatening or severe psychosocial consequences. The depressive phase of the illness has been associated with increased suicide, poor self-care, substance use, and disruption of important relationships [34].

Epidemiology

The bipolar spectrum disorders have a lifetime prevalence of approximately 1–4%, and there is an equal prevalence among men and women [35–38]. However, because the onset of illness occurs in women during their childbearing years, there is considerable risk associated with the disorder [35, 39]. During the peripartum period, women with bipolar disorder have an even higher risk of relapse than women with unipolar depression. In fact, women with bipolar disorder made up 22% of the women who screen positive for postpartum depressive symptoms in a study by Wisner et al. looking at a large urban population [11].

Currently, pregnancy is no longer thought to be protective in bipolar disorder despite some studies showing lower admission rates to inpatient psychiatric units and lower than expected rates of mood episodes during this period [40, 41]. Other studies have demonstrated the opposite, some with dramatic results: Freeman et al. showed higher than expected rates of mood episodes during pregnancy, and Viguera et al. found that 50–82% of women with untreated bipolar disorder experienced a relapse during pregnancy [39, 42]. Viguera et al. also found that women who relapsed tended to do so during the first trimester and spent an average of 40% of the time in an acute mood episode [42–45]. Women who continued medication during pregnancy had much lower rates of relapse (22.7–37%) [44, 45].

There is clear data that the postpartum period is very high risk for women with bipolar disorder. Approximately 85% of women who discontinued their mood stabilizers during pregnancy relapsed in the postpartum period and approximately 22% of women with bipolar disorder were hospitalized for a psychiatric emergency in the first 3 months postpartum [41, 45].

Risk Factors

As noted above, history of bipolar disorder is a major risk factor for a peripartum mood episode in and of itself, and the discontinuation of mood stabilizers increases this risk further [43].

Similarly, the rate of discontinuation of mood stabilizers can have significant impacts as well. Sixty-three percent of women who discontinued lithium rapidly (i.e., within 14 days) relapsed in the next 6 months compared to only 37% who discontinued the medication more gradually [42]. Many of the relapses occurred within the first few weeks after discontinuation [45]. This is particularly noteworthy because many women will immediately stop their medications upon learning that they are pregnant and this has significant risks associated with it.

Additionally, a personal history of prior postpartum mood episodes dramatically increases the risk of recurrence during a woman's subsequent pregnancies, just like unipolar depression [39]. Other notable risk factors associated with relapse during pregnancy and the postpartum period include younger age at illness onset, being unmarried, having a family history of postpartum mood disorders or bipolar disorder, being unemployed, having a history of rapid cycling, having a history of recent mood disorders prior to conception, and antidepressant use [39, 41, 42, 44, 46–49].

Clinical Course

Because of the risk of mood episodes associated with pregnancy and the postpartum period, it is a time where many women make their first contact with mental health professionals. Munk-Olsen et al. found that a significant proportion (14%) of women making their first contact with these providers have an underlying a bipolar disorder [50]. Women who experience their first depressive episode during the postpartum period are four times more likely to have bipolar disorder than if the first episode occurred outside of the peripartum period [11, 42]. To further complicate the picture, women with unipolar and bipolar depressive episodes often present similarly. However, women with bipolar depression may have more pronounced psychomotor retardation, cognitive difficulties, mood lability, and psychotic features than episodes of unipolar depression [51]. Because of the high prevalence, providers should screen women presenting with depressive episodes in the postpartum period for a history of manic or hypomanic symptoms before starting an antidepressant [52, 53].

Mood disorders in women with bipolar I disorder during pregnancy more commonly tend to be depressive (35%) and mixed (33%) in nature. Manic and hypomanic episodes make up approximately 25% of episodes reported. In the postpartum period, there is a much higher frequency of depressive episodes (50%), but 29% of these episodes are manic or hypomanic. Mixed episodes made up 19% of the episodes. Women with bipolar II disorder have a higher proportion of depressive episodes than are seen in bipolar I disorder [44]. Notably, there are high rates of hypomania – a sixfold increase – in the 1st week following delivery, but these symptoms are often misdiagnosed as normal euphoria following birth [54]. Women with bipolar disorder are at an elevated risk of postpartum psychosis as well [44].

Bipolar disorder has been associated with several adverse birth outcomes regardless of whether the women were treated or untreated during pregnancy. Women with bipolar disorder have been found to have more Caesarean sections, and have higher rates of preterm birth, gestational hypertension, and placenta previa than women without the disorder [55–58]. There have been mixed data about whether the infants born to women with bipolar disorder have a higher risk of small for gestational age or low birth weight [56–59]. There have not been any associations between the underlying disorder and stillbirth, fetal distress or infant mortality [57].

Postpartum Psychosis

Epidemiology

Postpartum psychosis is a psychotic state that occurs in the first several weeks following delivery. The disorder occurs in 1–2 women per 1000 live births [60] and is often associated with affective symptoms [61]. The rate of experiencing a psychotic or manic episode is 22-times higher in the 1st month following delivery than at any other point during a woman's life [62].

Risk Factors

The strongest risk factor for postpartum psychosis is history of an underlying bipolar disorder. In fact, Jones and colleagues found an incidence of 260 episodes per 1000 births in this population of women [63]. A family history of either bipolar disorder or postpartum psychosis carries morbidity risk between 10% and 50% [63–65]. Primiparity has also been associated with a higher risk of postpartum psychosis [66, 67]. However, this significant difference may be because women who experience severe postpartum episodes are less likely to have additional children [49]. There has not been a consistently established link between psychosocial stressors or obstetric outcomes and postpartum psychosis [67–69]. The relapse risk for women who have an episode of postpartum psychosis was approximately 18–37%, but prophylactic treatment during pregnancy results in significantly lower rates [65, 70]. Women diagnosed with a major depressive disorder with psychotic features and peripartum onset were less likely to experience additional relapses than women diagnosed with bipolar disorder [71].

Etiology

The etiology of postpartum psychosis remains unclear. Though hormonal fluctuations, particularly with estrogen, were suspected, hormonal supplementation has not been found to reduce rates of psychosis in at-risk women [72]. Bergink et al. found higher rates of inflammatory cells in women with postpartum psychosis suggesting a possible neuro-immunity trigger [73]. Another study by Bergink et al. found that one-fifth of women with postpartum psychosis had underlying autoimmune dysfunction involving the thyroid [74]. Sleep deprivation may also be responsible for the development of psychotic features in women who are already at risk [7]. One study found that women who had postpartum psychosis had longer deliveries that tended to occur later in the evening compared to women without the disorder [75].

Clinical Course

With postpartum psychosis, there are often early warning signs in the first few days following delivery. Between 50% and 75% of women with postpartum psychosis started to experience symptoms by day 3 post-delivery. Hypomanic symptoms, including elevated mood, decreased need for sleep, increased speech and increased energy were common, but mood lability and irritability have also been reported [62, 76, 77]. The symptoms rapidly progressed to more psychotic symptoms in the days that followed [17, 76]. Paranoid delusions, delusions of control, auditory hallucinations, manic symptoms, unusual behaviors, and poor self-care are common [76, 78–80]. Many women will have rapid cycling of their mood during this period [62]. However, some women present with striking cognitive impairments and appear delirious [78]. Less frequently, women may have delusions of altruistic homicide, and 4% of cases of postpartum psychosis result in infanticide [81]. Thus, screening for thoughts of harming herself or the infant is incredibly important. These thoughts are particularly worrisome if they are ego-syntonic, associated with psychotic beliefs or loss of reality testing, an inability to assess the consequences of such an action, and intent to act upon them [81].

Overall, postpartum psychosis carries a good prognosis with the vast majority of patients reporting good psychosocial functioning a year out [82]. However, a sizeable minority report ongoing symptoms 1 year out from delivery, and approximately 50–80% of women with postpartum psychosis are eventually diagnosed with bipolar disorder [49, 62, 65].

Evaluation and Treatment

Postpartum psychosis is a psychiatric emergency and should be treated with a high degree of alarm owing to the risk of infanticide. Typically, urgent psychiatric hospitalization is required.

In addition to stabilization with medications, women presenting with postpartum psychosis should be evaluated for medical etiologies for their symptoms. Common causes include infections, anemia, substance intoxication or withdrawal syndromes, autoimmune disease, and endocrine exacerbations [62]. Other rarer causes include anti-N-methyl-D-aspartate (NMDA) receptor encephalitis, late-onset disorders of metabolism, and primary hypoparathyroidism [62, 83]. Treatment options include benzodiazepines to regulate the sleep-wake cycle, antipsychotics for psychotic symptoms and a mood stabilizer, typically lithium. Electroconvulsive therapy (ECT) may be used as well. After improvement in symptoms, monotherapy with either an antipsychotic or lithium is common, though the latter had lower relapse rates than the former [84].

Screening During Pregnancy and Postpartum

Early diagnosis and treatment of postpartum depression is a major public health objective, and efforts to identify this disorder have increased worldwide. In the United States, screening for postpartum depression is now required by law in a few states, and several other states have funded initiatives to increase screening [85, 86]. In 2016, the United States Preventive Services Task Force expanded general screening recommendations for depression to include pregnant and postpartum women [87]. The American College of Obstetricians and Gynecologists (ACOG) recommends screening "at least once during the perinatal period for depression and anxiety symptoms using a standardized, validated tool" [88]. In their Bright Futures guidelines, the American Academy of Pediatrics (AAP) advises screening of all new mothers and notes the unique position of pediatricians, who are in contact with mothers routinely for well-baby visits [89]. However, the optimal timing and frequency of perinatal screens, consistent strategies to implement interventions, and acknowledgment of who should be responsible for screening perinatal women are the subjects of ongoing debate. Research toward integration of mental health care into obstetric and pediatric settings is emerging [90–92].

Numerous self- and clinician-administered screens exist though only a few were designed exclusively for perinatal women [93]. Currently, the most commonly used screens for postpartum depression include the Patient Health Questionnaire (PHQ) and the Edinburgh Postnatal Depression Scale (EPDS). The PHQ-9 is a screen commonly used in the general population that consists of nine questions examining symptoms over a 2-week period [94]. It has the advantages of being: (1) brief, (2) free, (3) easily scored, and (4) validated in numerous languages [94]. An abbreviated version of this scale (PHQ-2) may be asked verbally, with a positive screen meriting further screening with the PHQ-9 [95]. A positive PHQ-9 screen has a cutoff of 10 or more. Disadvantages of the PHQ include its emphasis on neurovegetative symptoms that are commonly found in pregnancy and postpartum, such as fatigue and disrupted sleep; this may result in overestimating peripartum depression [94]. The PHQ also does not capture anxiety symptoms, which tend to be highly correlated with perinatal mood disorders [11].

The EPDS is a 10-item self-report scale assessing symptoms over the past 7 days [93, 96]. It also has the advantages of being: (1) brief, (2) free, (3) easily scored, and (4) available in a variety of languages [97]. The EPDS has recommended cut-off points of scores >10 for settings with resources to assess women with positive screens and of scores >13 for places with limited clinical capacity for post-screening evaluation [96]. The AAP suggests a cut-off of >10 for assessing risk of postpartum depression which would allow for increased sensitivity in capturing at-risk women, but many primary care clinicians use the more conservative score of ≥13 to consume fewer post-screening resources for false positive screens [89, 96].

As a substantial minority of women who experience a postpartum depressive episode have bipolar disorder, screening with the Mood Disorder Questionnaire (MDQ) can improve diagnostic accuracy, and psychiatric referral is reasonable for a positive MDQ screen [11, 53, 98]. It is worth emphasizing that a positive screen is not diagnostic of a perinatal mood episode. Instead, it is an indication that further assessment by the clinician is warranted. Clinicians that initiate treatment based on a positive screen place may place some women at increased risks of side effects from unnecessary medications.

Treating the Perinatal Patient

Performing a Risk-Benefit Analysis

For patients considering pregnancy, a risk-benefit analysis should be performed by a treating or consulting clinician prior to conceiving. This should involve a determination of the patient's ideal timeline for pregnancy, interest in breastfeeding, her risk of illness during pregnancy, risk of relapse without treatment, all treatment options available to her (and her interest in those options) and depending on complexity, coordination of care involved with clinicians in other specialties (obstetrics, neonatology, etc.) [5]. If the desired timeline for conceiving allows, great pains should be taken to make sure the woman is euthymic or as close to euthymic as possible, ideally for some time before beginning trying to conceive.

While this conversation ideally would take place preconception, nearly half of pregnancies in the United States are unplanned [99]. Upon discovery of pregnancy, a patient may discontinue her medications, often with significant risk of relapse [100]. The risk-benefit analysis in these cases should emphasize that exposure to a medication has already occurred before discovery of the pregnancy.

The discerning patient may have preconceived notions of what is "safe" in pregnancy based on varying sources. While counseling such a patient that no medication should be considered "safe" in pregnancy, emphasis on the risks of untreated illness as they would apply to each patient should be taken into account as well. If a patient elects to begin or continue medication during pregnancy, it should be taken at the lowest, but effective dose. The well-intentioned woman who wishes to take a subtherapeutic dose of medication to minimize fetal exposure may become symptomatic, thus risking a double exposure to untreated illness and medications to the fetus [5]. We explore some of the literature regarding the more commonly prescribed agents below.

Navigating the literature on medication use in pregnancy can be challenging. There are numerous studies examining the safety profile of psychotropic medications compared to other medications in pregnancy, perhaps reflecting some of society's stigma against mental illness. Randomized controlled trials are not performed in this population because it is unethical to provide placebo treatment in this vulnerable population. As a result, numerous studies are derived from either retrospective case-control studies (which are limited by recall bias and low response rates), prospective cohort studies (which often have inadequate power to confidently determine associations and can be subject to reporter bias), and drug registry data studies (which are limited as medications prescribed by a clinician does not always equate to appropriate patient use) [101]. Many studies also are limited by confounders, often untreated illness [101]. Patients should be informed of the limitations in the literature but still made aware of the available studies when performing a risk-benefit analysis.

For the patient with mild depression, individual therapy alone is the first-line treatment during the peripartum, and for women with severe depression, a combination of medications and therapy is indicated. For women with moderate depression, determination of best treatment consists of individual therapy and possibly medications [5]. Given the risks of untreated bipolar disorder in pregnancy, medications are often recommended, though in select cases, women may be able to discontinue medications prior to conceiving [37].

Lactation Considerations

Current recommendations from the World Health Organization (WHO) and the American Academy of Pediatrics (AAP) are for exclusive breast feeding of an infant for the first 6 months of life [102, 103]. While the AAP advocates for ongoing exposure to breast milk for "one year or longer as mutually desired by mother and infant," the WHO recommends breastfeeding for up to 2 years or more. Breastfeeding can portend numerous benefits to the mother and infant. However, for women with mood disorders, the decision to breastfeed must take into account certain risks. Interruptions to sleep associated with nighttime nursing can be potentially destabilizing; this is especially true for women with bipolar disorder [1, 7, 81, 104]. In these women who elect to breastfeed, pumping milk for nighttime feedings by another individual should be considered [1]. For women who are taking medication, concern is given for potential toxicity through exposure to the breastmilk. Infant drug serum levels are influenced by several factors: drug levels upon birth (provided mother had exposed the fetus to medication during pregnancy), the rate of transmission of the drug into the breastmilk, the half-life of the medication and its metabolites, and speed of metabolizing and clearance of the drug in the newborn [105]. The relative infant dose (RID) is a useful measure that estimates the probable amount of exposure to the infant [105, 106]. The RID is equal to the infant dose in milk (mg/kg) divided by the maternal weight-adjusted dose (mg/kg). A RID of less than 10% is thought to reflect a level of minimal exposure to the infant and is accepted by the AAP as being compatible with breastfeeding; special considerations, however, must be paid to the premature or medically-complicated infant [105, 107].

The current consensus is that there is no clinical value from measuring antidepressant drug levels in milk or infant serum [106, 108]. Although this is not standard practice, there may be value in obtaining levels to provide relief in confirming that levels are low or even undetectable in order to prevent a woman from discontinuing her medication [106]. There are conflicting opinions regarding measuring mood stabilizer levels, in particular lithium [47]. Particular medications and their RIDs are discussed below.

Medications and Other Treatments in Pregnancy and Postpartum

Individual Psychotherapy

Numerous therapeutic modalities may be beneficial to the perinatal patient. However, interpersonal psychotherapy (IPT) and cognitive behavioral therapy (CBT) have the best evidence of efficacy in the peripartum population [109]. A patient already engaged in therapy with a provider who does not utilize these modalities may wish to continue owing to therapeutic bond as well as other practicalities.

Selective Serotonin Reuptake Inhibitors (SSRIs)

SSRIs are one of the best studied class of psychotropic medications in pregnancy as they are commonly prescribed in the general population. The literature is inconclusive regarding increased risk of miscarriage with SSRI use with several large, well-designed studies not finding an association [110–114]. Rates of major congenital malformations (MCMs) have been vigorously studied, and except paroxetine, no other SSRI has been consistently implicated with overall increased rates of malformations above the baseline risk in the general population (3%) or increased risks of a particular malformation [115]. First trimester use of paroxetine has been linked with an increased rate of cardiac anomalies in numerous studies, though not all (OR 1.5–2) [115–125].

Similar to the risks of untreated illness, SSRI use in pregnancy has been associated with low birth weight/small for gestational age as well as preterm birth [101, 126, 127]. With respect to neurodevelopmental outcomes, the literature is limited and inconclusive regarding long-term effects [101]. More recently, several studies have examined a potential link between SSRI use and risk of autism, with data in several positive studies being muddied by numerous confounders [128–134].

Third trimester use of SSRIs is associated with risks of postnatal adaptation syndrome (PNAS) and persistent pulmonary hypertension of the newborn (PPHN). PNAS, sometimes referred to as neonatal adaptation syndrome, is observed in 8–30% of infants born to mothers taking SSRIs [101]. Its mechanism is poorly understood although some patients will assert this is the result of antidepressant withdrawal in the newborn [101]. Symptoms consist of infant irritability, crying, poor feeding, tremor, jitteriness, lethargy, hypoglycemia and respiratory distress [101, 116, 135]. Symptoms often resolve within days up to 2 weeks, although case reports of symptoms lasting up to 6 weeks have been reported. Treatment is supportive, though, in some cases, closer observation may be required [101]. Persistent pulmonary hypertension of the newborn is a less common phenomenon (baseline risk of 1–2 in 1000 live births) but a serious complication in which there is a failure of relaxation in the fetal pulmonary vascular bed following delivery. PPHN can lead to long-term pulmonary and neurodevelopmental impairment, and mortality associated with PPHN can be as high as 10% [101]. Neonatal intensive care unit level of care is required for this condition. SSRIs were initially thought to increase risk of PPHN by up to six times though more recent stories that better controlled for confounders suggest less than a doubling of risk [136, 137]. While tapering antidepressants in the third trimester to mitigate this risk has been proposed, studies have not shown a decreased risk of PNAS or PPHN with this approach; moreover, doing so would increase a woman's vulnerability to relapse right as she approaches the vulnerable postpartum period [138].

Serotonin-Norepinephrine Reuptake Inhibitors (SNRIs)

The body of literature looking at SNRIs is much smaller than that of SSRIs. The risks appear similar to SSRIs, in particular with respect to lack of increased risk of MCMs and increased risks of preterm birth, low birth weight, PNAS and PPHN. Late third trimester use of SNRIs has been implicated in increasing risk of postpartum hemorrhage (OR 1.6–1.9) [139].

Other Antidepressants

There are also fewer studies examining other antidepressants in pregnancy. Mirtazapine use in the first trimester has not been linked with MCMs, but a postnatal adaptation syndrome has been described in up to 25% of cases [140]. Bupropion use has been linked with increased risk for cardiac malformations in two studies, though others have not found an association with this or other MCMs; there is no postnatal adaptation syndrome described with bupropion [141–143]. Two studies by the same team evaluating trazodone and nefazodone in the first trimester did not find an increased risk of MCMs [144, 145].

Studies evaluating tricyclic antidepressant (TCA) use in the first trimester have not shown an increased risk of MCMs [146–148]. Some TCAs have the benefit of having consistent therapeutic drug serum levels; because serum TCA levels often decline over the course of pregnancy given changes in plasma volume, increased renal clearance, and increased hepatic metabolism, dose adjustments may be needed to maintain a therapeutic level [148, 149]. The side effect profile of TCAs (especially more anticholinergic agents like clomipramine) may worsen already present symptoms of pregnancy, including hypotension and constipation [3]. PPHN has not been consistently linked to TCA use.

Lithium

Lithium is widely viewed as the gold standard treatment for bipolar disorder. Lithium has been found to significantly reduce manic and depressive episodes and is one of the few medications proven to reduce suicide risk [150]. During pregnancy, renal clearance of lithium nearly doubles, which can lead to lower therapeutic drug levels and increased risk of relapse if the dose of the medication is not increased [151]. Following delivery, preconception dosing of lithium can be continued, but a higher target plasma level (i.e., above 0.8) should be considered given the risk during the early postpartum [152].

Importantly, the benefits of the medication need to be weighed carefully against the risks for the mother and fetus. Lithium has been linked to cardiovascular malformations, particularly Ebstein's anomaly, in infants exposed to the medication in the first trimester, but newer data suggests that the risk may be smaller than originally stated [153–158]. Though relative risk (estimated between 10 and 20) is high, the absolute risk of Ebstein's anomaly after exposure in the first trimester is relatively small (0.05–0.1%) [43]. Because of the risk of Ebstein's anomaly and other cardiovascular malformations, it is recommended that women who are treated with lithium in the first trimester undergo fetal echocardiography and level-2 ultrasound [157].

At this time, there is not a clear link between lithium and adverse birth outcomes [55, 152]. However, gestational diabetes, large for gestational age, polyhydramnios, hypotonia, thyroid dysfunction, transient nephrogenic diabetes insipidus, polyuria, and polydipsia have been reported in exposed neonates – particularly with neonatal lithium toxicity [152, 159, 160]. Following delivery, the neonate should be monitored for central nervous system and neuromuscular complications, bradycardia, arrhythmias, hypothermia, fetal goiter, systolic murmur, tachypnea and poor suck reflex [152, 161].

Other Mood Stabilizers

Given the rate of relapse in untreated bipolar disorder during the postpartum period, mood stabilizers are often used to treat this population. However, there are many risks for MCMs associated with several drugs in this class. Therefore, it is recommended that all women of childbearing age who are taking an anticonvulsant medication have 4 mg/day of folic acid supplementation to reduce this risk [162].

Lamotrigine has been shown to be effective at reducing the number of total mood and depressive episodes experienced by patients with bipolar disorder but appears to have limited effectiveness at delaying manic episodes [163]. If used during pregnancy, glucuronidation of the medication (induced by estrogen) increases lamotrigine clearance during pregnancy, and many women require dose increases to maintain similar clinical efficacy [151]. In the postpartum period, the rate of drug clearance rapidly returns to its pre-pregnancy rate, which can lead to toxicity if dosage adjustments are not made. Signs of lamotrigine toxicity include diplopia, ataxia, nausea, and dizziness [164].

Lamotrigine was linked to an increased rate of isolated cleft lips or cleft palates in an early study, but upon reanalysis of the same data with a larger patient population, the association was not replicated. Additional studies have not found any association between lamotrigine and MCMs [165–168].

Valproate use in pregnancy is particularly problematic in the first few weeks of fetal development, a period where women may not realize they are pregnant. It has the highest associated congenital malformation rate (5–11%) of the antiepileptics. Neural tube defects, cleft lip, limb and cardiac malformations all have been linked with valproate use during the first trimester, with dose-dependent effects observed in several studies [169]. Children exposed to valproate in pregnancy were found to have lower IQ scores compared to nonexposed children as well [170]. Given the risks, the medication should not be used in pregnancy with rare exception [37, 171, 172]. Valproate has also been linked to heart rate decelerations and withdrawal symptoms, including irritability, difficulty feeding, jitteriness, and hypotonia [37]. Furthermore, its use has been associated with the development of polycystic ovarian syndrome, which can make conceiving more difficult [173].

Carbamazepine has been linked to increased malformation rates, including neural tube defects as well as craniofacial and digit malformations [171]. The medication has been associated with intrauterine growth restriction, transient neonatal hepatotoxicity, and direct hyperbilirubinemia in exposed infants [37]. Vitamin K deficiency in the neonate has been linked with carbamazepine use, and so supplementation with oral vitamin K in the last month of pregnancy is indicated [37]. Much like valproate, carbamazepine is generally avoided during pregnancy with infrequent exceptions.

Thus far, there have not been any studies linking oxcarbazepine to congenital malformations though there are fewer studies available; however, the shared properties with carbamazepine suggest providers may use caution with this drug [37, 169]. Oxcarbazepine during pregnancy has been noted in case reports to cause a transient neonatal adaptation syndrome characterized by jitteriness, increased muscle tone, irritability and limb shaking [174].

Antipsychotics

Treatment of mood disorders with antipsychotics has dramatically increased over the last several years [175]. The first-generation antipsychotics (FGAs) had been used many decades ago to treat hyperemesis gravidarum in pregnant women, which has provided us with a some data about their use in this population [37]. Though there was some initial concern about the effect that haloperidol may have on the fetal limb development, large studies have not found any association between the drug and any congenital malformation [176].

At present, there is not a consensus about the safety of second generation antipsychotics (SGAs) during pregnancy. Though most studies have not found an association between the SGAs and congenital malformations, one prospective cohort study found that infants exposed to SGAs had higher malformation rates than unexposed controls [47, 176–181]. However, there were several confounding variables for women taking SGA that could account for the findings [177]. The use of SGAs during pregnancy has been associated with higher rates of gestational diabetes, spontaneous and therapeutic abortions, and stillbirths, small and large for gestational age infants, preterm delivery, and Caesarean section [182]. Following delivery, there have been reports of neonatal extrapyramidal symptoms (EPS) and withdrawal syndromes characterized by irritability, abnormal muscle tone, insomnia, tremor, difficulty breathing, and difficulty feedings prompting a warning from the Food and Drug Administration; this finding is also reported with FGAs as well [183]. The Massachusetts General Hospital's National Pregnancy Registry for Atypical Antipsychotics is collecting additional data about the use of these drugs during pregnancy (www.womensmentalhealth.org/pregnancyregistry).

Antidepressants and Breastfeeding

For women who elect to breastfeed, Table 1 displays the following relative infant doses (RIDs) of the more common antidepressants in breastmilk. Fluoxetine, venlafaxine, and citalopram produce the highest relative infant doses while sertraline and paroxetine produce the lowest [107, 108, 184]. Case reports of breastfeeding mothers taking fluoxetine note babies with irritability, watery stools, and decreased feeding, and reports of mothers taking citalopram note babies with hypotonia, colic, poor sleep and decreased feeding [107, 184]. Two case reports of seizure, both occurring in 6-month-old infants born to mothers taking bupropion while breastfeeding have been reported; however, in one case, the mother was on dual antidepressant therapy, and in the other, the infant had a respiratory illness at the time of the seizure, and neither milk nor serum levels were reported [185, 186].

Table 1 Relative infant doses of common antidepressants

Medication (generic name)	Relative infant dose (%)
Sertraline	0.5–3
Paroxetine	0.5–3
Duloxetine	<1
Mirtazapine	0.5–3
Bupropion	2
Escitalopram	3–6
Citalopram	3–10
Venlafaxine	6–9
Fluoxetine	<12

[107]

Table 2 Relative infant doses of common mood stablizers

Medication (generic name)	Relative infant dose (%)
Lithium carbonate	33–69
Valproate sodium	0.1–3.9
Lamotrigine	17–32.5
Carbamazepine	15–65
Oxcarbazepine	0.1

[164, 184, 187–192]

Switching antidepressants based on RID in the postpartum is not advised owing to the potential for destabilizing a mother in the postpartum [106]. Sertraline and paroxetine are thought by some to be ideal first-options for a medication-naïve woman owing to their low RIDs, though the favorable profile of sertraline compared to paroxetine should the woman become interested in another pregnancy may be considered [108, 184]. However, clinical decision making may lead a clinician to start another antidepressant that would be best for a postpartum woman and still compatible with breastfeeding. Data evaluating long-term effects of medication exposure through breastmilk is limited [106, 108].

Mood Stabilizers and Breastfeeding

For women who wish to breastfeed, relative infant doses for mood stabilizers can be found below in Table 2.

Lithium is found in high levels in the breastmilk, with infant serum levels found to be up to one-quarter of the levels in maternal serum. Hypothyroidism, acute kidney failure, and lithium toxicity have been reported, and infants should be followed closely for changes [193]. Because lithium can be associated with significant effects in nursing infants, the AAP Committee on Drugs and the WHO recommend using extreme caution or avoiding breastfeeding altogether while on the medication [194, 195]. However, breastfeeding has been successful in motivated, adherent, and clinically stable patients when working closely with pediatricians who may elect to monitor serum levels in the infant [37, 193].

Valproate is found in very low levels in the breast milk and is generally compatible with breastfeeding. Infants should be monitored for jaundice [195]. There have been rare reports of thrombocytopenia, reticulocytosis, and anemia reported in breastfed-exposed infants [184, 187].

Carbamazepine is not found in low doses in the breast-milk but may be compatible with breastfeeding owing to favorable evidence showing effects on growth and development may be minimal. There have been very rare reports of hepatic dysfunction, and it is recommended that the infant is monitored for jaundice, drowsiness, poor suckling, vomiting and poor weight gain [187, 195].

The RID of lamotrigine has been found to be relatively high (17–32.5%) [164, 184, 187–189]. Because lamotrigine is cleared very slowly by neonatal glucuronidation, levels in the newborn can build up raising a theoretical risk of life-threatening Stevens-Johnson syndrome [196], though it is important to note that no cases of this have been reported [197]. Infants exposed to lamotrigine through the breastmilk should be monitored for signs of lamotrigine toxicity, including poor sucking and severe apnea [198].

Antipsychotic and Breastfeeding

Data related to breastfeeding and antipsychotics is primarily limited to various case reports. Because of the effect that the drugs can have on neurodevelopment and the lack of significant long-term follow-up on development, the AAP recommends caution when using these drugs during breastfeeding [194]. However, most antipsychotics tend to be found at relatively low doses in the breastmilk [184, 199]. In a study of olanzapine use in breastfeeding women, approximately 15% of infants experienced adverse events, including somnolence (3.9%), irritability (2%), tremor (2%), and insomnia (2%) [200]. Adverse events with most other antipsychotics occur at similar rates and are usually not severe [199]. One antipsychotic, clozapine, has been associated with agranulocytosis in one breastfed infant, and another drug, chlorpromazine, had been associated with drowsiness and delays in developmental scores. Both of these drugs should be avoided during breastfeeding [194, 201]. Given the relative lack of data with the class in general, all infants of women on antipsychotics should be monitored for signs of EPS, sedation, and developmental delay [201]. Relative infant doses of antipsychotics can be found in Table 3.

Lactation data for other medications is available through LactMed, a US database funded by the NIH.

ECT in Pregnancy

Electroconvulsive therapy (ECT) remains a rapid option for stabilization of the severely ill woman. Consideration for

Table 3 Relative infant doses of common antipsychotics

Medication name	Relative infant dose (%)
Haloperidol	0.2–9.6
Chlorpromazine	0.1–0.2
Perphenazine	0.1–0.2
Olanzapine	<0.1–4.0
Quetiapine	0.1–0.5
Risperidone	0.1–4.7
Aripiprazole	0.8
Ziprasidone	0.06
Clozapine	275–432

[184, 201–206]

ECT should be given to women with severe depression or mania including the presence of psychotic symptoms. Though some have suggested unique sensitivity of pregnant patients to ECT, more recent analyses show rates of response comparable to those of nonpregnant patients [207–209]. Limited current passes through the uterus during ECT as it is weakly innervated with parasympathetic fibers [209, 210]. Headaches, muscle aches, vaginal bleeding, abdominal pain, confusion and memory loss are common side effects for pregnant women [207, 208, 211, 212]. In the fetus, bradycardia arrhythmias (2.7–43%), premature contractions (3.5%), and preterm labor (28%) are among the most frequent common adverse events with ECT [207, 210, 212, 213]. A systematic review by Lieknes, et al. demonstrated a 7.1% fetal mortality rate associated with ECT [207] though other studies found lower rates [211, 212, 214]. Unique attention should be paid to selection of anesthetic agents as well as positioning of the gravid woman [207, 215]. There are no specific guidelines, though Walker et al. make several recommendations including routine fetal monitoring, such as non-stress tests and biophysical profiles. Tocolytic treatment may be considered to reduce the risk of premature labor, and intubation may be considered following the first trimester owing to the risk of aspiration [207–209, 215].

Complementary and Alternative Therapies

Patients hoping to avoid medication exposure may inquire about certain complementary and alternative therapies. Omega-3 fatty acids have promising evidence in adjunctive treatment for depression, but studies in the perinatal population have not shown consistent benefit [216]. Light therapy has mixed data regarding efficacy but may be helpful in women who experience disruption to the sleep-wake cycle owing to breastfeeding [1, 5, 216]. A meta-analysis of numerous randomized-controlled trials did find reduction of depressive symptoms with perinatal and infant massage [216]. Acupuncture has some data suggesting efficacy but safety data is lacking, and there are reports of isolated cervical ripening associated with use; further studies are needed [216, 217]. While postpartum placentophagy, ingestion of the placenta either in raw or processed form, more recently has been touted as having antidepressant properties by varying sources, there is no literature establishing its safety and no peer-reviewed studies showing benefit [218].

References

1. Ross LE, Murray BJ, Steiner M. Sleep and perinatal mood disorders: a critical review. J Psychiatry Neurosci. 2005;30(4):247–56.
2. Seyfried LS, Marcus SM. Postpartum mood disorders. Int Rev Psychiatry. 2003;15:231–42.
3. Meltzer-Brody S. New insights into perinatal depression: pathogenesis and treatment during pregnancy and postpartum. Dialogues Clin Neurosci. 2011;13:89–100.
4. Gavin N, Gaynes BN, Lohr K, Meltzer-Brody S, Gartlehner G, Swinson T. Perinatal depression: a systematic review of prevalence and incidence. Obstet Gynecol. 2005;106(5):1071–83.
5. Chaudron LH. Complex challenges in treating depression during pregnancy. Am J Psychiatry. 2013;170:12–20.
6. Gaynes BN, Gavin N, Meltzer-Brody S, Lohr KN, Swinson T, Gartlehner G, et al. Perinatal depression: prevalence, screening accuracy, and screening outcomes: summary. Rockville: Agency for Healthcare Research and Quality (US); 2005.. 119 p.
7. Sharma V, Mazmanian D. Sleep loss and postpartum psychosis. Bipolar Disord. 2003;5(2):98–105.
8. Fisher J, de Mello MC, Patel V, Rahman A, Tran T, Holton S, et al. Prevalence and determinants of common perinatal mental disorders in women in low- and lower-middle-income countries: a systematic review. Bull World Health Organ. 2012;90:139–149G.
9. Vesga-López O, Blanco C, Keyes K, Olfson M, Grant BF, Hasin DS. Psychiatric disorders in pregnant and postpartum women in the United States. Arch Gen Psychiatry. 2008;65(7):805–15.
10. Austin MP, Middleton P, Reilly NM, Highet NJ. Detection and management of mood disorders in the maternity setting: the Australian clinical practice guidelines. Women Birth. 2013;26(1):2–9.
11. Wisner KL, Sit DKY, McShea MC, Rizzo DM, Zoretich RA, Hughes CL, Eng HF, et al. Onset timing, thoughts of self-harm, and diagnoses in postpartum women with screen-positive depression findings. JAMA Psychiat. 2013;70(5):490–8.
12. Llewellyn AM, Stowe ZN, Nemeroff CB. Depression during pregnancy and the puerperium. J Clin Psychiatry. 1997;58(S15):26–32.
13. Beck CT, Records K, Rice M. Further development of the postpartum depression predictors inventory-revised. J Obstet Gynecol Neonatal Nurs. 2006;35(6):735–45.
14. O'Hara MW, Wisner KL. Perinatal mental illness: definition, description and aetiology. Best Pract Res Clin Obstet Gynaecol. 2014;28:3–12.
15. Bloch M, Schmidt PJ, Danaceau M, Murphy J, Nieman L, Rubinow DR. Effects of gonadal steroids in women with a history of postpartum depression. Am J Psychiatry. 2000;157:924–30.
16. Bloch M, Daly RC, Rubinow DR. Endocrine factors in the etiology of postpartum depression. Compr Psychiatry. 2003;44:234–46.
17. Wisner KL, Stowe ZN. Psychobiology of postpartum mood disorders. Semin Reprod Endocrinol. 1997;15(1):77–89.
18. Chrousos GP, Torpy DJ, Gold PW. Interactions between the hypothalamic-pituitary-adrenal axis and the female reproductive system: clinical implications. Ann Intern Med. 1998;129(3):229–40.
19. Sit DK, Wisner KL. The identification of postpartum depression. Clin Obstet Gynecol. 2009;52(3):456–68.
20. Bansil P, Kuklina EV, Meikle SF, Posner SF, Kourtis AP, Ellington SR, et al. Maternal and fetal outcomes among women with depression. J Women's Health. 2010;19(2):329–34.
21. Andersson L, Sundström-Poromaa I, Wulff M, Åström M, Bixo M. Implications of antenatal depression and anxiety for obstetric outcome. Obstet Gynecol. 2004;104:467–76.
22. Chung TKH, Lau TK, Yip ASK, Chiu HFK, Lee DTS. Antepartum depressive symptomatology is associated with adverse obstetric and neonatal outcomes. Psychosom Med. 2001;63:830–4.
23. Wu J, Viguera A, Riley L, Cohen L, Ecker J. Mood disturbance in pregnancy and the mode of delivery. Am J Obstet Gynecol. 2002;187(4):864–7.
24. Davalos DB, Yadon CA, Tregellas HC. Untreated prenatal maternal depression and the potential risks to offspring: a review. Arch Womens Ment Health. 2012;15:1–14.
25. Dayan J, Creveuil C, Marks MK, Conroy S, Herlicoviez M, Dreyfus M, et al. Prenatal depression, prenatal anxiety, and spontaneous preterm birth: a prospective cohort study among women with early and regular care. Psychosom Med. 2006;68(6):938–46.
26. Field T, Diego M, Hernandez-Reif M. Prenatal depression effects on the fetus and newborn: a review. Infant Behav Dev. 2011;34(1):1–14.
27. Jarde A, Morais M, Kingston D, Giallo R, MacQueen GM, Giglia L, et al. Neonatal outcomes in women with untreated antenatal depression compared with women without depression: a systematic review and meta-analysis. JAMA Psychiat. 2016;73(8):826–37.
28. Grigoriadis S, VonderPorten EH, Mamisashvili L, Tomlinson G, Dennis CL, Koren G, et al. The impact of maternal depression during pregnancy on perinatal outcomes: a systematic review and meta-analysis. J Clin Psychiatry. 2013;74(4):e321–41.
29. Lindahl V, Pearson JL, Colpe L. Prevalence of suicidality during pregnancy and the postpartum. Arch Womens Ment Health. 2005;8(2):77–87.
30. Mendez-Bustos P, Lopez-Castroman J, Baca-García E, Ceverino A. Life cycle and suicidal behavior among women. Sci World J. 2013;2013:485851.
31. Schiff MA, Grossman DC. Adverse perinatal outcomes and risk for postpartum suicide attempt in Washington state, 1987–2001. Pediatrics. 2006;118(3):e669–75.
32. Cooper PJ, Murray L. Course and recurrence of postnatal depression. Evidence for the specificity of the diagnostic concept. Br J Psychiatry. 1995;166(2):191–5.
33. Alaräisänen A, Miettunen J, Pouta A, Isohanni M, Räsänen P, Mäki P. Ante- and perinatal circumstances and risk of attempted suicides and suicides in offspring: the Northern Finland birth cohort 1966 study. Soc Psychiatry Psychiatr Epidemiol. 2012;47(11):1783–94.
34. Bassett DL. Risk assessment and management in bipolar disorders. Med J Aust. 2010;193(4 Suppl):S21–3.
35. Merikangas KR, Akiskal HS, Angst J, Greenberg PE, Hirschfeld RMA, Petukhova M, et al. Lifetime and 12-month prevalence of bipolar spectrum disorder in the national comorbidity survey replication. Arch Gen Psychiatry. 2007;64(5):543–52.
36. Kessler RC, Chiu WT, Demler O, Walters EE. Prevalence, severity, and comorbidity of 12-month DSM-IV disorders in the national comorbidity survey replication. Arch Gen Psychiatry. 2003;62:617–27.
37. Yonkers KA, Wisner KL, Stowe Z, Leibenluft E, Cohen L, Miller L, et al. Management of bipolar disorder during pregnancy and the postpartum period. Am J Psychiatry. 2004;161(4):608–20.
38. Leibenluft E. Women with bipolar illness: clinical and research illness. Am J Psychiatry. 1996;153(2):163–73.
39. Freeman MP, Smith KW, Freeman SA, McElroy SL, Kmetz GF, Wright R, et al. The impact of reproductive events on the course of bipolar disorder. J Clin Psychiatry. 2002;63(4):284–7.

40. Grof P, Robbins W, Alda M, Berghoefer A, Vojtechovsky M, Nilsson A, et al. Protective effect of pregnancy in women with lithium-responsive bipolar disorder. J Affect Disord. 2000;61(1–2):31–9.

41. Munk-Olsen T, Laursen TM, Mendelson T, Pedersen CB, Mors O, Moretnsen PB. Risks and predictors of readmission for a mental disorder during the postpartum period. Arch Gen Psychiatry. 2009;66(2):189–95.

42. Viguera AC, Nonacs R, Cohen LS, Tondo L, Murray A, Baldessarini RJ. Risk of recurrence of bipolar disorder in pregnant and nonpregnant women after discontinuing lithium maintenance. Am J Psychiatry. 2000;157(2):179–84.

43. Viguera AC, Cohen LS. The course and management of bipolar disorder during pregnancy. Psychopharmacol Bull. 1998;23(3):339–46.

44. Viguera AC, Tondo L, Koukopoulos AE, Reginaldi D, Lepri B, Balderssarini RJ. Episodes of mood disorders in 2,252 pregnancies and postpartum periods. Am J Psychiatry. 2011;168(11):1179–85.

45. Viguera AC, Whitifield T, Baldessarini RJ, Newport DJ, Stowe Z, Reminick A, et al. Risk of recurrence in women with bipolar disorder during pregnancy: prospective study of mood stabilizer discontinuation. Am J Psychiatry. 2007;164(12):1817–24.

46. Harlow BL, Vitonis AF, Sparen P, Cnattingius S, Joffe H, Hultman CM. Incidence of hospitalization for postpartum psychotic and bipolar episodes in women with and without prior prepregnancy or prenatal psychiatric hospitalizations. Arch Gen Psychiatry. 2007;64(1):42–8.

47. Khan SJ, Fersh ME, Ernst C, Klipstein K, Albertini ES, Lusskin SI. Bipolar disorder in pregnancy and postpartum: principles of management. Curr Psychiatry Rep. 2016;18(2):13.

48. Akdeniz F, Vahip S, Pirildar S, Vahip I, Doganer I, Bulut I. Childbearing-related episodes in women with bipolar disorder. Psychopathology. 2003;36(5):234–8.

49. Blackmore ER, Rubinow DR, O'Connor TG, Liu X, Tang W, Craddock N, et al. Reproductive outcomes and risk of subsequent illness in women diagnosed with postpartum psychosis. Bipolar Disord. 2013;15(4):394–404.

50. Munk-Olsen T, Laursen TM, Meltzer-Brody S, Mortensen PB, Jones I. Psychiatric disorders with postpartum onset. Arch Gen Psychiatry. 2012;69(4):428–34.

51. Mitchell PB, Goodwin GM, Johnson GF, Hirschfeld RM. Diagnostic guidelines for bipolar depression: a probabilistic approach. Bipolar Disord. 2008;10(1 Pt 2):144–52.

52. Sharma V, Penava D. Screening for bipolar disorder during pregnancy and the postpartum period. J Obstet Gynaecol Can. 2010;32(3):278–81.

53. Clark CT, Sit DK, Driscoll K, Eng HF, Confer AL, Luther JF, Wisniewski SR, Wisner KL. Does screening with the MDQ and EPDS improve identification of bipolar disorder in an obstetrical sample? Depress Anxiety. 2015;32:518–26.

54. Heron J, Haque S, Oyebode F, Craddock N, Jones I. A longitudinal study of hypomania and depression symptoms in pregnancy and the postpartum period. Bipolar Disord. 2009;11(4):410–7.

55. Boden R, Lundgren M, Brandt L, Reutfors J, Andersen M, Kieler H. Risk of adverse pregnancy and birth outcomes in women treated or not treated with mood stabilisers for bipolar disorder: population based cohort study. BMJ. 2012;345:e7085.

56. Mei-Dan E, Ray JG, Vigod SN. Perinatal outcomes among women with bipolar disorder: a population-based study. Am J Obstet Gynecol. 2015;212(3):367e1–7.

57. Rusner M, Berg M, Begley C. Bipolar disorder in pregnancy and childbirth: a systematic review of outcomes. BMC Pregnancy Childbirth. 2016;16(1):331.

58. Jablensky AV, Morgan V, Zubrick SR, Bower C, Yellachich LA. Pregnancy, delivery, and neonatal complications in a popu-lation cohort of women with schizophrenia and major affective disorders. Am J Psychiatry. 2005;162(1):79–91.

59. Lee HC, Lin HC. Maternal bipolar disorder increased low birth-weight and preterm births: a nationwide population-based study. J Affect Disord. 2010;121(1–2):100–5.

60. Kendell RE, Chalmers JC, Platz C. Epidemiology of puerperal psychoses. Br J Psychiatry. 1987;150:662–73.

61. Terp IM, Mortensen PB. Clinical diagnoses and relative risk of admission after parturition. Br J Psychiatry. 1998;172:521–6.

62. Bergink V, Rasgon N, Wisner KL. Postpartum psychosis: madness, mania, and melancholic in motherhood. Am J Psychiatry. 2016;173(12):1179–88.

63. Jones I, Craddock N. Familiality of the puerperal trigger in bipolar disorder: results of a family study. Am J Psychiatry. 2001;158(6):913–7.

64. Jones I, Craddock N. Do puerperal psychotic episodes identify a more familial subtype of bipolar disorder? Results of a family history study. Psychiatr Genet. 2002;12(3):143–53.

65. Chaudron LH, Pies RW. The relationship between postpartum psychosis and bipolar disorder: a review. J Clin Psychiatry. 2003;64(11):1284–92.

66. Videbech P, Gouliaev G. First admission with puerperal psychosis: 7–14 years of follow-up. Acta Psychiatr Scand. 1995;91(3):167–73.

67. Blackmore ER, Jones I, Doshi M, Haque S, Holder R, Brockington I, et al. Obstetric variables associated with bipolar affective puerperal psychosis. Br J Psychiatry. 2006;188:32–6.

68. Jones I, Chandra PS, Dazzan P, Howard LM. Bipolar disorder, affective psychosis, and schizophrenia is pregnancy and the postpartum period. Lancet. 2014;384:1789–99.

69. McNeil TF. A prospective study of postpartum psychoses in a high-risk group. Acta Psychiatr Scand. 1988;78(5):613–7.

70. Wesseloo R, Kamperman AM, Munk-Olsen T, Pop VJ, Kushner SA, Bergink V. Risk of postpartum relapse in bipolar disorder an postpartum psychosis: a systematic review and meta-analysis. Am J Psychiatry. 2016;173(2):117–27.

71. Robling SA, Paykel ES, Dunn VJ, Abbott R, Katona C. Long-term outcome of severe puerperal psychiatric illness: a 23 year follow-up study. Psychol Med. 2000;30:1263–71.

72. Kumar C, McIvor RJ, Davies T, Brown N, Papdopoulos A, Wieck A, et al. Estrogen administration does not reduce the rate of recurrence of affective psychosis after childbirth. J Clin Psychiatry. 2003;64(2):112–8.

73. Bergink V, Burgerhout KM, Weigelt K, Pop VJ, de Wit H, Drexhage RC, et al. Immune system dysregulation in first-onset postpartum psychosis. Biol Psychiatry. 2013;73(10):1000–7.

74. Bergink V, Kushner SA, Pop V, Kuijipens H, Lambregtse-van den Berg MP, Drehage RC, et al. Prevalence of autoimmune thyroid dysfunction in postpartum psychosis. Br J Psychiatry. 2011;198(4):262–8.

75. Sharma V, Smith A, Khan M. The relationship between duration of labour, time of delivery, and puerperal psychosis. J Affect Disord. 2004;83(2–3):215–20.

76. Heron J, Blackmore ER, McGuinness M, Craddock N, Jones I. No 'latent period' in the onset of bipolar affective puerperal psychosis. Arch Womens Ment Health. 2007;10(2):79–81.

77. Heron J, McGuinness M, Blackmore ER, Craddock N, Jones I. Early postpartum symptoms in puerperal psychosis. BJOG. 2008;115(3):348–53.

78. Wisner KL, Peindl K, Hanusa BH. Symptomatology of affective and psychotic illness related to childbearing. J Affect Disord. 1994;30(2):77–87.

79. Oosthuizen P, Russouw H, Roberts M. Is puerperal psychosis bipolar mood disorder? A phenomenological comparison. Compr Psychiatry. 1995;36:77–81.

80. Brockington IF, Cernik KF, Schofield EM, Downing AR, Francis AF, Keelan C. Puerperal psychosis: phenomena and diagnosis. Arch Gen Psychiatry. 1981;38(7):829–33.

81. Spinelli MG. Postpartum psychosis: detection of risk and management. Am J Psychiatry. 2009;166(4):405–8.

82. Burgerhout KM, Kamperman AM, Roza SJ, Lambregtse-Van den Berg MP, Koorengevel KM, Hoogendijk WJ, et al. Functional recovery after postpartum psychosis: a prospective longitudinal study. J Clin Psychiatry. 2017;78(1):122–8.

83. Sit D, Rothschild AJ, Wisner KL. A review of postpartum psychosis. J Womens Health (Larchmt). 2006;15(4):352–68.

84. Bergink V, Burgerhout KM, Koorengevel KM, Kamperman AM, Hoogendijk WJ, Labregtse-van den Berg MP, et al. Treatment of psychosis and mania in the postpartum period. Am J Psychiatry. 2015;172(2):115–23.

85. Rhodes AM, Segre LS. Perinatal depression: a review of US legislation and law. Arch Womens Ment Health. 2013;16:259–70.

86. Haran C, van Driel M, Mitchell BL, Brodribb WE. Clinical guidelines for postpartum women and infants in primary care—a systematic review. BMC Pregnancy Childbirth. 2014;14:51.

87. Siu AL, US Preventive Services Task Force (USPSTF). Screening for depression in adults: US preventive services task force recommendation statement. JAMA. 2016;315:380–7.

88. American College of Obstetricians and Gynecologists Committee on Obstetric Practice. The American College of Obstetricians and Gynecologists Committee opinion no. 630. Screening for perinatal depression. Obstet Gynecol. 2015;125:1268–71.

89. Earls MF, The Committee on Psychosocial Aspects of Child and Family Health. Clinical report: incorporating recognition and management of perinatal and postpartum depression into pediatric practice. Pediatrics. 2010;126:1032–9.

90. Liberto TL. Screening for depression and help-seeking in postpartum women during well-baby pediatric visits: an integrated review. J Pediatr Health Care. 2012;26:109–17.

91. Melville JL, Reed SD, Russo J, Croicu CA, Ludman E, LaRocco-Cockburn A, et al. Improving care for depression in obstetrics and gynecology: a randomized controlled trial. Obstet Gynecol. 2014;123:1237–46.

92. Coverdale J, Roberts LW, Balon R, Beresin EV. Pedagogical implications of partnerships between psychiatry and obstetrics-gynecology in caring for patients with major mental disorders. Acad Psychiatry. 2015;39:430–6.

93. Boyd RC, Le HN, Somberg R. Review of screening instruments for postpartum depression. Arch Womens Ment Health. 2005;8(3):141–53.

94. Kroenke K, Spitzer RL, Williams JB. The PHQ-9: validity of a brief depression severity measure. J Gen Intern Med. 2001;16(9):606–13.

95. Kroenke K, Spitzer RL, Williams JB. The patient health questionnaire-2: validity of a two-item depression screener. Med Care. 2003;41(11):1284–92.

96. Cox J, Holden J. Perinatal mental health: a guide to the Edinburgh postnatal depression scale (EPDS). Glasgow: Bell & Bain Ltd; 2003.

97. Gibson J, McKenzie-McHarg K, Shakespeare J, Price J, Gray R. A systematic review of studies validating the Edinburgh postnatal depression scale in antepartum and postpartum women. Acta Psychiatr Scand. 2009;119(5):350–64.

98. Hirschfeld RM, Williams JBW, Spitzer RL, Calabrese JR, Flynn L, Keck PE, Lewis L, McElroy SL, Post RM, Rapport DJ, Russell JM, Sachs GS, Zajecka J. Development and validation of a screening instrument for bipolar spectrum disorder: the mood disorder questionnaire. Am J Psychiatry. 2000;157(11):1873–5.

99. Finer LB, Zolna MR. Unintended pregnancy in the United States: incidence and disparities, 2006. Contraception. 2011;84(5):478–85.

100. Einarson A, Selby P, Koren G. Abrupt discontinuation of psychotropic drugs during pregnancy: fear of teratogenic risk and impact of counselling. J Psychiatry Neurosci. 2001;26(1):44–8.

101. Byatt N, Deligiannidis KM, Freeman MP. Antidepressant use in pregnancy: a critical review focused on risks and controversies. Acta Psychiatr Scand. 2013;127(2):94–114.

102. American Academy of Pediatrics Section on Breastfeeding. Breastfeeding and the use of human milk. Pediatrics. 2012;129(3):e827–41.

103. World Health Organization. The optimal duration of exclusive breastfeeding: report of an expert consultation. Geneva: World Health Organization; 2001.. 10 p.

104. Tham EK, Tan J, Chong YS, Kwek K, Saw SM, Teoh OH, et al. Associations between poor subjective prenatal sleep quality and postnatal depression and anxiety symptoms. J Affect Disord. 2016;202:91–4.

105. Austin MP, Mitchell PB. Use of psychotropic medications in breastfeeding women: acute and prophylactic treatment. Aust N Z J Psychiatry. 1998;32(6):778–84.

106. Chad L, Pupco A, Bozzo P, Koren G. Update on antidepressant use during breastfeeding. Can Fam Physician. 2013;59(6):633–4.

107. Berle JO, Spigset O. Antidepressant use during breastfeeding. Curr Womens Health Rev. 2011;7(1):28–34.

108. Lanza di Scalea T, Wisner KL. Antidepressant medication use during breastfeeding. Clin Obstet Gynecol. 2009;52(3):483–97.

109. Spinelli MG, Endicott J. Controlled clinical trial of interpersonal psychotherapy versus parenting education program for depressed pregnant women. Am J Psychiatry. 2003;160(3):555–62.

110. Andersen JT, Andersen NL, Horwitz H, Poulsen HE, Jimenez-Solem E. Exposure to selective serotonin reuptake inhibitors in early pregnancy and the risk of miscarriage. Obstet Gynecol. 2014;124(4):655–61.

111. Hemels ME, Einarson A, Koren G, Lanctôt KL, Einarson TR. Antidepressant use during pregnancy and the rates of spontaneous abortions: a meta-analysis. Ann Pharmacother. 2005;39(5):803–9.

112. Einarson A, Choi J, Einarson TR, Koren G. Rates of spontaneous and therapeutic abortions following use of antidepressants in pregnancy: results from a large prospective database. J Obstet Gynaecol Can. 2009;31(5):452–6.

113. Robinson GE. Psychopharmacology in pregnancy and postpartum. Focus. 2012;10:3–14.

114. Jimenez-Solem E, Andersen JT, Petersen M, Broedbaek K, Lander AR, Afzal S, et al. SSRI use during pregnancy and risk of stillbirth and neonatal mortality. Am J Psychiatry. 2013;170(3):299–304.

115. Reefhuis J, Devine O, Friedman JM, Louik C, Honein MA. Specific SSRIs and birth defects: bayesian analysis to interpret new data in the context of previous reports. BMJ. 2015;351:h3190.

116. Yonkers KA, Wisner KL, Stewart DE, Oberlander TF, Dell DL, Stotland N, et al. The management of depression during pregnancy: a report from the American Psychiatric Association and the American College of Obstetricians and Gynecologists. Gen Hosp Psychiatry. 2009;31(5):403–13.

117. Wogelius P, Nørgaard M, Gislum M, Pedersen L, Munk E, Mortensen PB, et al. Maternal use of selective serotonin reuptake inhibitors and risk of congenital malformations. Epidemiology. 2006;17(6):701–4.

118. Davis RL, Rubanowice D, McPhillips H, Raebel MA, Andrade SE, Smith D, HMO Research Network Center for Education, Research in Therapeutics, et al. Risks of congenital malformations and perinatal events among infants exposed to antidepressant medications during pregnancy. Pharmacoepidemiol Drug Saf. 2007;16(10):1086–94.

119. Wichman CL, Moore KM, Lang TR, St Sauver JL, Heise RH Jr, Watson WJ. Congenital heart disease associated with selective serotonin reuptake inhibitor use during pregnancy. Mayo Clin Proc. 2009;84(1):23–7.

120. Källén BA, Otterblad Olausson P. Maternal use of selective serotonin re-uptake inhibitors in early pregnancy and infant congenital malformations. Birth Defects Res A Clin Mol Teratol. 2007;79(4):301–8.

121. Louik C, Lin AE, Werler MM, Hernandez-Diaz S, Mitchell AA. First-trimester use of selective serotonin-reuptake inhibitors and the risk of birth defects. N Engl J Med. 2007;356:2675–83.

122. Cole JA, Ephross SA, Cosmatos IS, Walker AM. Paroxetine in the first trimester and the prevalence of congenital malformations. Pharmacoepidemiol Drug Saf. 2007;16:1075–85.

123. Williams M, Wooltron E. Paroxetine (Paxil) and congenital malformations. CMAJ. 2005;173:1320–1.

124. Wurst KE, Poole C, Ephross SA, Olshan AF. First trimester paroxetine use and the prevalence of congenital, specifically cardiac, defects: a meta-analysis of epidemiological studies. Birth Defects Res A Clin Mol Teratol. 2010;88:159–70.

125. Malm H, Artama M, Gissler M, Ritvanen A. Selective serotonin reuptake inhibiton and risk for major congenital anomalies. Obstet Gynecol. 2011;118:111–20.

126. Wisner KL, Sit DK, Hanusa BH, Moses-Kolko EL, Bogen DL, Hunker DF, et al. Major depression and antidepressant treatment: impact on pregnancy and neonatal outcomes. Am J Psychiatry. 2009;166(5):557–66.

127. Wisner KL, Bogen DL, Sit D, McShea M, Hughes C, Rizzo D, et al. Does fetal exposure to SSRIs or maternal depression impact infant growth? Am J Psychiatry. 2013;170(5):485–93.

128. Boukhris T, Sheehy O, Mottron L, Bérard A. Antidepressant use during pregnancy and the risk of autism spectrum disorder in children. JAMA Pediatr. 2016;170(2):117–24.

129. Brown HK, Ray JG, Wilton AS, Lunsky Y, Gomes T, Vigod SN. Association between serotonergic antidepressant use during pregnancy and autism spectrum disorder in children. JAMA. 2017;317(15):1544–52.

130. Clements CC, Castro VM, Blumenthal SR, Rosenfield HR, Murphy SN, Fava M, et al. Prenatal antidepressant exposure is associated with risk for attention-deficit hyperactivity disorder but not autism spectrum disorder in a large health system. Mol Psychiatry. 2015;20(6):727–34.

131. Croen LA, Grether JK, Yoshida CK, Odouli R, Hendrick V. Antidepressant use during pregnancy and childhood autism spectrum disorders. Arch Gen Psychiatry. 2011;68(11):1104–12.

132. Rai D, Lee BK, Dalman C, Golding J, Lewis G, Magnusson C. Parental depression, maternal antidepressant use during pregnancy, and risk of autism spectrum disorders: population based case-control study. BMJ. 2013;346:f2059.

133. Sørensen MJ, Grønborg TK, Christensen J, Parner ET, Vestergaard M, Schendel D, et al. Antidepressant exposure in pregnancy and risk of autism spectrum disorders. Clin Epidemiol. 2013;5:449–59.

134. Sujan AC, Rickert ME, Öberg AS, Quinn PD, Hernández-Díaz S, Almqvist C, et al. Associations of maternal antidepressant use during the first trimester of pregnancy with preterm birth, small for gestational age, autism spectrum disorder, and attention-deficit/hyperactivity disorder in offspring. JAMA. 2017;317(15):1553–62.

135. Lorenzo L, Byers B, Einarson A. Antidepressant use in pregnancy. Expert Opin Drug Saf. 2011;10(6):883–9.

136. Chambers CD, Hernandez-Diaz S, Van Marter LJ, Werler MM, Louik C, Jones KL, et al. Selective serotonin-reuptake inhibitors and risk of persistent pulmonary hypertension of the newborn. New Engl J Med. 2006;354(6):579–87.

137. Occhiogrosso M, Omran SS, Altemus M. Persistent pulmonary hypertension of the newborn and selective serotonin reuptake inhibitors: lessons from clinical and translational studies. Am J Psychiatry. 2012;169(2):134–40.

138. Warburton W, Hertzman C, Oberlander TF. A register study of the impact of stopping third trimester selective serotonin reuptake inhibitor exposure on neonatal health. Acta Psychiatr Scand. 2010;121(6):471–9.

139. Hanley GE, Smolina K, Mintzes B, Oberlander TF, Morgan SG. Postpartum hemorrhage and use of serotonin reuptake inhibitor antidepressants in pregnancy. Obstet Gynecol. 2016;127(3):553–61.

140. Smit M, Wennink H, Heres M, Dolman KM, Honig A. Mirtazapine in pregnancy and lactation: data from a case series. J Clin Psychopharmacol. 2015;35(2):163–7.

141. Cole JA, Modell JG, Haight BR, Cosmatos IS, Stoler JM, Walker AM. Bupropion in pregnancy and the prevalence of congenital malformations. Pharmacoepidemiol Drug Saf. 2007;16(5):474–84.

142. Chun-Fai-Chan B, Koren G, Fayez I, Kalra S, Voyer-Lavigne S, Boshier A, et al. Pregnancy outcome of women exposed to bupropion during pregnancy: a prospective comparative study. Am J Obstet Gynecol. 2005;192(3):932–6.

143. Louik C, Kerr S, Mitchell AA. First-trimester exposure to bupropion and risk of cardiac malformations. Pharmacoepidemiol Drug Saf. 2014;23(10):1066–75.

144. Einarson A, Bonari L, Voyer-Lavigne S, Addis A, Matsui D, Johnson Y, et al. A multicentre prospective controlled study to determine the safety of trazodone and nefazodone use during pregnancy. Can J Psychiatr. 2003;48(2):106–10.

145. Einarson A, Choi J, Einarson TR, Koren G. Incidence of major malformations in infants following antidepressant exposure in pregnancy: results of a large prospective cohort study. Can J Psychiatr. 2009;54(4):242–6.

146. Misri S, Sivertz K. Tricyclic drugs in pregnancy and lactation: a preliminary report. Int J Psychiatry Med. 1991;21(2):157–71.

147. Osborne LM, Birndorf CA, Szkodny LE, Wisner KL. Returning to tricyclic antidepressants for depression during childbearing: clinical and dosing challenges. Arch Womens Ment Health. 2014;17(3):239–46.

148. Altshuler LL, Cohen L, Szuba MP, Burt VK, Gitlin M, Mintz J. Pharmacologic management of psychiatric illness during pregnancy: dilemmas and guidelines. Am J Psychiatry. 1996;153(5):592–606.

149. Wisner KL, Perel JM, Wheeler SB. Tricyclic dose requirements across pregnancy. Am J Psychiatry. 1993;150(10):1541–2.

150. Cipriani A, Pretty H, Hawton K, Geddes JR. Lithium in the prevention of suicidal behavior and all-cause mortality in patients with mood disorders: a systematic review of randomized trials. Am J Psychiatry. 2005;162(10):1805–19.

151. Deligiannidis KM. Therapeutic drug monitoring in pregnant and postpartum women: recommendations for SSRIs, lamotrigine, and lithium. J Clin Psychiatry. 2010;71(5):649–50.

152. Bergink V, Kushner SA. Lithium during pregnancy. Am J Psychiatry. 2014;171(7):712–5.

153. Weinstein MR, Goldfield M. Cardiovascular malformations with lithium use during pregnancy. Am J Psychiatry. 1975;132(5):529–31.

154. Schou M, Goldfield MD, Weinstein MR, Villeneuve A. Lithium and pregnancy—I. Report from the register of lithium babies. Br Med J. 1973;2(5859):135–6.

155. Kallen B, Tandberg A. Lithium and pregnancy. A cohort study on manic-depressive women. Acta Psychiatr Scand. 1983;68(2):134–9.

156. Jacobson SJ, Jones K, Johnson K, Ceolin L, Kaur P, Sahn D, Donnenfeld AE, et al. Prospective multicenter study of pregnancy outcome after lithium exposure during first trimester. Lancet. 1992;339(8792):530–3.

157. Diav-Citrin O, Shechtman S, Tahover E, Finkel-Pekarsky V, Arnon J, Kennedy D, et al. Pregnancy outcome following in utero exposure to lithium: a prospective, comparative, observational study. Am J Psychiatry. 2014;171(7):785–94.

158. Patorno E, Huybrechts KF, Bateman BT, Cohen JM, Desai RJ, Mogun H, et al. Lithium use in pregnancy and the risk of cardiac malformations. NEJM. 2017;376(23):2245–54.

159. Mizrahi EM, Hobbs JF, Goldsmith DI. Nephrogenic diabetes insipidus in transplacental lithium intoxication. J Pediatr. 1979;94(3):493–5.

160. Pinelli JM, Symington AJ, Cunningham KA, Paes BA. Case report and review of perinatal implications of maternal lithium use. Am J Obstet Gynecol. 2002;197:245–9.

161. Newport DJ, Viguera AC, Beach AJ, Ritchie JC, Cohen LS, Stowe ZN. Lithium placental passage and obstetrical outcome: implications for clinical management during late pregnancy. Am J Psychiatry. 2005;162(11):2162–70.

162. Cheschier N, American College of Obstetrics and Gynecologists (ACOG) Committee on Practice Bulletins-Obstetrics. Neural tube defects. Int J Gynaecol Obstet. 2003;83(1):123–33.

163. Bowden CL, Calabrese JR, Sachs G, Yatham LN, Asghar SA, Hompland M, Montgomery P, Earl N, Smoot TM, DeVeaugh-Geiss J, Lamictal 606 Study Group. A placebo-controlled 18-month trial of lamotrigine and lithium maintenance treatment in recently manic or hypomanic patients with bipolar I disorder. Arch Gen Psychiatry. 2003;60(4):392–400.

164. Clark CT, Klein AM, Perel JM, Helsel J, Wisner KL. Lamotrigine dosing for pregnant patients with bipolar disorder. Am J Psychiatry. 2013;170(11):1240–7.

165. Morrow J, Russell A, Guthrie E, Parsons L, Robertson I, Waddell R, et al. Malformation risks of antiepileptic drugs in pregnancy: a prospective study from the UK Epilepsy and Pregnancy Register. J Neurol Neurosurg Psychiatry. 2006;77(2):193–8.

166. Holmes LB, Baldwin EJ, Smith CR, Habecker E, Glassman L, Wong SL, et al. Increased frequency of isolated cleft palate in infants exposed to lamotrigine during pregnancy. Neurology. 2008;70(22):2152–8.

167. Tennis P, Eldridge RR, International Lamotrigine Pregnancy Registry Scientific Advisory Committee. Preliminary results on pregnancy outcomes in women using lamotrigine. Epilepsia. 2002;43(10):1161–7.

168. Cunnington M, Tennis P, International Lamotrigine Pregnancy Registry Scientific Advisory Committee. Lamotrigine and the risk of malformations in pregnancy. Neurology. 2005;64(6):955–60.

169. Weston J, Bromley R, Jackson CF, Adab N, Clayton-Smith J, Greenhalgh J, et al. Monotherapy treatment of epilepsy in pregnancy: congenital malformation outcomes in the child. Cochrane Database Syst Rev. 2016;11(CD010224):1–348.

170. Banach R, Boskovic R, Einarson T, Koren G. Long-term developmental outcome of children of women with epilepsy, unexposed or exposed prenatally to antiepileptic drugs: a meta-analysis of cohort studies. Drug Saf. 2010;33(1):73–9.

171. Iqbal MM, Sohhan T, Mahmud SZ. The effects of lithium, valproic acid, and carbamazepine during pregnancy and lactation. J Toxicol Clin Toxicol. 2001;39(4):381–92.

172. Meador K, Reynolds MW, Crean S, Fahrback K, Probst C. Pregnancy outcomes in women with epilepsy: a systematic review and meta-analysis of published pregnancy registries and cohorts. Epilepsy Res. 2008;81(1):1–13.

173. Joffe H, Cohen LS, Suppes T, Hwang CH, Molay F, Adams JM, Sachs GS, Hall JE. Longitudinal follow-up of reproductive and metabolic features of valproate-associated polycystic ovarian syndrome features: a preliminary report. Biol Psychiatry. 2006;60(12):1378–81.

174. Chen CY, Li X, Ma LY, Zhou Y, Feng Q, Cui YM. In utero oxcarbazepine exposure and neonatal abstinence syndrome: case report and brief review of literature. Pharmacotherapy. 2017;37(7):e71–5.

175. Hayes J, Prah P, Nazareth I, King M, Walters K, Petersen I, et al. Prescribing trends in bipolar disorder: cohort study in the United Kingdom THIN primary care database 1995–2009. PLoS One. 2011;6(12):e28725.

176. Cohen LS, Viguera AC, McInerney KA, Freeman MP, Sosinsky AZ, Moustafa D, et al. Reproductive safety of second-generation antipsychotics: current data from the Massachusetts General Hospital National Pregnancy Registry for Atypical Antipsychotics. Am J Psychiatry. 2016;172(3):263–70.

177. Habermann F, Fritzsche J, Fuhlbruck F, Wacker E, Alignol A, Weber-Schoendorfer C, et al. Atypical antipsychotic drugs and pregnancy outcome: a prospective, cohort study. J Clin Psychopharmacol. 2013;33(4):453–62.

178. Coughlin CG, Blackwell KA, Bartley C, Hay M, Yonkers KA, Bloch MH. Obstetric and neonatal outcomes after antipsychotic medication exposure in pregnancy. Obstet Gynecol. 2015;125(5):1224–35.

179. Ennis ZN, Damkier P. Pregnancy exposure to olanzapine, quetiapine, risperidone, aripiprazole and risk of congenital malformations. A systematic review. Basic Clin Pharmacol Toxicol. 2015;116(4):315–20.

180. McKenna K, Korea G, Tetelbaum M, Wilton L, Shakir S, Diav-Citrin O, et al. Pregnancy outcome of women using atypical antipsychotic drugs: a prospective comparative study. J Clin Psychiatry. 2005;66(4):444–9.

181. Reis M, Kallen B. Maternal use of antipsychotics in early pregnancy and delivery outcome. J Clin Psychopharmacol. 2008;28(3):279–88.

182. Tosato S, Albert U, Tomassi S, Iasevoli F, Carmassi C, Ferrari S, et al. A systematized review of atypical antipsychotics in pregnant women: balancing between risks of untreated illness and risks of drug-related adverse effects. J Clin Psychiatry. 2017;78(5):e477–89.

183. United States Food and Drug Administration. FDA Drug Safety Communication: antipsychotic drug labels updated on use during pregnancy and risk of abnormal muscle movements and withdrawal symptoms in newborns. Washington (US). United States Food and Drug Administration; 2011.

184. Fortinguerra F, Clavenna A, Bonati M. Psychotropic drug use during breastfeeding: a review of the evidence. Pediatrics. 2009;124(4):e547–56.

185. Chaudron LH, Schoenecker CJ. Bupropion and breastfeeding: a case of a possible infant seizure. J Clin Psychiatry. 2004;65(6):881–2.

186. Neuman G, Colantonio D, Delaney S, Szynkaruk M, Ito S. Bupropion and escitalopram during lactation. Ann Pharmacother. 2014;48(7):928–31.

187. Pennell PB, Gidal BE, Sabers A, Gordon J, Perucca E. Pharmacology of antiepileptic drugs during pregnancy and lactation. Epilepsy Behav. 2007;11(3):263–9.

188. Newport DJ, Pennell PB, Calamaras MR, Ritchie JC, Newman M, Knight B, et al. Lamotrigine in breast milk and nursing infants: determination of exposure. Pediatrics. 2008;122(1):e223–31.

189. Ohman I, Vitols S, Tomson T. Lamotrigine in pregnancy: pharmacokinetics during delivery, in the neonate and during lactation. Epilepsia. 2000;41(6):709–13.

190. Schou M, Amdisen A. Lithium and pregnancy – III, lithium ingestion by children breast-fed by women on lithium treatment. BMJ. 1973;2(5859):138.

191. Wisner KL, Perel JM. Serum levels of valproate and carbamazepine in breastfeeding mother-infant pairs. J Clin Psychopharmacol. 1998;18(2):167–9.

192. Kaneko S, Sato T, Suzuki K. The levels of anticonvulsants in breast milk. Br J Clin Pharmacol. 1979;7(6):624–7.

193. Viguera AC, Newport DJ, Ritchie J, Stowe Z, Whitfield T, Mogielnicki J, et al. Lithium in breast milk and nursing infants: clinical implications. Am J Psychiatry. 2007;164(2):342–5.

194. American Academy of Pediatrics Committee on Drugs. Transfer of drugs and other chemicals into human milk. Pediatrics. 2001;108(3):776–89.

195. World Health Organization. Breastfeeding and maternal medication: recommendations for drugs in the Eleventh WHO Model List of Essential Drugs. Geneva: World Health Organization; 2003. 43 p.

196. Ito S. Drug therapy for breast-feeding women. NEJM. 2000;343(2):119–26.

197. Chaudron LH, Jefferson JW. Mood stabilizers during breastfeeding: a review. J Clin Psychiatry. 2000;61(2):79–90.

198. Nordmo E, Aronsen L, Wasland K, Smabrekka L, Vorren S. Severe apnea in an infant exposed to lamotrigine in breast milk. Ann Pharmacother. 2009;43(11):1983–7.

199. Uguz F. Second-generation antipsychotics during the lactation period: a comparative systematic review on infant safety. J Clin Psychopharmacol. 2016;36(3):233–52.

200. Brunner E, Falk DM, Jones M, Dey DK, Shatapathy CC. Olanzapine in pregnancy and breastfeeding: a review of data from global safety surveillance. BMC Pharmacol Toxicol. 2013;14:38.

201. Winans EA. Antipsychotics and breastfeeding. J Hum Lact. 2001;17(4):344–7.

202. Gardiner SJ, Kristensen JF, Begg EJ, Hackett LP, Wilson DA, Ilett KF, et al. Transfer of olanzapine into breast milk, calculation of infant drug dose, and effect on breast-fed infants. Am J Psychiatry. 2003;160(8):1428–31.

203. Rampono J, Kristensen JF, Ilett KF, Hackett LP, Kohan R. Quetiapine and breast feeding. Ann Pharmacother. 2007;41(4):711–4.

204. Lee A, Giesbrecht E, Dunn E, Ito S. Excretion of quetiapine in breast milk. Am J Psychiatry. 2004;161(9):1715–6.

205. Gentile S. Clinical utilization of atypical antipsychotics in pregnancy and lactation. Ann Pharmacother. 2004;38(7–8):1264–71.

206. Schlotterbeck P, Saur R, Hiemke C, Gründer G, Vehren T, Kircher T, et al. Low concentration of ziprasidone in human milk: a case report. Int J Neuropsychopharmacol. 2009;12(3):437–8. https://doi.org/10.1017/S1461145709009936.. Epub 2009 Feb 10.

207. Leiknes KA, Cooke MJ, Jarosch-von Schweder L, Harboe I, Høie B. Electroconvulsive therapy during pregnancy: a systematic review of case studies. Arch Womens Ment Health. 2015;18(1):1–39.

208. Reed P, Sermin N, Appleby L, Faragher B. A comparison of clinical response to electroconvulsive therapy in puerperal and non-puerperal psychoses. J Affect Disord. 1999;54(3):255–60.

209. Walker R, Swartz CM. Electroconvulsive therapy during high-risk pregnancy. Gen Hosp Psychiatry. 1994;16(5):348–53.

210. Anderson EL, Reti IM. ECT in pregnancy: a review of the literature from 1941 to 2007. Psychosom Med. 2009;71(2):235–42.

211. Calaway K, Coshal S, Jones K, Coverdale J, Livingston R. A systematic review of the safety of electroconvulsive therapy use during the first trimester of pregnancy. J ECT. 2016;32(4):230–5.

212. Miller LJ. Use of electroconvulsive therapy during pregnancy. Hosp Community Psychiatry. 1994;45(5):444–50.

213. Bhatia SC, Baldwin SA, Bhatia SK. Electroconvulsive therapy during the third trimester of pregnancy. J ECT. 1999;15(4):270–4.

214. Sinha P, Goyal P, Andrade C. A meta-review of the safety of electroconvulsive therapy in pregnancy. J ECT. 2017;33(2):81–8.

215. Saatcioglu O, Tomruk NB. The use of electroconvulsive therapy in pregnancy: a review. Isr J Psychiatry Relat Sci. 2011;48(1):6–11.

216. Deligiannidis KM, Freeman MP. Complementary and alternative medicine therapies for perinatal depression. Best Pract Res Clin Obstet Gynaecol. 2014;28(1):85–95.

217. Manber R, Schnyer RN, Lyell D, Chambers AS, Caughey AB, Druzin M, et al. Acupuncture for depression during pregnancy: a randomized controlled trial. Obstet Gynecol. 2010;115(3):511–20.

218. Schuette SA, Brown KM, Cuthbert DA, Coyle CW, Wisner KL, Hoffman MC, et al. Perspectives from patients and healthcare providers on the practice of maternal placentophagy. J Altern Complement Med. 2017;23(1):60–7.

Postpartum Neuropathy

Janet F. R. Waters

One of the most frequent scenarios where neurologists are called to the bedside of a postpartum patient takes place when the patient develops leg weakness after delivery. Neuraxial anesthesia is often blamed for the complication, but this in fact is rarely the case. Obstetrical nerve injuries due to compression or stretching of a vulnerable nerve is more common and occurs in 1% of deliveries [1]. This chapter will review the various clinical presentations of obstetrical nerve injuries and will then discuss how to distinguish these relatively benign injuries from more serious complications such as retroperitoneal hematoma, epidural hematoma, and conus and cauda equine injuries.

The most common lower extremity nerve injuries associated with pregnancy and delivery involve in descending order, the lateral femoral cutaneous nerve, femoral nerve, peroneal nerve, lumbosacral plexus, sciatic nerve and obturator nerve [2–4]. Use of epidural anesthesia in management of labor pain may increase risk of nerve injury due to a tendency to contribute to prolonged second stage of labor. Absence of sensation prevents women from sensing pressure and adjusting their position. Other risk factors for obstetrical nerve injury include nulliparity, short stature, large fetus, excessive weight gain and instrumental delivery (See Table 1).

The most commonly injured nerve in pregnancy is the lateral cutaneous femoral nerve [5]. During pregnancy, it may be stretched or compressed by the expanding abdomen. Injury is associated with hyperglycemia, excessive weight gain and large fetal size, and can be a complication of gestational diabetes. Women with this neuropathy complain of painful paresthesias in the lateral thigh. Meralgia paresthetica in pregnancy may be treated by avoidance of tight clothing and positions that aggravate the condition. Most resolve after delivery. There is no motor component to the nerve and it is not a source of postpartum leg weakness.

Femoral nerve injury is the most common cause of postpartum leg weakness [6]. It occurs in 2.8 per 100,000 deliveries. In 25% of patients, injury is bilateral causing significant impairment of mobility in new mothers. The femoral nerve arises from the lumbar plexus where nerve roots L2-4 are joined. It passes between the iliacus and psoas muscles then courses under the inguinal ligament. During vaginal delivery, the femoral nerve may be compressed by the fetal head at the level of the inguinal ligament. It may also undergo a stretch injury due to hip abduction and external rotation. A prolonged period of time spent in lithotomy position can increase the risk of femoral nerve injury.

Injury to the femoral nerve produces weakness in the quadriceps femoris and in the iliopsoas muscle if the injury occurs proximal to the inguinal ligament. Sensory loss and anesthesia occurs in the distribution of the femoral nerve in the anteromedial thigh. Knee jerk will be reduced or absent. Diagnosis of femoral neuropathy can often be made at the bedside by obtaining a thorough history and clinical exam. Most injuries are demyelinative and improve within days to weeks. Treatment includes knee brace and physical therapy. Patients whose symptoms do not improve within 3 weeks may undergo Electromyography and Nerve Conduction Studies for confirmation and prognostication. Axonal injuries may take up to 6–12 months to improve and recovery may be incomplete.

Case 1

Chief Complaint: The patient is a 33 year old female G1P1 who was noted to have bilateral lower extremity weakness following vaginal delivery.

Table 1 Risk factors for obstetrical nerve injury

Large fetus
Short stature
Nulliparity
Prolonged second stage of labor
Instrumental delivery
Epidural anesthesia

J. F. R. Waters (✉)
University of Pittsburgh Medical Center, Pittsburgh, PA, USA
e-mail: watersjf@upmc.edu

© Springer Nature Switzerland AG 2019
M. A. O'Neal (ed.), *Neurology and Psychiatry of Women*, https://doi.org/10.1007/978-3-030-04245-5_19

History of Present Illness

The patient presented with spontaneous rupture of membranes with meconium stained fluid, followed by onset of contractions. Epidural anesthesia was placed with uneventful insertion at the first attempt. The patient progressed to complete dilatation. Labor required augmentation with Pitocin in the second stage for spaced contractions. After pushing for approximately 2.5–3 h, the patient gave birth to a healthy female infant, Apgar's 9/9, weight 7 lb, 3 oz. Epidural infusion was stopped 1 h after delivery and the catheter was removed. Shortly after delivery, her anesthesiologist was called to the bedside due to the patient's complaint of lower extremity weakness. The patient reported weakness in her legs bilaterally. She found that her legs buckled when she attempted to walk. She noted pins and needles sensation in the medial upper thighs and knees. The patient was not experiencing back pain. She reported no bowel or bladder incontinence. Neurology was consulted for further care.

Exam

General examination revealed a well appearing 5 ft 6 in. female in no acute distress. Back examinations revealed an epidural catheter insertion site which was unremarkable without firmness or tenderness.

Mental status exam was normal

Cranial nerves were intact

Motor exam revealed Normal bulk and tone throughout. Upper extremity power was normal, 5/5 at deltoids, biceps, triceps, wrist flexors, wrist extensors, and hand grip bilaterally. Right lower extremity power was diminished 4/5 at the iliopsoas, 5/5 hamstrings, 3/5 quadriceps, 5/5 tibialis anterior, gastrocnemius, and extensor hallucis longus. Left lower extremity power was 4/5 at the iliopsoas, 5/5 hamstrings, 2+/5 quadriceps, 5/5 tibialis anterior, gastrocnemius, and extensor hallucis longus.

Sensory exam was intact to temperature, vibration and pinprick throughout.

Reflexes were 2+ at biceps, triceps, brachioradialis, 0 patella, and 2+ achilles bilaterally. Toes were down going bilaterally.

Gait examination could not be assessed due to leg weakness.

MRI of the lumbosacral spine was normal. CT scan of the pelvis revealed no evidence of retroperitoneal hematoma.

Weakness improved but was still present after 3 weeks. EMG confirmed bilateral femoral neuropathy. Symptoms continued to improve with physical therapy and total recovery occurred. The patient ran in the Pittsburgh marathon 1 year after delivery.

While the diagnosis of femoral neuropathy can often be made at the bedside, the bilateral presentation in this patient prompted imaging as noted above. The absence of radicular pain makes the diagnosis of radiculopathy less likely, and the distribution of weakness and sensory loss is more consistent with femoral neuropathy than plexopathy.

Fibular neuropathy (previously known as common peroneal neuropathy) may be caused by compression of the nerve at the fibular head. In the obstetrical population it has been attributed to prolonged knee flexion while squatting, lithotomy position, or by pressure on the fibular head with stirrups during delivery. Patients with fibular nerve compression develop foot drop due to weakness in the tibialis anterior, extensor hallucis longus and moderate weakness in foot eversion. Patients will have decreased sensation to pinprick on the dorsum of the foot, most pronounced between the first and second toes [7]. Awareness of the vulnerability to injury has lead to appropriate repositioning and decreased frequency of injury.

Case 2

The patient is a 29 year old female G1 P1 who delivered a healthy baby boy 8 lbs, 10 oz via vaginal delivery after 24 h of labor. Epidural was placed without complications prior to delivery. The patient was not placed in stirrups but was in a squatting position during labor. Epidural catheter was removed. Several hours later, the patient attempted to walk to the bathroom and noted a right foot drop. Anesthesiology was called to the bedside and contacted Neurology for further evaluation. In addition to weakness, the patient complained of numbness and paresthesia in the right foot. She had no complaint of back pain or bowel and bladder symptoms.

Examination revealed 0/5 power in the right tibialis anterior and extensor hallicus muscles. Weakness 3/5 was present in the right foot evertors. Power was otherwise normal including right foot invertors and gastrocnemius muscle. The patient had relatively decreased pinprick on the dorsal surface of the foot and lateral calf. Absent pinprick was noted between the first and second toes. The remainder of the neurologic exam was normal. Fibular nerve compression was diagnosed at the bedside. Over the next 72 h, symptoms resolved.

The absence of weakness in the gastrocnemius muscles, hamstrings and foot invertors distinguish this injury from a sciatic nerve injury.

Injuries to the lumbosacral plexus can occur during delivery due to compression from the fetal head or forceps at the pelvic brim. Symptoms are dependent upon the nerve roots involved. Muscles innervated by L4 and L5 nerve roots are most affected causing weakness in ankle dorsiflexion, inversion and eversion. Sensory impairment is predominantly in the distribution of the L5 dermatome. Achilles reflex is often preserved. Risk factors include large fetal size, small maternal size, fetal malposition and instrumental delivery.

Obturator neuropathy is rare. It represents less than 4.7% of all postpartum neuropathies. Patients will present with weakness of thigh adduction and sensory loss of the upper third of the medial thigh. Patients with this disorder will have a wide based gait with circumduction. Risk factors include cephalopelvic disproportion and instrumental vaginal delivery. Patients are treated supportively with physical therapy [8].

Obstetrical sciatic nerve injuries are rare in the United States. They occur more frequently abroad where intramuscular injections of pain medication or methergine are administered in the gluteal region. Sciatic nerve injury can result in a wide range of symptoms which vary from minor sensory disturbances to disabling paralysis of the foot. The sciatic nerve is formed from the anterior and posterior divisions of L4, L5, S1 and S2 spinal nerves and the anterior division of S3. The anterior divisions becomes the tibial division and the posterior division becomes the peroneal division. They pass through the pyriformis muscle. The peroneal portion lies lateral to the tibial portion. Injections into the gluteal region should be administered to the upper lateral quadrant of the gluteus muscle to avoid injury. Risk of injury is increased in underweight patients. Mechanical injury to the nerve by the needle produces pain which alerts the provider to avoid injection of the agent. Mechanical injuries are generally minor. Intrafascicular injection into the nerve by a neurotoxic agent can cause severe nerve injury. After injection of a neurotoxic agent, the nerve appears pale with areas of petechial hemorrhage and splitting and fragmentation of myelin. This is followed by axonal degeneration and scar formation. Sciatic nerve injury produces weakness in the tibialis anterior, extensor hallucis longus, foot everters and inverters and gastrocnemius muscles and hamstrings. Paresthesias and loss of pain and temperature may occur and are located on the dorsal and plantar surfaces of the foot and lateral calf. Sensory loss may include vibration and joint position sense. Absent Achilles tendon reflex will be found on exam.

The differential diagnosis for leg weakness in the postpartum patient is broad and it is important to distinguish neuropathies from other more ominous disorders [9, 10]. Epidural hematoma is an extremely rare but serious cause of postpartum leg weakness. It occurs in one in 200,000 patients after spinal anesthesia and one in 150,000 patients who receive epidural anesthesia [11, 12]. Patients will complain of back pain and tenderness, prolonged anesthesia with numbness and weakness and will have sphincter dysfunction. Risk factors include use of antiplatelet agents and anticoagulants, inherited clotting dysfunction, low platelet count, and the presence of spine and nerve root tumors (See Table 2). Imaging with MRI confirms the diagnosis and treatment with urgent surgical decompression is indicated to prevent permanent neurologic deficit [13].

Retroperitoneal hematoma can occur postoperatively following cesarean section in the setting of bleeding diathesis or trauma. Spontaneous rupture of the uterine artery may also produce retroperitoneal hematoma. Patients will complain of pain in the back, hip, groin and abdomen. Leg weakness is caused by compression of the femoral nerve at the iliopsoas gutter. Diagnosis is made with CT of the abdomen and pelvis.

Injury to the conus medullaris during administration of neuraxial block is extremely rare. It occurs if there is inad-

Table 2 Predisposing factor for epidural hematoma

Iatrogenic clotting dysfunction
Spinal cord and nerve root tumor (neurofibromatosis)
Gestational thrombocytopenia
Preeclampsia/eclampsia/HELLP
Inherited clotting dysfunction

Case 3

The patient is a 20 year old female G1 P1 who delivered her first infant via vaginal delivery in a maternity hospital in Serbia. She received epidural anesthesia prior to delivery. She had uterine atony after delivery and while anesthetized with the epidural, was treated with an IM shot of methergine in the left gluteus maximus muscle. She did not experience pain during the injection. The epidural catheter was removed. The patient developed severe pain in the right leg and numbness and paralysis of the distal lower extremity. The patient was assured that her symptoms would resolve and she was discharged to home. The patient returned for a post-partum visit the following week. She presented in a wheel chair due to inability to walk. Pain had improved but was still present. Examination revealed loss of pin prick in the left foot and lateral calf. Vibration and position sense were absent. She had 0/5 power in the left tibialis anterior, extensor hallucis longus, foot invertors, foot evertors and gastrocnemius muscles. Weakness 3/5 was present in the left hamstring and ankle jerks were two on the right and absent on the left. She underwent a CT of the pelvis which revealed an enlarged sciatic nerve on the left. Weakness and sensory loss were unimproved when seen in follow up 6 months later.

Table 3 Differential diagnosis for postpartum leg weakness

Femoral nerve injury
Fibular nerve injury
Lumbosacral plexopathy
Sciatic nerve injury
Obturator nerve injury
Retroperitoneal hematoma
Epidural hematoma
Direct spinal cord/cauda equina injury
Anterior spinal artery syndrome

vertent placement of the catheter at a higher level than L2. Patients will complain of pain in the lower limbs, saddle anesthesia and bowel and bladder dysfunction. Chemical injury to the cauda equine by local anesthetic agents has been reported and causes lower extremity weakness, polyradicular pain, numbness and diminished reflexes. Changes in the anesthetic agents used today has virtually eradicated this complication.

Anterior Spinal Artery syndrome is an extremely rare entity that can occur in the setting of prolonged hypotension. Lack of perfusion in the anterior spinal artery leads to paraplegia, loss of pain and temperature sensation and bowel and bladder dysfunction. Proprioception, light touch and vibratory sense are spared. The presence of bowel and bladder dysfunction and the diffuse weakness and sensory loss distinguish this injury from bilateral neuropathies [14].

Postpartum leg weakness after delivery is not an expected event. Yet it occurs in 1% of women after childbirth. It takes place most often as a result of compression of the femoral nerve, fibular nerve or lumbosacral plexus during delivery. It rarely occurs as a complication of epidural or spinal anesthesia through direct injury to the cauda equine or conus medullaris, or to the development of an epidural hematoma (See Table 3). When an epidural hematoma does occur, it is cru-

cial to make the diagnosis promptly so that surgical intervention can take place prior to permanent injury. A thorough history and neurologic examination at the bedside is paramount to localizing the injury.

References

1. O'Neal A, Chang L, Salajeghi K. Postpartum spinal cord, root, plexus and peripheral nerve injuries involving lower extremities: a practical approach. Anesth Analg. 2014;XXX:1–8.
2. Massey EW, Guidon AC. Peripheral neuropathies in pregnancy. Continuum Neurol. 2014;20(1):100–14.
3. Massey EW, Stolp KA. Peripheral neuropathy in pregnancy. Phys Med Rehabil Clin N Am. 2008;19:149–62.
4. Wong CA, Scavone BM, Dugan S, Smith JC, Prather H, Ganchiff JN, McCarthy RJ. Incidence of postpartum lumbosacral spine and lower extremity nerve injuries. Obstet Gynecol. 2003;101:279–88.
5. Van Diver T, Camann W. Meralgia paresthetica in the parturient. Int J Obstet Anesth. 1995;4:109–12.
6. O'Neal A. What do I do Now? Women's Neurol:115–8.
7. Blumenfeld H. Neuroanatomy through clinical cases. 2002; 339–360.
8. Nogajski JH, Shnier RC, Zagami AS. Postpartum obturator neuropathy. Neurology. 2004;63:2450–1.
9. Kowe O, Waters JH. Neurologic complications in the patient receiving obstetric anesthesia. Neurol Clin. 2012;30:823–33.
10. Christie IW, McCabe S. Major complications of epidural analgesia after surgery: results of a six-year survey. Anaesthesia. 2007;62:335–41.
11. Waters JH. Neurologic complications in the obstetrical anesthesia patient, chapter 4. In: Neurologic illness in pregnancy. Oxford: Wiley; 2015.
12. Ruppen W, Derry S, McQuay H, Moore RA. Incidence of epidural hematoma, infection, and neurologic injury in obstetric patients with epidural analgesia/anesthesia. Anesthesiology. 2006;105:394–9.
13. Lawton MT, Porter RW, Heiserman JE, Jacobowitz R, Sonntag VK, Dickman CA. Surgical management of spinal epidural hematoma: relationship between surgical timing and neurologicaloutcome. J Neurosurg. 1995;83:1–7.
14. Dunn DW, Ellison J. Anterior spinal artery syndrome during the postpartum period. Arch Neurol. 1981;38:263.

Myasthenia Gravis and Pregnancy

Christyn Edmundson and Mohammad Kian Salajegheh

Overview of Myasthenia Gravis

Myasthenia Gravis (MG) is caused by antibody-mediated damage to the post-synaptic neuromuscular junction in skeletal muscle. In the ocular form of the disease, weakness affects the periocular muscles, causing fluctuating ptosis and diplopia. In the generalized form of disease, weakness may also involve oropharyngeal, respiratory and limb muscles. The weakness appears, or worsens, with activity of involved muscles and improves with rest. Patients with severe bulbar and respiratory weakness are diagnosed as having "myasthenic crisis" and require intensive care unit admission (ICU) and emergent therapy [1]. Acetylcholine receptor (AChR) antibodies are present in 85% of patients with generalized MG and 40–60% of patients with the ocular form of disease [1]. Antibodies to muscle-specific kinase (MuSK) and receptor-related low-density lipoprotein-4 (LRP-4) are found in a smaller proportion of MG patients. MG can be exacerbated by a variety of triggers, including certain medications, surgery, infection, pregnancy and other emotional and physical stressors. Treatment modalities include pyridostigmine, corticosteroids, other immunosuppressive (IS) agents, intravenous immunoglobulin (IVIG), plasma exchange (PLEX) and thymectomy [2] (see Table 1).

Hormonal Effects and Myasthenia Gravis

Sex hormones can influence the development and severity of autoimmune disorders [3] including MG [4]. Not only do women experience earlier onset and increased incidence of MG in comparison with men [4], but MG symptoms may worsen during menstruation [5], oral contraceptives and ovulatory suppression may mitigate symptoms of MG [6, 7] and MG can fluctuate during the course of pregnancy [8]. In an animal model of MG, treatment with estrogen enhanced production of acetylcholine receptor antibodies and increased the severity of MG symptoms in mice [9]. Experimental data also suggest that short-term elevations in estrogen may impair neuromuscular transmission [10].

Symptoms of MG first appear during pregnancy or the post-partum period in 11–18% of women with MG, with the greatest risk of symptom onset in the first 6 months post-partum [11]. Symptoms typical of MG should prompt further workup, starting with testing for AChR, MuSK or LRP-4 antibodies. If antibodies are unrevealing, nerve conduction studies with repetitive nerve stimulation or the more sensitive single fiber electromyography (EMG) may be safely performed in pregnancy. In non-pregnant patients with newly diagnosed MG with AChR antibodies, computed tomography (CT) of the chest should be performed to assess for thymoma. However, in pregnant patient with MG, radiation exposure should be avoided and thymic imaging can generally be delayed until after pregnancy. In cases where there is a strong clinical suspicion for thymoma, chest magnetic resonance imaging (MRI) is preferred over chest CT during pregnancy [12].

In women known to have MG, symptoms worsen in 20–50% during pregnancy and are stable or improved in the remainder [8, 13–15]. Exacerbations appear to be relatively more common in the first trimester, third trimester and 6–8 weeks post-partum, with fewer exacerbations occurring in the second trimester [14]. In addition to hormonal and immunological changes after delivery, sleep deprivation and physical fatigue related to caring for an infant can precipitate symptomatic exacerbation post-partum. Patients should be educated regarding the potential for disease exacerbation so that expectant mothers can arrange for support in childcare and their own activities of daily living.

C. Edmundson
Division of Neuromuscular Medicine, Department of Neurology, Hospital of the University of Pennsylvania, Philadelphia, PA, USA
e-mail: Christyn.Edmundson@uphs.upenn.edu

M. K. Salajegheh (✉)
Neuromuscular Center & EMG Laboratory, Department of Neurology, VA Boston Healthcare System, Harvard Medical School, Boston, MA, USA
e-mail: msalajegheh@bwh.harvard.edu

© Springer Nature Switzerland AG 2019
M. A. O'Neal (ed.), *Neurology and Psychiatry of Women*, https://doi.org/10.1007/978-3-030-04245-5_20

Table 1 Medications used to treat myasthnia gravis, pregnancy and lactation [2, 12, 16, 18, 41, 42]

Medication	Dose range	Adverse reactions (partial list)	Pregnancy category (FDA)	Teratogenicity	Lactation
First line therapies					
Pryridostigmine	60–600 mg per day (divided every 4–6 h)	Increased respiratory secretion, diarrhea, muscle twitching, bradycardia	C	No clear data. Has been successfully used in pregnancy	Considered compatible with breastfeeding
Prednisone	Varies significantly. 5–1 mg/kg per day	Hypertension, hyperglycemia, weight gain, gastrointestinal ulcers, osteoporosis	C	Possible risk of cleft palate. Use lowest effective dose in pregnancy	Considered compatible with breastfeeding
Rapid acting therapies					
IV immunoglobulin	Varies. Innitial treatment often 2 g/kg, divided over 5 days	Venous thrombosis (including PE), stroke, aseptic meningitis, anaphylaxis, kidney injury	C	Has been successfully used in pregnancy	No significant data. Assess risk and benefit in individual case
Plasma exchange	Varies. Typically 5 exchanges of 3–5 L over 7–14 days	Electrolyte and fluid imbalance, sepsis, hypotension	NA	Has been successfully used in pregnancy	No significant data
Immunosuppressives					
Azathioprine	50–200 mg per day	Bone marrow suppression, infection, heaptotoxicity	D	May cause congenital defects. Considered immunosuppresive of choice in Europe	Likely to adversely affect infant
Cylcosporine	2.5–4 mg/kg per day, divided BID	Hypertension, renal toxicity, seizure, infection	C	May cause premature birth or low birth weight	Likely to adversely affect infant
Eculizumab	900 mg IV weekly – 1200 mg IV weekly	Infection, hypertension, anemia	C	No significant data	No significant data
Methotrexate	7.5–25 mg per week	Hepatotoxicity, pulmonary toxicity, gastrointestinal toxicity, infection	X	May cause fetal death or congenital defects	Likely to adversely affect infant
Mycophenolate mofetil	1000–200 mg per day, divided BID	Bone marrow suppression, infection, nausea/diarrhea	D	May cause congential defects	No significant data
Rituximab	375 mg/m² weekly for 4 weeks, or 1000 mg every 2 weeks ×2	Hepatitis B reactivation, infection, fever, infection, progressive multifocal leukoencephalopathy	C	May cause B-cell lymphocytopenia in infant, usually lasting <6 months	No significant data

FDA pregnancy categories
  A=No risk in controlled human studies
  B=No evidence of risk in studies
  C=Risk cannot be ruled out
  D=Positive evidence of risk
  X=Contraindicated in pregnancy
The FDA has discontinued this rating system, though it is still commonly used in practice. These categories have been replaced with a summary of the risks of using a drug during pregnancy and breastfeeding
FDA United States Food and Drug Administration, *NA* Not Applicable

Pregnancy Considerations and Treatment

Pre-pregnancy planning for women with MG should begin well in advance of conception in order to optimize disease control prior to pregnancy [2]. Women with MG considering pregnancy should be cared for by a multidisciplinary team that includes input from neurology, obstetrics and anesthesiology [2, 16]. While most women with well controlled MG remain more or less stable during pregnancy and experience uncomplicated delivery of healthy infants, pregnancy complications and infant outcomes remain a significant concern for patients and providers, and a diagnosis of MG may impact family planning [2, 16]. In women with poorly controlled MG, there may be significant risks to both the mother and fetus, and such patients should be counseled to delay conception until MG can be better controlled. In one cohort, half of women who had not intentionally completed child bearing at the time of MG diagnosis abstained from further pregnancies because of their MG [17]. Given the personal nature of decisions regarding child-bearing, cases may arise in which ideal medical management is in conflict with patient preference, necessitating an open and trusting dialogue between patients and medical providers.

Because MG does not reduce female fertility, contraceptive use should be addressed with all women with MG of childbearing age, particularly prior to starting immunosuppressive (IS), some of which have teratogenic effects as discussed below. In women with childbearing potential, contraception should be started at least 4 weeks prior to IS, continued for the duration of therapy [12] and for at least 3 months after discontinuation of IS [16]. Of note, mycophenolate mofetil, which carries a high risk of teratogenicity, reduces the serum concentration of oral contraceptives [18]. Women with childbearing potential taking mycophenolate mofetil should use two forms of highly effective birth control, unless total abstinence is chosen.

First-Line Therapies

Oral pyridostigmine is considered first-line for treatment of MG during pregnancy. Intravenous (IV) cholinesterase inhibitors should not be used due to the risk of producing uterine contractions [2]. If oral pyridostigmine does not adequately control MG symptoms, corticosteroids (CS) at the lowest effective dose are the preferred immunosuppressive agent in pregnancy [2, 16]. CS may increase the risk of gestational diabetes mellitus, infection and preterm deliveries [16]. While CS were previously thought to increase the risk of cleft palate in infants [19, 20], more recent studies did not show an increase cleft palate with prenatal exposure to CS [21, 22].

Rapid-Acting Therapies

In instances of severe MG symptoms or MG crisis in pregnancy, IVIG and PLEX may be used in an attempt to promptly, though temporarily, modify disease severity [2, 23]. While the safety of IVIG or PLEX for MG in pregnancy has not been investigated, both have been frequently used during pregnancy and are generally well tolerated [23, 24]. When using IVIG in pregnancy, particular attention should be given to possible side effects of hyperviscosity and fluid overload. When using PLEX in pregnancy, fetal monitoring is recommended during the third trimester. Additional attention to fluid balance and positioning the mother in the left lateral decubitus position are recommended [25].

Immunosuppressives

Immunosuppressives (IS) other than corticosteroids are avoided in pregnancy when possible due to potential harm to the fetus. However, this must be carefully weighed against the risk of an MG exacerbation or crisis caused by withholding them. Particularly if an unintended pregnancy occurs,

drug withdrawal may occur too late to avoid teratogenesis. Patients taking IS during pregnancy should be included in drug specific registries, which can be found at www.fda.gov.

In patients with MG that is not adequately controlled by corticosteroids, recent international consensus guidelines suggest that azathioprine and cyclosporine are relatively safe in pregnancy [2]. In Europe, azathioprine is the nonsteroidal IS of choice for MG in pregnancy [16], though the US Food and Drug Administration (FDA) recommends against its use in pregnancy [18]. Azathioprine is metabolized to 6-mercaptopurine, which is then converted intracellularly to active nucleotides. Because the fetal liver does not express the enzyme responsible for converting azathioprine to its active metabolites, the fetus is theoretically protected from potential teratogenic effects of the drug [16]. However, there are no well-controlled studies of azathioprine in pregnant women and observational studies have produced conflicting results. Similarly, cyclosporine has not been studied prospectively in pregnancy. While not considered teratogenic, cyclosporine may increase the risk of prematurity and low birth weight [18].

Rituximab has been used to treat MG and may be particularly effective in patients with anti-MuSK antibodies [2, 26]. However, no prospective studies of its efficacy in MG or its safety in pregnancy have been published to date. In women with MG treated with Rituximab, there are reports of uncomplicated pregnancies resulting in the birth of healthy infants, though rituximab was not used for >12 months prior to pregnancy in these cases [27]. Eculizumab is a newly available complement inhibitor used to treat MG. There is no human data available regarding the effects of eculizumab on pregnancy [18].

Mycophenolate mofetil and methotrexate are teratogenic and are contraindicated in pregnancy. Both drugs should be discontinued at least 3 months prior to conception when possible [16].

Thymectomy

Thymectomy is considered standard of care in patients with MG and thymoma [2] and may also benefit patients with non-thymomatous, AChR antibody positive, generalized MG [28]. Because the therapeutic benefit of thymectomy is delayed, and surgery presents an immediate risk of causing MG crisis or exacerbation, thymectomy should preferably be postponed until after pregnancy [2].

Pregnancy Complications

Eclampsia and preeclampsia complicate 2–8% of pregnancies in the United States [29]. While these hypertensive disorders of pregnancy do not appear to be more common in

Table 2 Treatment of eclampsia and preeclampsia in myasthenia gravis [2, 30–32]

Treatment	Potential complications
Traditional first line treatment	
IV magnesium sulfate	Likely to cause exacerbation of MG. If used prepare to provide ventilatory support
Other antihypertensives	
Methyldopa	
Hydralazine	
β-blockers	Often causes exacerbation of MG. Consider use under close observation
Other anticonvulsants	
Barbiturates	May cause respiratory suppression
Benzodiazepines	May cause respiratory suppression
Phenytoin	Occasionally causes exacerbation of MG
Levetiracetam	

MG Myasthenia Gravis

Table 3 Medications that may exacerbate myasthenia gravis [1, 14]

Drug class	Examples
Antiarrhythmic agents	Lidocaine, quinidine, quinine and procainamide
Antimicrobial agents	Aminoglycosides, fluoroquinolones, macrolides, colistin and polymyxin B
Beta-blockers	Propranolol, metoprolol, carvedilol, etc.
Calcium channel blockers	Verapamil, diltiazem, amlodipine, etc.
Corticosteroids	
Iodinated contrast agents	
Magnesium (parenteral)	
Neuromuscular blocking agents	Succinylcholine, vecuronium and botulism toxin
D-pennicillamine	
α-interferon	

For an extensive review of medications and myasthenia gravis, see:
Myasthenia Gravis Foundation of America "Medications and Myasthenia Gravis, A Reference for Healthcare Professionals." http://www.myasthenia.org/portals/0/draft_medications_and_myasthenia_gravis_for_MGFA_website_8%2010%2012.pdf

women with MG, their management is complicated in the patients (see Table 2). The first line treatment for hypertensive disorders of pregnancy, intravenous (IV) magnesium sulfate, is known to cause exacerbations of MG by reducing acetylcholine release. Magnesium sulfate should be used only when its potential benefits outweigh risks, such as when a patient is actively experiencing eclamptic seizures. In such cases, the treating team should be prepared to manage an exacerbation of MG, which may require ventilatory support [30]. Methyldopa and hydralazine can also be considered for management hypertension in these disorders [30, 31]. Calcium channel blockers and β-blockers should also be avoided due to the risk of MG exacerbation, though there are some reports of labetalol being used successfully under close observation [30]. Barbiturates, benzodiazepines, phenytoin and levetiracetam may be used for seizure prevention and control in preeclampsia and eclampsia [2, 30, 32].

Infections during pregnancy, such as urinary tract infections, may cause MG exacerbations. Such infections should be treated promptly with antibiotics appropriate for use in both MG (see Table 3) and in pregnancy.

Labor and Delivery

MG is unlikely to affect the manner and timing of delivery [2, 16]. Women with MG in labor should be cared for at a center with the capacity to provide intensive care and access to specialists in obstetrics, anesthesiology, neonatology and neurology. Spontaneous vaginal delivery is the objective in any pregnancy and should be actively encouraged in MG patients [2]. If women are on long term steroids at doses greater than 7.5 mg prednisone daily, expert opinion suggests that stress dose parenteral hydrocortisone (100 mg IV) should be given in the first stage of labor [16]. Because MG affects only striated or skeletal muscle, the first stage of

labor, which depends primarily on smooth muscle contraction of the myometrium, is typically not affected. In the second stage of labor striated muscle becomes involved in the voluntary expulsive effort and fatigability due to MG may be pronounced. Cholinesterase inhibitors can be used to help manage muscle fatigability. The obstetrician should be prepared to assist vaginal delivery with the use of vacuum or forceps if fatigue occurs. Cesarean section should only be performed for standard obstetric indications [12, 16].

Regarding anesthetic use in labor, expert opinion favors epidural or combined spinal-epidural anesthesia in vaginal delivery, as it may protect against prolonged overexertion and fatigue [16]. However, regional anesthesia may also exacerbate underlying skeletal muscle weakness and those who receive high levels of regional anesthesia may experience decreased respiratory function. Regional anesthesia is also recommended for cesarean delivery [16]. Narcotics should be avoided as they may cause respiratory depression in both the mother and fetus. General anesthesia and neuromuscular blockade should be avoided whenever possible. Patients with MG are exquisitely sensitive to non-depolarizing neuromuscular blocking agents and if their use cannot be avoided, the function of the neuromuscular junction should be closely monitored using peripheral nerve stimulation [12, 16].

Fetal Considerations

While the rate of severe birth defects is not significantly higher in infants of mothers with MG, transplacental passage of antibodies during pregnancy can cause transient neonatal MG (TNMG). Because of this, delivery should take place in a facility with immediate access to neonatal resuscitation and intensive care [2]. The incidence of TNMG in infants born to mothers with MG ranges from 10% to 30% [8, 13, 15, 33]. TNMG is characterized by generalized hypotonia, poor sucking and feeding, weak cry and respiratory difficulties. Symptoms typically occur within hours, but are sometimes delayed several days after birth, and resolve within 1–7 weeks [34]. While this syndrome was initially recognized in infants of mothers with anti-AChR positive MG, it has also been reported in anti-MuSK positive MG and in seronegative MG [35–38]. Diagnosis is made though examination of the infant and mother, and must be distinguished from congenital myasthenic syndromes, which are caused by genetic mutations affecting various components of the neuromuscular junction. Treatment is primarily supportive, using nasogastric feeding, ventilatory support and acetylcholinesterase inhibitors, particularly before feedings. In severe cases IVIG and PLEX may be considered [16]. Infants born to mothers with MG should be monitored for symptoms of TNMG [2] and some experts recommend an inpatient observation period of at least 2 days [16].

In rare cases, infants born to mothers with high levels of antibodies to the fetal γ-subunit of the AChR have persistent complications, collectively labeled fetal AChR inactivation syndrome. It is hypothesized that such deficits are due to inactivation of the AChR, primarily in muscle but possibly in other tissues, during critical periods of intrauterine development. The most severe manifestation is arthrogryposis multiplex congenita (AMC). AMC is a potentially fatal syndrome characterized by multiple joint contractures, polyhydramnios, pulmonary hypoplasia and other anomalies which may result from reduced intrauterine movements. Because of the risk of AMC, a fetal scan should be offered at 13 and 20 weeks and women with MG should be encouraged to monitor fetal movements [16]. In milder cases, infants may have mild facial weakness, high arched palate, hearing loss, or variable myopathic features [39, 40]. While case reports suggest that treatment of maternal MG may modify the severity of fetal AChR inactivation syndrome, data is limited [40].

Lactation

Breastfeeding is not contraindicated in women with MG. While maternal antibodies are present in breast milk, there is no evidence reported in the literature that breastfeeding increases the risk of myasthenic symptoms in newborns. Most medications used to treat MG are secreted in breast milk, and their impact on the newborn should be carefully considered. Prednisone, prednisolone and pyridostigmine are considered compatible with breast feeding [41]. The US Food and Drug Administration (FDA) labels both methotrexate and azathioprine as contraindicated in breast feeding.

However, as with its use in pregnancy, azathioprine is generally considered safe in breast feeding in European practice [16]. Cyclosporine is found in breast milk, and because of possible immunosuppression and growth delay in the infant it is contraindicated in breast feeding [42]. Mycophenolate mofetil is excreted in milk in animal studies, but it is not known whether its active metabolite is excreted in human breast milk, thus its safety in breast feeding is unknown [12, 41]. The safety of rituximab and IVIG in breast feeding is unknown. Human studies have not been performed to assess whether rituximab, eculizumab and IVIG are excreted in human breast milk [18]. See Table 1 for further information.

Other General Considerations in Women with Myasthenia Gravis

Bone density should be routinely addressed in women with MG. Corticosteroids (CS) have been shown to increase the risk of osteoporosis in MG patients [43]. Additionally, MG patients may be at increased risk of bone fracture, though data from two large cohort studies are conflicting on this point [44, 45]. As with all individuals treated with CS, MG patients on CS should undergo screening for osteoporosis and be offered prophylactic intervention to improve bone health when indicated [46].

Body image and cosmetic concerns should also be considered in women with MG, although there is no literature explicitly addressing this issue. The effect of MG on facial appearance, alterations in body habitus and hair patterns from CS use, scarring from thymectomy and the cosmetic effect of ports or long term IV lines may all influence quality of life for individual patients.

References

1. Amato AA, Russell JA. Neuromuscular disorders. 2nd ed. New York: McGraw-Hill Medical; 2016.
2. Sanders DB, Wolfe GI, Benatar M, Evoli A, Gilhus NE, Illa I, et al. International consensus guidance for management of myasthenia gravis: executive summary. Neurology. 2016;87(4):419–25.
3. Cutolo M, Capellino S, Straub RH. Oestrogens in rheumatic diseases: friend or foe? Rheumatology (Oxford). 2008;47(Suppl 3):iii2–5.
4. Mays J, Butts CL. Intercommunication between the neuroendocrine and immune systems: focus on myasthenia gravis. Neuroimmunomodulation. 2011;18(5):320–7.
5. Leker RR, Karni A, Abramsky O. Exacerbation of myasthenia gravis during the menstrual period. J Neurol Sci. 1998;156(1):107–11.
6. Frenkel M. Treatment of myasthenia gravis by ovulatory suppression. Arch Neurol. 1964;11:613–7.
7. Stickler DE, Stickler LL. Single-fiber electromyography during menstrual exacerbation and ovulatory suppression in MuSK antibody-positive myasthenia gravis. Muscle Nerve. 2007;35(6):808–11.

8. Djelmis J, Sostarko M, Mayer D, Ivanisevic M. Myasthenia gravis in pregnancy: report on 69 cases. Eur J Obstet Gynecol Reprod Biol. 2002;104(1):21–5.

9. Delpy L, Douin-Echinard V, Garidou L, Bruand C, Saoudi A, Guery JC. Estrogen enhances susceptibility to experimental autoimmune myasthenia gravis by promoting type 1-polarized immune responses. J Immunol. 2005;175(8):5050–7.

10. Wu KH, Tobias ML, Kelley DB. Estrogen and laryngeal synaptic strength in *Xenopus laevis*: opposite effects of acute and chronic exposure. Neuroendocrinology. 2001;74(1):22–32.

11. Boldingh MI, Maniaol AH, Brunborg C, Weedon-Fekjaer H, Verschuuren JJ, Tallaksen CM. Increased risk for clinical onset of myasthenia gravis during the postpartum period. Neurology. 2016;87(20):2139–45.

12. Massey JM, De Jesus-Acosta C. Pregnancy and myasthenia gravis. Continuum (Minneap Minn). 2014;20(1):115–27.

13. Batocchi AP, Majolini L, Evoli A, Lino MM, Minisci C, Tonali P. Course and treatment of myasthenia gravis during pregnancy. Neurology. 1999;52(3):447–52.

14. Braga AC, Pinto C, Santos E, Braga J. Myasthenia gravis in pregnancy: experience of a portuguese center. Muscle Nerve. 2016;54(4):715–20.

15. Ducci RD, Lorenzoni PJ, Kay CS, Werneck LC, Scola RH. Clinical follow-up of pregnancy in myasthenia gravis patients. Neuromuscul Disord. 2017;27(4):352–7.

16. Norwood F, Dhanjal M, Hill M, James N, Jungbluth H, Kyle P, et al. Myasthenia in pregnancy: best practice guidelines from a U.K. multispecialty working group. J Neurol Neurosurg Psychiatry. 2014;85(5):538–43.

17. Ohlraun S, Hoffmann S, Klehmet J, Kohler S, Grittner U, Schneider A, et al. Impact of myasthenia gravis on family planning: how do women with myasthenia gravis decide and why? Muscle Nerve. 2015;52(3):371–9.

18. US Food and Drug Administration pregnancy categories, drug safety and availability. www.accessdata.fda.gov/scripts/cder/daf/. Accessed 15 Nov 2017.

19. Park-Wyllie L, Mazzotta P, Pastuszak A, Moretti ME, Beique L, Hunnisett L, et al. Birth defects after maternal exposure to corticosteroids: prospective cohort study and meta-analysis of epidemiological studies. Teratology. 2000;62(6):385–92.

20. Carmichael SL, Shaw GM, Ma C, Werler MM, Rasmussen SA, Lammer EJ, et al. Maternal corticosteroid use and orofacial clefts. Am J Obstet Gynecol. 2007;197(6):585 e1–7. discussion 683–4, e1–7

21. Hviid A, Molgaard-Nielsen D. Corticosteroid use during pregnancy and risk of orofacial clefts. CMAJ. 2011;183(7):796–804.

22. Skuladottir H, Wilcox AJ, Ma C, Lammer EJ, Rasmussen SA, Werler MM, et al. Corticosteroid use and risk of orofacial clefts. Birth Defects Res A Clin Mol Teratol. 2014;100(6):499–506.

23. Guidon AC, Massey EW. Neuromuscular disorders in pregnancy. Neurol Clin. 2012;30(3):889–911.

24. Clark AL. Clinical uses of intravenous immunoglobulin in pregnancy. Clin Obstet Gynecol. 1999;42(2):368–80.

25. Ciafaloni E, Massey JM. Myasthenia gravis and pregnancy. Neurol Clin. 2004;22(4):771–82.

26. Hehir MK, Hobson-Webb LD, Benatar M, Barnett C, Silvestri NJ, Howard JF Jr, et al. Rituximab as treatment for anti-MuSK myasthenia gravis: multicenter blinded prospective review. Neurology. 2017;89(10):1069–77.

27. Stieglbauer K, Pichler R, Topakian R. 10-year-outcomes after rituximab for myasthenia gravis: efficacy, safety, costs of inhospital care, and impact on childbearing potential. J Neurol Sci. 2017;375:241–4.

28. Wolfe GI, Kaminski HJ, Aban IB, Minisman G, Kuo HC, Marx A, et al. Randomized trial of thymectomy in myasthenia gravis. N Engl J Med. 2016;375(6):511–22.

29. Duley L. The global impact of pre-eclampsia and eclampsia. Semin Perinatol. 2009;33(3):130–7.

30. Lake AJ, Al Khabbaz A, Keeney R. Severe preeclampsia in the setting of myasthenia gravis. Case Rep Obstet Gynecol. 2017;2017:9204930.

31. Ozcan J, Balson IF, Dennis AT. New diagnosis myasthenia gravis and preeclampsia in late pregnancy. BMJ Case Rep. 2015;1–4.

32. Haider B, von Oertzen J. Neurological disorders. Best Pract Res Clin Obstet Gynaecol. 2013;27(6):867–75.

33. Hoff JM, Daltveit AK, Gilhus NE. Myasthenia gravis in pregnancy and birth: identifying risk factors, optimising care. Eur J Neurol. 2007;14(1):38–43.

34. Ahlsten G, Lefvert AK, Osterman PO, Stalberg E, Safwenberg J. Follow-up study of muscle function in children of mothers with myasthenia gravis during pregnancy. J Child Neurol. 1992;7(3):264–9.

35. O'Carroll P, Bertorini TE, Jacob G, Mitchell CW, Graff J. Transient neonatal myasthenia gravis in a baby born to a mother with new-onset anti-MuSK-mediated myasthenia gravis. J Clin Neuromuscul Dis. 2009;11(2):69–71.

36. Niks EH, Verrips A, Semmekrot BA, Prick MJ, Vincent A, van Tol MJ, et al. A transient neonatal myasthenic syndrome with anti-musk antibodies. Neurology. 2008;70(14):1215–6.

37. Lee JY, Min JH, Han SH, Han J. Transient neonatal myasthenia gravis due to a mother with ocular onset of anti-muscle specific kinase myasthenia gravis. Neuromuscul Disord. 2017;27(7):655–7.

38. Townsel C, Keller R, Johnson K, Hussain N, Campbell WA. Seronegative maternal ocular myasthenia gravis and delayed transient neonatal myasthenia gravis. AJP Rep. 2016;6(1):e133–6.

39. D'Amico A, Bertini E, Bianco F, Papacci P, Jacobson L, Vincent A, et al. Fetal acetylcholine receptor inactivation syndrome and maternal myasthenia gravis: a case report. Neuromuscul Disord. 2012;22(6):546–8.

40. Hacohen Y, Jacobson LW, Byrne S, Norwood F, Lall A, Robb S, et al. Fetal acetylcholine receptor inactivation syndrome: a myopathy due to maternal antibodies. Neurol Neuroimmunol Neuroinflamm. 2015;2(1):e57.

41. Ressel G. AAP updates statement for transfer of drugs and other chemicals into breast milk. American Academy of Pediatrics. Am Fam Physician. 2002;65(5):979–80.

42. American Academy of Pediatrics Committee on D. Transfer of drugs and other chemicals into human milk. Pediatrics. 2001;108(3):776–89.

43. Wakata N, Nemoto H, Sugimoto H, Nomoto N, Konno S, Hayashi N, et al. Bone density in myasthenia gravis patients receiving long-term prednisolone therapy. Clin Neurol Neurosurg. 2004;106(2):139–41.

44. Pouwels S, de Boer A, Javaid MK, Hilton-Jones D, Verschuuren J, Cooper C, et al. Fracture rate in patients with myasthenia gravis: the general practice research database. Osteoporos Int. 2013;24(2):467–76.

45. Yeh JH, Chen HJ, Chen YK, Chiu HC, Kao CH. Increased risk of osteoporosis in patients with myasthenia gravis: a population-based cohort study. Neurology. 2014;83(12):1075–9.

46. Grossman JM, Gordon R, Ranganath VK, Deal C, Caplan L, Chen W, et al. American College of Rheumatology 2010 recommendations for the prevention and treatment of glucocorticoid-induced osteoporosis. Arthritis Care Res. 2010;62(11):1515–26.

Ethical Decisions in Pregnancy

Thomas I. Cochrane

The Pregnant Woman with Brain Injury

A 35-year-old woman presented to our emergency room with severe headache and right hemiparesis in the 17th week of pregnancy. A cerebral arteriovenous malformation (AVM) had ruptured, causing a left frontal hemorrhage, subarachnoid hemorrhage (SAH) and intraventricular hemorrhage (IVH). She was treated with hyperosmolar therapy but soon required hemicraniectomy, and the AVM was resected. Four weeks later she suffered recurrent hemorrhage, now with more extensive IVH. She underwent surgical evacuation of the parenchymal hemorrhage, clipping of perinidal aneurysms, and placement of bilateral external ventricular drains. Two weeks later, she remained comatose, with intracerebral pressure (ICP) remaining elevated at 30 cm H2O or higher. She retained some brainstem reflexes, including a corneal response, a gag reflex, and some spontaneous respiratory drive. She was not expected to ever recover consciousness, and was most likely to remain in a vegetative state permanently. Her neurologists predicted that even if she did regain some awareness, she would remain cognitively devastated, incapable of meaningful communication or self-care—likely in the Minimally Conscious State (MCS) at best.

At 24 3/7 weeks, ultrasound showed the fetus' weight was in the 15–20th percentile, and fetal scalp edema suggested generalized fetal edema (hydrops fetalis). Neonatologists and maternal-fetal medicine specialists estimated odds of survival for the fetus were 20–40%. If the fetus survived, the odds of survival without severe neurodevelopmental impairment were estimated at 10%. Risks of continuing the pregnancy included preterm delivery, intrauterine growth retardation, pre-eclampsia, placental abruption, and intrauterine fetal demise. They also expressed concern that statistics regarding hydrops fetalis could overestimate the odds of a good outcome, because the hypernatremia and hyperosmolality being used to control the mother's intracranial pressure would increase the risk of fetal venous sinus thrombosis, cerebral hemorrhage, and cerebral infarction.

This case involves decisions on behalf of a newly incapacitated pregnant woman, and decisions on behalf of a never-previously-capable mid-term fetus. The standards for decision-making in each situation differ but are well agreed-upon, and not too difficult to describe. Naturally, however, when the two types of cases become combined, as in this case, the complexity increases. It will be worth reviewing the standards for decision-making in each type of case separately, because when discussing and contemplating cases like this, it is important to try and remain clear about which concepts and principles are being invoked or relied upon.

Decision-Making for the Incapacitated, Previously-Competent Patient

If a (non-pregnant) competent adult woman suffers an incapacitating brain injury, then the standards for making decisions on her behalf would generally be invoked as follows. The list is ordered by ethical priority, with the first generally having the highest priority and the last having the least [1].

1. *Previously-expressed wishes/advance directives*
2. *Substituted judgement*, whereby someone familiar with the patient tries to make the decision they think the patient would have made
3. *Best-interests standard*, whereby efforts are made to assess what would be best for the patient, in the face of a lack of information about what this specific patient would want

First and foremost, we turn to the patient's own directly-expressed thoughts and wishes, in the form of advance directives or previous expressions regarding the situation at hand. These can be more formal (e.g. living wills) or less formal

T. I. Cochrane (✉)
Brigham and Women's Hospital, Center for Bioethics, Harvard Medical School, Boston, MA, USA
e-mail: tcochrane@bwh.harvard.edu

© Springer Nature Switzerland AG 2019
M. A. O'Neal (ed.), *Neurology and Psychiatry of Women*, https://doi.org/10.1007/978-3-030-04245-5_21

(e.g. discussions with family members or friends). The more formally-expressed the wish, generally speaking, the more reliable the expression should be considered [1]. Recent expressions tend to carry more weight than more remote expressions. And obviously, the closer the fit between the previous expression and the current circumstances, the more reliable the expression should be considered. For example, if a family remembers a conversation in which the patient said: "I'd never want to be kept alive on machines" in the context of watching a television show about an elderly patient with untreatable cancer, this would not be considered a reliable indicator of the patient's wishes if she was otherwise healthy but then suffered encephalitis associated with a reasonably good prognosis.

When helpful or decisive advance directives are unavailable, the next best standard is the substituted judgement standard. Someone who knows the patient well enough can use their knowledge of the patient's values and preferences, to try and make the decision that the patient would have made—if only they had been able. The degree to which one can exercise substituted judgement depends on the extent of one's personal knowledge of the patient and her preferences. Therefore, there is an order of priority among surrogates who could potentially exercise substituted judgement, whereby greater deference is given to those surrogates with greater knowledge of the patient. In some states, the order of priority is written into statute. In other states, the order of priority is less formal, but is often to be found by consulting precedent and case law. For our purposes, it is enough to begin by describing the typical ethical priority that is followed [1, 2]:

1. Someone who the patient has designated as their surrogate. This is often done legally by granting someone *durable power of attorney for healthcare* or appointing someone the *health care proxy agent*.
2. The patient's spouse.
3. The patient's adult children.
4. The patient's other immediate family (parents, siblings).
5. The patient's extended family.
6. The patient's friends and acquaintances.

Note that this is a default list and a starting point. It is not a definitive guide to identifying a surrogate in a particular case. In many cases, the default ordering cannot be followed for practical reasons (e.g. difficulty communicating with someone higher on the list), and in others it should not be followed. For example, one might have good reason to believe that the surrogate with priority lacks capacity himself, or might have ulterior motives that compromise his ability to exercise substituted judgement on the patient's behalf. Sometimes, a surrogate who would ordinarily have priority by default might delegate his responsibility to another surrogate, because he finds himself psychologically incapable of exercising substituted judgement, or has a reason to believe that another would do a better job. As an example, in our institution it is not uncommon for family members to defer to a close friend of the patient, because they believed he or she had a much clearer sense of the patient's values and preferences.

Although it is usually possible to find at least some information to use in exercising substituted judgement, some patients have no advance directives or previously known wishes, and no surrogate who can exercise substituted judgement on their behalf. In these cases, caregivers must use the best interests standard, whereby they try to assess what type of care would be best for their patient—all things considered—and provide that care.

When it comes to very important and irreversible decisions, such as a decision about whether to withhold or withdraw life-sustaining therapy (LST), the best interests standard is fraught with some ethical and legal difficulties. *All things considered* is meant to highlight the fact that the best interests standard cannot be applied by simply assessing the "medical" facts of a case—the patient's entire life circumstances must be considered. This is one reason why medical professionals should generally avoid making this type of decision unilaterally, and should seek broad counsel and consensus about the best interests of a patient with no advance directives or surrogates. In many institutions, ethics consultation is required when withholding or withdrawing LST in these circumstances. In our institution, ethics consultants will facilitate efforts to find anyone who knew the patient (e.g. outpatient providers, prior coworkers, staff at a nursing home or homeless shelter, etc.). Even if these individuals do not know the patient well enough to exercise substituted judgement, the information they provide about the patient's life circumstances, personality, and interactions with healthcare can provide a much-needed context for decision making. Medical providers should exercise humility and recognize that their expertise does not necessarily extend to evaluation of the entire context of a patient's life. They should seek help from social workers, community patient advocates, spiritual consultants, or others, as appropriate to the individual patient.

Decision-Making on Behalf of a Fetus

Perhaps obviously, one cannot rely on previously expressed wishes when it comes to making decisions for a fetus. Almost as obviously, one cannot exercise substituted judgement on behalf of a fetus, since there can be no knowledge of the patient's values or preferences. One is therefore compelled to resort to the best interests standard when it comes to this type of patient—the never-previously-competent patient. The question can usually be formulated as: "what, all things considered, is in the best interests of this fetus?" Although this question sounds simple enough in theory, it leads to other questions: Do fetuses have interests? If so, of what type and at what gestational age? If fetuses do have interests, who is best situated to evaluate and represent those interests? How should disagreement or disputes about the best interests of a fetus be resolved? These are difficult questions, and they don't even address the public or political implications of the answers (for example, if fetuses do have interests, and if those interests arise at an early gestational age, then this could have implications for other sorts of decision-making about fetuses, like elective abortion or fetal surgery). These further implications are beyond the scope of this chapter, so after briefly addressing the main questions just raised, we will focus on practical advice and general principles regarding this type of decision-making.

Do Fetuses Have Interests and If so, at What Gestational Age?

This question is obviously a philosophical and ethical question, and cannot be answered on strictly medical grounds. But we can start with some basics, by acknowledging some uncontroversial facts that bear on these questions. First: it should be uncontroversial that a healthy fetus at full term has the same *interests* as a newborn baby. If one accepts this, then we've established that at the far end of the gestational continuum, a fetus' interests must be considered to the same extent to which a newborn baby's interests are considered—which is to say, a very great deal [3].

Second, let's look at the other end of the gestational continuum—the very beginning. This end is more controversial, but let us for now simply acknowledge that most observers would say that a just-fertilized egg does not have interests in anything like the same sense that a full-term healthy fetus, or a newborn, does. That is, most observers would not say that a just-fertilized egg has interests that must be given considerable weight when it comes to decisions that could affect its future.

If one accepts this framework, then in theory one must agree that interests are something that develop over the course of normal gestation, from little-to-no-interests at conception, to same-interests-as-a-newborn at full term. This is why rules that restrict abortion are associated with a gestational age cutoff. It is simply obvious to most that the full term healthy fetus cannot be aborted without violating the same norms that would be violated in killing a healthy newborn, but it is also obvious to most that destroying a just-fertilized egg would not violate those norms. This means that

there must be some sort of continuum of interests that develop over the course of gestation.[1]

If it is true that fetal interests develop along a continuum, then we must admit that any lines we wish to draw (e.g. "after week X of pregnancy, it is not morally permissible to deliberately harm a healthy fetus") are semi-arbitrary. This raises a difficulty for analyzing individual cases. For example, the case description above begins with a fetus of 17 weeks, and ends with a fetus of 24 3/7 weeks. What interests does a fetus have during these weeks of the second trimester? How much have they changed between those time points? Do those interests have anything to do with the limits of fetal viability, which range somewhere between 22 and 24 weeks in most institutions? These are difficult questions, and cannot be answered satisfyingly in the abstract. For the moment, suffice it to say that most observers, caregivers, and parents would agree that the closer to term a fetus is, the greater its interest in survival. In a moment we will return to the case, and describe how the analysis played out, to see how the above principles were applied.

But before we return to the case, let us try to answer the third question raised above: *who is best situated to evaluate and represent the interests of a fetus?* This is another question that is simple on the surface, but complex in practice. In general, it is easiest to start by recognizing that prospective parents deserve a great deal of deference and respect when it comes to making decisions for fetuses. This is primarily because parents are assumed to have the best interests of their fetuses or their children in mind, and are usually the most emotionally committed to the flourishing of the developing fetus. However, parental discretion is not unlimited, and others can lay some claim to representing the best interests of the fetus as well [4–6]. For example, imagine that our case had involved a woman whose severe brain injury occurred at 34 5/7 weeks, and that the fetus appeared unharmed. In such a case, if the patient's family requested withdrawal of the mother's LST (and refused to allow delivery of the fetus), then caregivers would have strong ethical reasons to question, and likely resist, the request. At a minimum, caregivers would be ethically obliged to try and persuade the family to allow them to deliver the fetus before stopping the mother's LST. If the family could not be persuaded, the caregivers' obligations would very likely extend further, possibly even to the point of seeking a court decision regarding whether the fetus must be delivered before life

---

[1] People from some religious traditions *do* in fact claim that a just-fertilized egg has the same interests as a newborn baby, and that destroying a just-fertilized egg would violate the same norms that are violated if one were to kill a healthy newborn. Holding such a viewpoint would dramatically alter the ethical analysis involving life-sustaining therapies for pregnant women. Analysis of cases from this viewpoint, and analysis of the full ethical implications of such a viewpoint, are beyond the scope of this chapter.

support is discontinued. The general point is that while parents and families deserve the greatest say when analyzing best interests of a fetus, they do not have unlimited ethical (or legal) authority. The closer the fetus is to full term, and the better the medical and neurological prognosis of the fetus, the greater the weight that must be given to its interests.

Now that we have reviewed the principles of decision-making for brain-injured adults and for fetuses, we can return to the specific case. The ethics consultants, facing a complex web of interrelated questions, began by analyzing some simpler hypothetical questions. First: would this mother want us to continue her LST if she had suffered this same brain injury but were not pregnant? And then second: what if the mother were healthy, but the fetus were in the same condition as in the case (hydrops fetalis, with odds of survival and a good neurological outcome around 2–4%)? If we can answer the hypothetical question about the mother, it will help us understand whether there is a rationale for continuing LST independent from the effect of LST on the fetus, and the second question helps us analyze the case from the perspective of the fetus' best interests, separate from the mother's interests.

Analysis of the first question was straightforward. The patient did not have any advance directives, but she had appointed her husband her Massachusetts Health Care Proxy Agent. This made it easy to determine that the person best placed to exercise substituted judgement on her behalf was her husband. Happily, her parents were also involved, and fully supportive of her husband's role as surrogate. Furthermore, they were unanimous in their assessment that, given her extremely grim neurological prognosis, the patient would not want LST continued if she were not pregnant. They were able to describe their position in terms of the patient's values, reassuring the clinicians and ethics consultants that they were exercising substituted judgement on her behalf, rather than representing their own personal perspectives or wishes. Having this question answered in such clear and convincing fashion allowed the stakeholders to turn to the second question, about the best interests of the fetus.

Analysis of the second question was harder than the first. This was partly because the family was being asked to use the best interests standard rather than the substituted judgement standard. When exercising substituted judgement, it is sometimes easier to be confident that one is truly pursuing the right course, because it seems clear what the patient would want. But in best interests analyses, there is always a bit of extra uncertainty: "we *think* this is in the patient's best interests, but how can anyone know whether the patient would agree?" Furthermore, in the case of the fetus, there remained some residual hope of an acceptably good outcome, although the odds of achieving it were low (on the order of 2–4%). It is not obvious how to weigh probabilities

like this when performing a best interests analysis, so our institution has adopted a practice of careful deliberation among all the stakeholders when contemplating end-of-life decisions, using the best interests standard, in the face of prognostic uncertainty. In practice, this involves meetings facilitated by the Ethics Consultation Service—meetings which include surrogates and family members, medical providers (especially doctors and nurses, but sometimes including physical or occupational therapists), and sometimes representatives of Chaplaincy, Social Work, the Palliative Care Service, or others. In this case, the father, the parents of the mother, the attending physician and primary nurse, two ethics consultants, and the consulting neurologists (one adult, one pediatric) were involved in the ethics consultation discussion.

The question faced in this case, simply put, was whether the fetus in this case had a good enough prognosis that continued life was in its best interests. This question occasionally strikes some as strange when discussing fetuses or even neonates—how could it be that life is *not* in its best interests? The answer is that some lives are characterized by such poor quality that continued life would be worse than death. Most observers can probably agree that a life characterized by severe suffering, no meaningful human interactions, *and* no hope of improvement could be worse than simply dying. So the task faced by the stakeholders was to decide whether this fetus' prospects for a meaningful life were so poor, or whether its odds of severe suffering were so high, that it would have little or no interest in continued life.

After carefully reviewing the medical facts regarding the fetus, and after a long discussion of the possible neurological outcomes and the quality of life (or lack thereof) expected for a child with this fetus' expected neurological and cognitive disabilities, the father of the fetus and the mother's parents were convinced that the best course of action from the fetus' perspective was to be allowed to die when life support was withdrawn from the mother.

There was at least some discomfort with this idea among members of the medical staff, who observed that a 2–4% probability of an acceptably good neurological outcome could not be considered extremely remote. If one re-describes 4% as "a 1 in 25 chance", it is easy to appreciate the plausibility of this observation. And because there is no "objective" standard for evaluating best interests, or for deciding how unlikely an acceptable outcome must be before it is defensible to forego life support, the ethics consultants thought it was important to assess the degree of discomfort among all the team members, and reach consensus if possible.

The team members who had expressed discomfort were asked to describe their feelings in more detail. Some questions that were helpful included: Do you feel that withdrawal of life support from the mother (and by extension, the fetus) would be morally *impermissible*? How strongly do you feel about it—strongly enough to seek an administrative or legal remedy such as going to court? In this case, the team members with concerns did not feel very strongly about the matter, and eventually indicated that they thought withdrawal of LST would be *permissible*, even if they might not have made the same decision, had they been the surrogates. As a way of expressing their ambivalence, they indicated that they would definitely have supported the family if they had decided to pursue continued life support. In other words, they thought that a wide range of possible actions would have been morally and ethically defensible—but for the most part, they simply wanted to make sure that the appropriate level of deliberation had gone into the irreversible decision to withdraw LST.

In this case, consensus had been reached—the mother would have wanted her LST discontinued, and most agreed that the fetus' interests were best served by allowing it to die when the LST was stopped. The few stakeholders with misgivings did not feel strongly, and did endorse the plan to withdraw LST in the end.

Conclusion

Decisions regarding life support for a pregnant woman who has lost the ability to make choices for herself and her fetus are complex, because they involve making decisions on behalf of a previously-competent adult and on behalf of a never-competent fetus, whose medical fates are intertwined. The decision-making standards for previously-competent adults differ from decision-making standards for the never-competent fetus, which can lead to some confusion. For this reason, ethics consultation should be strongly considered whenever end-of-life decisions involve pregnant women. Clarity can sometimes be aided by considering the mother's perspective and the fetus' interests separately.

Decision-making for an incapacitated pregnant woman involves the same principles that are used for other previously-capable adults. Advance directives and directly expressed wishes of the patient are given the highest priority. When such directives or expressions are unavailable or inadequate, surrogates who know the patient can try to exercise substituted judgement, whereby they try to make the decision

that they think the patient would have made. When surrogates are unavailable, unable, or unwilling to exercise substituted judgement, stakeholders must resort to a best-interests analysis whereby an attempt is made to evaluate what is in the patient's best interests, all things considered. The patient's best interests should be evaluated from the widest possible perspective, and deliberations should involve as many care providers and disciplines as can be arranged.

When making decisions for the fetus, who has never previously had decision-making capacity, one must always resort to a best-interests analysis, because there are no advance directives and no previously-known values or preferences that could be used in substituted judgement. In the case of fetuses and children, parents and family are generally given a great deal of leeway and authority to determine what constitutes the best interests of the child, and their judgement should generally be respected unless it obviously runs counter to the interests of the child.

Because decision-making for others is always fraught with uncertainty, and because "objective" standards for making choices about LST in these situations simply do not exist, providers and institutions are best served by adopting a model that involves consultation, careful deliberation involving multiple perspectives, and a strong desire to seek consensus among all the stakeholders—patients, families and surrogates, and medical professionals.

References

1. Beauchamp TL, Childress JF. A framework of standards for surrogate decision making. In: Pierce J, Randels G, editors. Contemporary bioethics. New York: Oxford University Press; 2012.
2. Beauchamp TL, Childress JF. Principles of biomedical ethics. 7th ed. New York: Oxford University Press; 2012.
3. Ringer S. Neonatal Intensive Care Unit (NICU) ethics. In: Toy E, Raine SP, Cochrane T, editors. Case files: medical ethics and professionalism. New York: McGraw Hill; 2015. p. 267–277.
4. Hagen EM, Therkelsen OB, Forde R, Aasland O, Janvier A, Hansen TW. Challenges in reconciling best interest and parental exercise of autonomy in pediatric life-or-death situations. J Pediatr. 2012;161:146–51.
5. Harrison H. The offer they can't refuse: parents and perinatal treatment decisions. Semin Fetal Neonatal Med. 2008;13:329–34.
6. McHaffie HE, Laing IA, Parker M, McMillan J. Deciding for imperiled newborns: medical authority or parental autonomy? J Med Ethics. 2001;27:104–9.

Part III

Women's Health and Aging

Menopausal Hot Flashes, Sleep and Mood Disturbances

Geena Athappilly and Margo Nathan

Defining Menopause

Varying and inconsistent characterizations of menopause have led to historic difficulties in formulating a uniform, standard definition of menopause [1]. In more recent years, many clinicians and researchers alike are using the Stages of Reproductive Aging Workshop (STRAW) Criteria as well as recent revisions; namely, the revised STRAW +10 Staging System to define and designate the various stages of menopause [2]. According to the STRAW +10 Staging System, menstrual cycle characteristics constitute the principal criteria and hormonal markers (FSH (follicle-stimulating hormone) AMH (antimullerian (has umlaut) hormone), AFC (antral follicle count) and inhibin-B) the supportive criteria in designating the various phases and stages of menopause [2]. The phases of the menstrual cycle have been roughly divided into reproductive, menopausal transition, and postmenopause. Although the STRAW +10 Staging System addresses many populations, the criteria may have limited applicability in certain populations including those with premature ovarian failure [3], HIV/AIDS [4, 5], women who have undergone cancer treatment [6], or a hysterectomy [7].

Reproductive: The reproductive stage is divided into an early, peak and late stage. For the majority of the reproductive stage, menstrual cycles are regular and hormonal markers are normal [8]. However, the late reproductive stage heralds changes in hormonal markers namely, low AMH and AFC [2]. As the late reproductive stage progresses, subtle changes in menstrual cycle length begin accompanied by low levels of AMH, inhibin-B, and AFC. FSH levels during the early follicular phase are also typically higher and more variable [2, 9, 10].

Menopausal Transition: The menopausal transition is divided into an early and late stage. The average duration of the menopausal transition is believed to be approximately 4 years with an average age of onset of 47.5 years [11]. Early menopausal transition is marked by variability in menstrual cycle length by greater than 7 days over ten consecutive cycles. The late menopausal transition is marked by an even greater variability in hormonal fluctuations as well as menstrual cycle length including the occurrence of at least 60 but less than 360 consecutive days without a menses. FSH levels during this phase, albeit with great fluctuation, often rise above 25 IU/L [12]. Menopausal transition is to be differentiated from perimenopause. Perimenopause is defined as the period of time that extends from the onset of menopausal transition to 1 year after the final cessation of menses [2, 8].

Postmenopause: Postmenopause is divided into an early and late postmenopause. The inception of early postmenopause is marked by final menstrual period. The first 2 years of early postmenopause is marked by a steady elevation in FSH levels and steady decline in estradiol level [13]. In the ensuing 3–6 years of early postmenopause, elevated FSH and decreased estradiol levels start to equilibrate [2]. During late postmenopause, the menstrual and endocrinological realms are marked by less change although some studies suggest a further decline in FSH in later stages of aging [14].

This chapter will describe the epidemiology, risk factors, identification, and treatment of symptoms many women experience during the menopausal transition, including affective symptoms such as depression and psychological distress, as well as hot flashes and sleep disturbance.

G. Athappilly (✉)
Harvard Medical School, Boston, MA, USA

Edith Nourse Rogers Memorial Veterans Hospital, Bedford, MA, USA

Site Director for Boston University Family Medicine Residency at Edith Nourse Rogers Memorial Veteran Affairs Hospital, Boston, MA, USA
e-mail: Geena.Athappilly@va.gov

M. Nathan
Division of Women's Mental Health and Department of Psychiatry, Harvard Medical School, Brigham and Women's Hospital, Boston, MA, USA
e-mail: mdnathan@bwh.harvard.edu

© Springer Nature Switzerland AG 2019
M. A. O'Neal (ed.), *Neurology and Psychiatry of Women*, https://doi.org/10.1007/978-3-030-04245-5_22

Depression During Menopause

Historically, lack of uniformity in defining depression and menopause as well as variations in choice of assessment scales have led to some difficulty in characterizing and managing depression during the menopause [1, 15]. However, with the advent of the STRAW criteria and STRAW +10 Staging System for staging menopause as well as efforts to characterize the various severities/subgroups of depression; there has been greater precision in determining epidemiology, risk factors, clinical presentation, diagnosis, and treatment of depression and other psychiatric symptoms during the menopause [1, 16]. These subgroups of depression are defined below:

Major Depression: when five or more symptoms such as depressed mood, loss of appetite, worthlessness, hypersomnia or insomnia, loss of interest, among others are present for at least a 2-week period [17].

Depressive Symptoms (subsyndromal depression): Subsyndromal Depression is defined as exhibiting one to four symptoms of major depression with concurrent functional impairment or distress [18].

Psychological Distress: this term was coined to describe the presence of feelings of tension/nervousness, feelings of depression or blues, and feelings of irritability/grouchiness for a period of 2 weeks and was described in extrapolations of The Study of Women's Health across the Nation (SWAN) [19].

Epidemiology

Major Depression: Epidemiological studies have not demonstrated an increased prevalence of depression during the menopause [20]. However, with some convergence, cross-sectional and longitudinal studies have demonstrated an increased prevalence of major depression during the menopausal transition [21] or both during menopausal transition and early postmenopause [22]. Women who experience major depression during the menopausal transition often have suffered from previous episodes of major depression [23]. Although new onset major depression during menopausal transition is thought to be less common [23], some studies have demonstrated an increased prevalence of first episode major depression during menopausal transition [18, 24].

Depressive Symptoms: Several cross-sectional studies, adjusted for confounding variables, as well as longitudinal studies have demonstrated an increased risk of depressive symptoms during the menopause as compared to premenopause [24–26]. Longitudinal studies have been able to further parse out prevalence of depression per stage of menopause with results demonstrating an increased risk of depressive symptoms during the early and late menopausal transition [25–28]. As with major depression, an increased risk of depressive symptoms during the menopausal transition has been correlated with previous depressive symptoms [29]. However, more than one longitudinal study has demonstrated an increased risk of depressive symptoms independent of previous history [24, 27, 30].

Psychological Distress: Psychological distress was found to be more common during the early (28.9%) and late menopause (25.6%) as compared to premenopause (20.9%) and postmenopause (22%) [19].

Risk Factors

- Demographic Factors

Major Depression: More studies are needed to parse out demographic risk factors for major depression during the menopause. However, more than one longitudinal study has demonstrated decreased age at menopause [23, 31] as well as African American race as risk factors for major depression during the menopause [30, 31].

Depressive Symptoms: Studies have correlated financial difficulties [28, 32] and unemployment [30, 32] with depressive symptoms during the menopause. Younger age has also been demonstrated by several studies to be associated with depressive symptoms during the menopause [25, 26, 31]. Ethnic risk factors for depressive symptoms during the menopause have been suggested; however, the results are inconsistent [25, 30].

Psychological Distress: Financial limitations have been associated with increased risk of psychological distress during the menopause. Moreover, minority races including African American, Hispanic, Chinese, and Japanese were noted to have a decreased odds ratio for psychological distress in the menopause as compared to Caucasians [19].

- *Psychiatric Factors*

Major Depression: Major depression during the menopause has also been associated with a prior history of depressive symptoms [23, 33, 34] and premenstrual symptoms [33]. Prior history of an anxiety disorder has also been demonstrated as a risk factor for major depression [23, 34].

Depressive Symptoms: Prior history of depressive episodes or major depression is one of the most studied risk factors for depressive symptoms during the menopause [30, 32, 33, 35]. Family history of depression also has a demonstrated interrelationship with depressive symptoms during the menopause [26]. Moreover, studies have shown, with increased convergence, an association of premenstrual symptoms with depressive symptoms during menopause [29, 30, 33, 36, 37].

- *Psychological Factors*

Major Depression: Anxious personality temperaments [23, 34] as well as self-consciousness [23] have also been correlated with major depression during menopause.

Depressive Symptoms: Negative perceptions of aging have been correlated with depressive symptoms during the menopause in more than one study [28, 36].

Psychological Distress: Negative perceptions of health have also been associated with increased odds ratio of psychological distress during the menopause [19].

- *Psychosocial Factors*

Major Depression: Distressing life events have been correlated with major depression during the menopause [16, 31].

Depressive Symptoms: Distressing life events including losses have also been associated with depressive symptoms during the menopause [26, 28, 32].

Psychological Distress: Limited social support has also been associated with increased odds ratio of psychological distress during the menopause [19].

- *Medical Factors*

Major Depression: A lifetime medical condition [23], vasomotor symptoms and sleep disturbances have been linked to major depression during the menopause [30].

Depressive Symptoms: Vasomotor Symptoms as well as sleep disturbances have been linked with depressive symptoms during the menopause [38].

Psychological Distress: Vasomotor symptoms, sleep impairment and health concerns have also been associated with psychological distress during this stage [19].

- *Lifestyle Factors*

Major Depression: Smoking and increased BMI have been demonstrated by at least one study to be risk factors for major depression during the menopause [31].

Depressive Symptoms: More than one study has connected smoking and increased BMI with depressive symptoms during the menopause [25, 26, 31].

Psychological Distress: Smoking has also been associated with an increased risk of psychological distress during the menopause [19].

Clinical Presentation

Although diagnostic criteria for the major mood disorders are similar both during menopause and otherwise, the clinical course is unique because of the presence of coinciding and complicating symptoms of menopause as well as psychological and daily life challenges specific to stage [39, 40].

- *Coinciding Symptoms*

Fatigue: Fatigue may be present during a major depressive episode as well as during the menopause. The dual effect may be additive or the symptom may be solely contributed by one phenomenon, though it may be difficult to disentangle the etiology [39, 41, 42].

Concentration: Cognitive complaints are not uncommon during the menopause. Longitudinal studies have supported this subjective complaint with findings of impaired learning during the menopausal transition, a measure that is believed to improve in the postmenopause [43]. In addition, depression during menopause may itself present with decreased concentration which can compound existing cognitive changes and ensuing distress [44, 45].

Difficulty Sleeping: Sleep disturbances are common during the menopause [46]. Difficulty sleeping is a common symptom of depression that may overlap with inherent sleep difficulties during the menopause [39].

Sexual Dysfunction: During the menopause and postmenopause, vaginal atrophy and associated pain during intercourse may affect sexual function and desire [47]. Moreover, decreased sex drive may be a common symptom of depression [48]. Therefore, the individual contributions may complicate and magnify sexual dysfunction during midlife [49].

Weight Gain: Increased appetite and ensuing weight gain may co-occur in a neurovegetative depression as well as in menopause [39, 41].

- *Complicating Symptoms and Challenges*

Hot Flashes: Several Studies have implicated vasomotor symptoms as a risk factor for depression, although causation has not been consistently demonstrated [38, 50, 51]. Despite this lack of clarity, the presence of vasomotor symptoms complicates the clinical picture of depression during midlife as outlined in further detail in subsequent sections.

Psychological and Daily Life Challenges: Previous theories suggested menopause leads to a depressive state of "involutional melancholia" [52] related to the departure of children from the home previously coined "empty nest" syndrome [53].These theories have since been refuted by empiric studies [54]. However, the menopause and menopausal transition are periods replete with psychosocial challenges. Women are often contending with a myriad of changes and demands both in the external world as well as in the internal body. Women often bear the burden of juggling care of elderly parents, children, household chores, work demands amidst possible mood changes, hot flashes, sleep disturbances, and medical comorbidities [39, 40].

Differential Diagnosis

When assessing mood symptoms during menopause, it is important to consider bipolar and unipolar depression (as well as subtypes of depression). The differential diagnosis includes psychological distress, adjustment disorder, bereavement, subsyndromal depression, major depressive disorder, and bipolar disorder [40]. Psychological distress is defined as a feeling of being nervous, dysphoric, or irritable for 2 weeks and demonstrated to be relatively common during menopause [19]. Adjustment disorder is distinct from psychological distress as it requires a distinct stressor that precipitates symptoms which can include caring for parents, sometimes amidst caring for children, facing new medical comorbidities, and juggling career demands [17]. Bereavement also follows a stressor that involves a loss, which is commonly encountered during this stage [17]. Subsyndromal Depression is defined as exhibiting one to four symptoms of major depression with concurrent functional impairment or distress [18]. This to be differentiated from Major depression in which five to six symptoms are necessary to meet the criteria for major depression with concurrent functional impairment [17]. Mood swings and irritability have been described during the menopause and may be independent symptom clusters or may be part of a Bipolar Disorder Diathesis [55].

Assessment Scales

An independent mood disorder assessment scale specific to menopause has not yet been designed. However, general validated measures including the PHQ-9, are often used to diagnose depression, anxiety and other mood disorders during menopause [56]. Whilst a menopause specific mood disorder scale is not available, validated menopause-specific quality of life and general symptom measure scales may be useful in disentangling symptoms common to menopause and depression [42]. The Menopause Rating Scale assesses various parameters during the menopause including but not exclusive to mood, libido, and vaginal dryness [57]. The Menopause-Specific Quality of Life Scale both assessed various parameters of menopause and qualifies their impact on quality of life [58]. It is important to note that neither the Menopause Rating Scale or the Menopause-Specific Quality of Life Scale is diagnostic for mood or anxiety disorders during the menopause [57, 58].

Treatment

- *Major Depression*

Nonpharmacological Interventions
CBT: Cognitive behavioral therapy (CBT) has been demonstrated to be effective in the treatment of depressive symptoms in the general population [59]. There is a paucity of studies exploring effects of CBT on depressive symptoms during the menopause; nonetheless, some do suggest efficacy of CBT for depressive symptoms during the menopause and menopausal transition [60].

IPT: Although there is a scarcity of studies exploring the effects of interpersonal therapy on depressive symptoms during the menopausal transition, interpersonal therapy (IPT) may be uniquely suited to addressing role transitions during the menopause and has a robust evidence base in the general population as a stand-alone therapy or in conjunction with antidepressants [61].

Pharmacological Interventions
Antidepressants: Randomized double blind controlled studies have demonstrated benefit of serotonin norepinephrine reuptake inhibitors (SNRI's) in the treatment of depressive symptoms during the menopausal transition [15, 62]. These results are supported by several open label studies demonstrating treatment benefit with both SNRI's as well as selective serotonin reuptake inhibitors (SSRI's) during the menopausal transition [63, 64]. Although some studies have found a less robust treatment response to antidepressants in the postmenopause as compared to the premenopause [65, 66]; these results have not been universally replicated [67]. In our review of the literature, a differential effect of one antidepressant over the other in the treatment of depressive symptoms during the menopausal transition has not yet been systematically established [68].

Hormone Therapy: Hormone Therapy (HT) is not FDA approved for the treatment of major depression [40, 69]. However, in a limited number of studies, estrogen therapy, as a sole agent as well as an adjunct to antidepressants, has been demonstrated to have positive effects on depressive symptoms during the perimenopause; however, not during the postmenopause [70–72]. A recent study has demonstrated efficacy of HT in prevention of depressive symptoms in perimenopausal and early postmenopausal women [73]. Risk benefit analysis surrounding Hormone Therapy will be addressed in subsequent subsections.

- *Subsyndromal Depression/Depressive Symptoms*

CBT and IPT may be effective in addressing subsyndromal depressive symptoms as well as major depression [60, 61].

- *Psychological Distress*

Although not systematically studied, psychological distress during the menopause may respond to more supportive measures including symptom reduction of the manifestation of menopause, mobilization of resources, supportive therapy, exercise, optimization of diet, and relaxation techniques [40].

- *Bereavement*

Individual and group therapy targeting grief and loss may be effective in managing bereavement, providing support and recognizing signs of complicated grief [74].

- *Adjustment Disorder*

Although there is a lack of studies specifically addressing IPT and CBT in adjustment disorder during the menopause, IPT may potentially address distress surrounding role transitions in the menopause as it does in other populations [75]. Likewise, CBT may target negative beliefs that may potentially arise from the myriad of internal and external changes that take place during the menopause as it does so in other populations [76].

Hot Flashes

Epidemiology

Many women experience vasomotor symptoms (hot flashes and night sweats) during the menopausal transition. They are described as intense heat along with flushing and sweating, generally localized to the head and trunk. Vasomotor symptoms are linked with sleep disturbance, mood symptoms, and reduced quality of life [77–79]. Additionally, they are a primary reason women seek medical treatment during the menopausal transition [80]. Although severity can vary, studies have shown that as many as 85% of women experience vasomotor symptoms at some point during midlife [81, 82]. Around half of women will experience these symptoms even before noticing any irregularities in their menstrual cycle [83], though vasomotor symptoms generally peak in intensity around the late perimenopause [84].

Time Course

Previously vasomotor symptoms were thought to last 4–5 years; however, recent research has shown that there is substantial heterogeneity in the intensity and duration of vasomotor symptoms among women during the menopausal transition [85]. Around 25% of women will continue to have hot flashes for 5 years or more after their last menstrual period [86]. Around 30% of women will experience more intense and frequent hot flashes that persist as long as 10 years after their final menstrual period [87, 88].

Physiology

The presence of vasomotor symptoms coincides with the decline in estradiol and rise in follicular stimulating hormone (FSH) characteristic of the menopausal transition [89]. However, the underlying pathophysiology of vasomotor symptom is not fully understood. They are thought to originate in the central nervous system and to be associated with a lower thermoregulatory set point. This theory of the etiology of vasomotor symptoms is referred to as the 'Thermoregulatory Model' [89].

Risk Factors

- *Age and Menopausal Stage:* Younger women (age <40) and onset of symptoms during the early or late pre-menopausal by STRAW criteria are linked to longer duration and intensity of hot flashes [90].
- *Race:* Higher levels of vasomotor symptoms have been reported in African-American women [82] compared to women from other ethnic groups.
- *Metabolic:* Previously it was postulated that increased body fat was protective against the development of vasomotor symptoms as androstenedione, present in adipose tissue or peripheral body fat, is aromatized into estrone, which is an additional source of estrogen for the body [91]. Thus, it was thought that thinner women who have less adipose tissue would be more likely to have hot flashes; this theory was called the "Thin Hypothesis." Recent research has shown that increased body fat maybe related to increased frequency of vasomotor symptoms [92]. Adipose tissue has a strong insulating capacity, which is thought to make it harder for women with vasomotor symptoms to dissipate heat [92, 93]. Epidemiological studies have also shown that higher Body Mass index (BMI) is correlated with increasing frequency of vasomotor symptoms [94].

- *Smoking:* Current cigarette smoking is linked with the presence of daily hot flashes and longer-duration of cigarette use is associated with increasing frequency and severity of hot flashes [94]. The pathophysiology behind the increase in hot flashes among smokers is not fully clear, it is thought that cigarettes may affect estrogen metabolism [95]. Additionally, cigarette smoking has also been linked to earlier onset of menopause [96].
- *Anxiety:* The presence of anxiety both prior to the onset of vasomotor symptoms and during the menopausal transition has been linked with more frequent and intense vasomotor symptoms [97, 98].
- *Caffeine:* Although studies have varied, higher caffeine use is associated with more bothersome hot flashes during the menopausal transition [99].
- *Early Childhood Adversity:* Exposure to childhood trauma has also been linked with higher levels of vasomotor symptoms during midlife [100].

Cardiovascular Disease and Bone Health Risk

Vasomotor symptoms have been associated with underlying vascular changes linked to subclinical cardiovascular disease and greater risk of coronary heart disease [101, 102]. Vasomotor symptoms have also been linked to increased risk for osteoporosis [103].

Assessment Scales

The Hot Flash Related Daily Interference Scale (HFRDIS) is a ten-item questionnaire designed to assess how much hot flashes bother women on a day-to-day basis [104]. It is used both in clinical and research settings to track symptoms both observationally and in response to treatment. It has also been adapted into a shorter scale the Hot Flash Interference Scale (HFI) to be more usable in clinical settings [105].

Treatment

Nonpharmacological Interventions
Supportive Tools: Several lifestyle changes can be helpful to manage vasomotor symptoms, including avoiding caffeine, dressing in layers, and the use of cooling pillows. Additionally, aerobic exercise may be helpful to manage some of the repercussions of hot flashes (insomnia and low mood primarily), though studies evaluating its effect on hot flash severity and frequency have had mixed findings [106]. Similarly, yoga and mindfulness have been studied as well and may have benefit for some patients [107]. Acupuncture has also been shown to have some benefit, particularly when hot flashes are related to treatment with anti-estrogen therapy for breast cancer [108].

Cognitive Behavioral Therapy: Cognitive Behavioral Therapy (CBT) has been shown to be effective at modifying negative and catastrophic beliefs related to hot flashes. Further, this form of therapy addresses anxiety and stress that are often linked to more bothersome symptoms [109, 110]. CBT can be delivered on an individual or group basis [110], and recently has been adapted to both telephone and online versions to make this form of treatment more accessible [111].

Pharmacological Interventions
Hormone Therapy: Hormone therapy (HT) was the primary treatment of vasomotor symptoms until 2002 the Women's Health Initiative HT treatment study for cardiovascular disease prevention was stopped early due to concerns about increased risk of invasive breast cancer [69] and later identified to be associated with hypercoagulable events such as ischemic stroke [112]. However, in younger healthy women with no medical contraindications (prior malignancy, history of hypercoagulability) hormone based therapy such as estrogen replacement can be an effective treatment for vasomotor symptoms [69]. If a woman has an intact uterus, estrogen is given concomitantly with progesterone to prevent thickening of the endometrium which can become cancerous [113]. Any decision to start a hormone-based therapy should be discussed with a woman's gynecologist to make sure she is a good candidate for this treatment.

Serotonergic agents: Serotonergic agents such as selective serotonin reuptake inhibitor (SSRI) or serotonin norepinephrine reuptake inhibitor (SNRI) antidepressants have been shown to reduce hot flashes and are great options for women who are not candidates for hormone based therapy or who have co-occurring disorders (depression or anxiety) which may also benefit from the use of these medications. Many of the SSRIs including but not exclusive to Citalopram [114], Escitalopram [115], and Paroxetine [116] and SNRI Venlafaxine [117] have been shown to be effective at reducing hot flash frequency, though any serotonergic agent can be effective. When considering using an antidepressant for hot flashes, the potential for medication interactions should be considered as they are metabolized by the cytochrome p450 (CYP) system and can interact with other medications typically used during this time-period (for example tamoxifen).

Other: Gabapentin has been shown to reduce the severity and frequency of hot flashes in prior randomized trials [118, 119]. Additionally, the herbal supplement black cohosh has been used to reduce hot flash frequency, though prior research has shown mixed efficacy [120]. However, caution should be used as some studies have shown a potential relationship between black cohosh and increased risk of breast cancer.

Sleep Disturbances

Epidemiology

Around 30–60% women suffer from insomnia symptoms during the menopausal transition [121]. Often sleep disruption during the menopausal transition coincides with hot flashes [122], though not always. Women are at increased risk for sleep disturbance during this period even in the absence of hot flashes [123]. Menopausal related sleep disruption has been related to increased healthcare utilization, reduced quality of life, mood symptoms and reduced functioning [124]. Along with vasomotor symptoms, it is a common reason women seek out medical care during midlife. Although research in this area has been mixed, studies have shown that the transition between late reproductive and early perimenopause [125, 126] and between late perimenopause and post-menopause coincide with reports of more severe insomnia symptoms [126].

Clinical Presentation

Sleep disturbance during the menopausal transition is typically a problem of sleep maintenance rather than a problem of sleep onset or early morning awakening [125]. Specifically, women will have higher numbers of awakenings overnight as well as more time spent awake overnight. This combination of increased awakenings and wake-time after sleep onset (WASO) is referred to as 'sleep fragmentation.' Additionally, sleep efficiency (defined as the total amount of time spent asleep over the total amount of time spent in bed) will also be decreased in this population.

In addition to being a period of increased risk for sleep fragmentation, the menopausal transition is also a period of increased risk for other primary sleep disorders. The prevalence of obstructive sleep apnea and periodic leg movements increases with age [127, 128] and it is important to assess for these disorders when women in midlife report sleep disturbance.

Risk Factors

• *Vasomotor Symptoms:* As above, poor sleep during the menopausal transition is frequently attributed to vasomotor symptoms [129, 130]. In studies that have experimentally induced menopause by giving leuprolide, a gonadotropin releasing hormone agonist (GnRHa) to premenopausal women, reports of nighttime vasomotor symptoms have correlated with reports of poor sleep (primarily evidenced by higher WASO and spending more time in the lighter stages of sleep) both on subjective assessments and more objective assessments such as polysomnography [131]. The relationship between vasomotor symptoms and insomnia symptoms also varies per menopausal stage, suggesting that vasomotor symptoms alone likely do not account for all sleep disturbance reported during the menopausal transition [129]. Specifically, when comparing ratios of vasomotor symptoms to reported sleep disturbance during the post-menopause, studies have shown that women report continued sleep disturbance although the absolute numbers of vasomotor symptoms have often decreased during this time. Similarly, during the perimenopause, some studies have shown that more women report incidents of vasomotor symptoms than insomnia symptoms [129]. Additionally, often it is the severity of vasomotor symptoms that corresponds with sleep disturbance, rather than the frequency of vasomotor events [122, 123, 132]. However, there is substantial variability as mentioned above which points to the fact that the etiology of sleep disturbance during the menopausal transition is likely multifactorial.

• *Cultural Variations:* studies have shown that African-American women report worse sleep during the midlife as compared to Caucasian and Asian women [133]. This finding has also been replicated during studies that used polysomnography [133]. Specifically, African-American women spend more time in lighter sleep stages as compared to other races [134], though the etiology of this is not fully understood.

• *Depression and Anxiety:* Overall women are more likely to have depression as compared to men, and the menopausal transition is a time when women are particularly vulnerable to mood disturbance [27, 28, 135] as above. Often depressive symptoms and insomnia symptoms coincide, though it is unclear whether the latter is a consequence or cause of the former [28, 39]. Anxiety is another factor that may be related to both depressive symptoms and sleep disturbance [136]. The interrelationship between depressive symptoms, sleep disturbance and anxiety during the menopausal transition is difficult to parse although given the frequent co-occurrence it is important to screen for each of them during this time. Further, the treatment of each is likely to have some overlapping benefit (e.g. the treatment of depression is likely to improve sleep).

• *Metabolic:* As with hot flashes, increasing BMI has also been associated with sleep disturbance during midlife. In a study of BMI in postmenopausal women, higher BMI (in the obesity range; BMI >30) was linked with lower sleep efficiency and spending less time in the deep stages of sleep [127]. However, this relationship may largely be explained by the increased rate of obstructive sleep apnea as age and BMI increase.

Assessment Scales

There are no validated scales to specifically assess sleep in menopause. However, there are several standardized scales which can be helpful to assess the degree and impact of sleep disturbance in this population. The Insomnia Severity Index (ISI) assesses distress related to sleep disturbance [137] and the Pittsburgh Sleep Quality Index (PSQI) assesses sleep quality and disturbance over a 1 month period [138]. Although often used in research settings, these instruments can be used clinically as well.

Treatment

Nonpharmacological Interventions

Sleep Hygiene: Lifestyle changes such as maintaining a regular bed and wake time, avoiding naps, and limiting TV and phone use within a few hours of bed can be helpful for sleep disruption regardless of the etiology [139]. Additionally, avoiding caffeine use late in the evening or alcohol, using cooling pillows, and dressing in layers can be helpful for menopausal related sleep disruption. However, these strategies alone are not sufficient for many women.

Cognitive Behavioral Therapy (CBT): CBT is an evidence-based form of psychotherapy that can be effective for both insomnia and difficulty tolerating hot flashes [140]. This form of therapy is manualized and divided into a finite number of sessions and involves helping patients change distressing thoughts linked to poor sleep and provides patients with skills to reduce suffering related to these symptoms. This form of treatment can be particularly helpful for women with comorbid insomnia and depression [140].

Pharmacological Interventions

Anti-depressants: As in the treatment of vasomotor symptoms, the use of serotonergic antidepressants (SSRI, SNRI) can be helpful, particularly to address nighttime hot flashes which could be a cause of sleep disturbance.

Sedatives/hypnotics: Hypnotic agents such as zolpidem [141] and eszopiclone [142] have been studied for menopausal sleep disruption and shown to be helpful with short term use. However, there have not been studies that have examined whether these benefits are long lasting. Potential side effects of these medications and the consequences of long-term use (such as dependence or tolerance) should be considered as well.

Other: as discussed above, gabapentin can be helpful to address hot flashes, which can therefore improve sleep. Additionally, if there are any restless leg symptoms this medication can be useful.

Putting It All Together: Interrelationship of Depression, Hot Flashes, and Sleep

The domino theory is often referenced in the literature as a way of explaining the correlation of mood, hot flashes, and sleep. According to this theory, night sweats lend way to difficulty sleeping, which, in turn, may result in depressive symptoms [143]. Since the development of this theory, several studies have attempted to further explore the interrelationship of mood, hot flashes, and sleep. It is important to note that lack of uniformity in defining depression (i.e. major depression vs subsyndromal depression vs depressive symptoms) have led to inconsistencies in findings in the existing literature [46]. Prospective and other studies have found a causative relationship between hot flashes/night sweats and sleep [24, 131]. Randomized double-blind placebo controlled studies have demonstrated an association between improvements in sleep and subsequent improvement in depressive symptoms [50]. However, improvements in hot flashes, measured over a period of 24 h, were not associated with a subsequent improvement in depressive symptoms [50]. These results are consistent with other epidemiological data demonstrating a lack of correlation of hot flashes to recurrent major depression [38]; however, inconsistent with other studies that have demonstrated an association between vasomotor symptoms and depressive symptoms [38, 51] as well as new onset major depression [23]. Other studies have questioned the domino theory cascade suggesting that sleep does not mediate the role between hot flashes and mood [144]. Fluctuations in estradiol levels have been posited as a possible underlying etiology for depressive symptoms during the menopausal transition [24, 30]; albeit, not consistently demonstrated in all studies [23].

Conclusion

When approaching mood, sleep and hot flashes during the menopause, it is first important to delineate the stage of menopause as prevalence and management may differ depending on stage of menopause [1, 2, 15]. Menopausal transition is the stage in which depressive symptoms, sleep changes, and vasomotor symptoms are most likely to take place [23, 24, 81, 82, 121]. Clinical evaluation and use of certain scales can aid in diagnosing mood symptoms, sleep disturbance, or vasomotor changes during the menopause. As the triad of symptoms often co-occur and treatment interventions may overlap, a clinician may approach the triad of symptoms of mild severity with a cadre of non-pharmacological interventions including but not exclusive of sleep hygiene [139], supportive measures [106, 107], and CBT [59, 60, 140]. For moderate to severe triad of symptoms that are not sufficiently addressed by non-pharmacological measures, SSRI's/SNRI's [15, 62, 114–116] and/or Hormone Therapy [69–72]may be considered. Additionally, gabapentin can be used as a non-serotonergic option for the management of vasomotor symptoms and sleep [118, 119]. Of relevance, Hormone Therapy is only FDA approved for the treatment of moderate to severe hot flashes [69]. As it has been shown to be beneficial in the treatment of depressive symptoms during the menopausal transition [71, 72], there may be a role for Hormone Therapy for the triad of symptoms that are moderate to severe (vasomotor symptoms must be moderate to severe) and/or treatment refractory to above stated interventions. Initiation of Hormone Therapy will entail a careful risk benefit analyses with a woman's gynecologist.

References

1. Harsh V, Meltzer-Brody S, Rubinow DR, Schmidt PJ. Reproductive aging, sex steroids, and mood disorders. Harv Rev Psychiatry. 2009;17(2):87–102.
2. Harlow SD, Gass M, Hall JE, Lobo R, Maki P, Rebar RW, et al. Executive summary of the Stages of Reproductive Aging Workshop + 10: addressing the unfinished agenda of staging reproductive aging. J Clin Endocrinol Metab. 2012;97(4):1159–68.
3. Bidet M, Bachelot A, Bissauge E, Golmard JL, Gricourt S, Dulon J, et al. Resumption of ovarian function and pregnancies in 358 patients with premature ovarian failure. J Clin Endocrinol Metab. 2011;96(12):3864–72.
4. Santoro N, Arnsten JH, Buono D, Howard AA, Schoenbaum EE. Impact of street drug use, HIV infection, and highly active antiretroviral therapy on reproductive hormones in middle-aged women. J Women's Health (Larchmt). 2005;14(10):898–905.
5. Santoro N, Lo Y, Moskaleva G, Arnsten JH, Floris-Moore M, Howard AA, et al. Factors affecting reproductive hormones in HIV-infected, substance-using middle-aged women. Menopause. 2007;14(5):859–65.
6. Welt CK, Pagan YL, Smith PC, Rado KB, Hall JE. Control of follicle-stimulating hormone by estradiol and the inhibins: critical role of estradiol at the hypothalamus during the luteal-follicular transition. J Clin Endocrinol Metab. 2003;88(4):1766–71.
7. Johnson BD, Merz CN, Braunstein GD, Berga SL, Bittner V, Hodgson TK, et al. Determination of menopausal status in women: the NHLBI-sponsored Women's Ischemia Syndrome Evaluation (WISE) study. J Women's Health (Larchmt). 2004;13(8):872–87.
8. Harlow SD, Gass M, Hall JE, Lobo R, Maki P, Rebar RW, et al. Executive summary of the Stages of Reproductive Aging Workshop +10: addressing the unfinished agenda of staging reproductive aging. Climacteric. 2012;15(2):105–14.
9. Van Voorhis BJ, Santoro N, Harlow S, Crawford SL, Randolph J. The relationship of bleeding patterns to daily reproductive hormones in women approaching menopause. Obstet Gynecol. 2008;112(1):101–8.
10. Mitchell ES, Woods NF, Mariella A. Three stages of the menopausal transition from the Seattle Midlife Women's Health Study: toward a more precise definition. Menopause. 2000;7(5):334–49.
11. McKinlay SM, Brambilla DJ, Posner JG. The normal menopause transition. Maturitas. 1992;14(2):103–15.
12. Stricker R, Eberhart R, Chevailler MC, Quinn FA, Bischof P. Establishment of detailed reference values for luteinizing hormone, follicle stimulating hormone, estradiol, and progesterone during different phases of the menstrual cycle on the Abbott ARCHITECT analyzer. Clin Chem Lab Med. 2006;44(7):883–7.
13. Randolph JF, Zheng H, Sowers MR, Crandall C, Crawford S, Gold EB, et al. Change in follicle-stimulating hormone and estradiol across the menopausal transition: effect of age at the final menstrual period. J Clin Endocrinol Metab. 2011;96(3):746–54.
14. Hall JE, Lavoie HB, Marsh EE, Martin KA. Decrease in gonadotropin-releasing hormone (GnRH) pulse frequency with aging in postmenopausal women. J Clin Endocrinol Metab. 2000;85(5):1794–800.
15. Kornstein SG, Young EA, Harvey AT, Wisniewski SR, Barkin JL, Thase ME, et al. The influence of menopause status and postmenopausal use of hormone therapy on presentation of major depression in women. Menopause. 2010;17(4):828–39.
16. Bromberger JT, Kravitz HM, Chang YF, Cyranowski JM, Brown C, Matthews KA. Major depression during and after the menopausal transition: Study of Women's Health Across the Nation (SWAN). Psychol Med. 2011;41(9):1879–88.
17. Diagnostic and statistical manual of mental disorders. 5th ed. American Psychiatric Association; 2013.
18. Schmidt PJ, Haq N, Rubinow DR. A longitudinal evaluation of the relationship between reproductive status and mood in perimenopausal women. Am J Psychiatry. 2004;161(12):2238–44.
19. Bromberger JT, Meyer PM, Kravitz HM, Sommer B, Cordal A, Powell L, et al. Psychologic distress and natural menopause: a multiethnic community study. Am J Public Health. 2001;91(9):1435–42.
20. Kessler RC, McGonagle KA, Swartz M, Blazer DG, Nelson CB. Sex and depression in the National Comorbidity Survey. I: lifetime prevalence, chronicity and recurrence. J Affect Disord. 1993;29(2–3):85–96.
21. Zainal NZ. Depressive symptoms in middle-aged women in peninsular Malaysia. Asia Pac J Public Health. 2008;20(4):360–9.
22. Bromberger JT, Kravitz HM. Mood and menopause: findings from the Study of Women's Health Across the Nation (SWAN) over 10 years. Obstet Gynecol Clin N Am. 2011;38(3):609–25.
23. Bromberger JT, Schott L, Kravitz HM, Joffe H. Risk factors for major depression during midlife among a community sample of women with and without prior major depression: are they the same or different? Psychol Med. 2015;45(8):1653–64.
24. Freeman EW, Sammel MD, Lin H, Nelson DB. Associations of hormones and menopausal status with depressed mood in women with no history of depression. Arch Gen Psychiatry. 2006;63(4):375–82.
25. Bromberger JT, Schott LL, Kravitz HM, Sowers M, Avis NE, Gold EB, et al. Longitudinal change in reproductive hormones and depressive symptoms across the menopausal transition: results from the Study of Women's Health Across the Nation (SWAN). Arch Gen Psychiatry. 2010;67(6):598–607.
26. Woods NF, Smith-DiJulio K, Percival DB, Tao EY, Mariella A, Mitchell S. Depressed mood during the menopausal transition and early postmenopause: observations from the Seattle Midlife Women's Health Study. Menopause. 2008;15(2):223–32.
27. Cohen LS, Soares CN, Vitonis AF, Otto MW, Harlow BL. Risk for new onset of depression during the menopausal transition: the Harvard study of moods and cycles. Arch Gen Psychiatry. 2006;63(4):385–90.
28. Bromberger JT, Matthews KA, Schott LL, Brockwell S, Avis NE, Kravitz HM, et al. Depressive symptoms during the menopausal transition: the Study of Women's Health Across the Nation (SWAN). J Affect Disord. 2007;103(1–3):267–72.
29. Avis NE, Brambilla D, McKinlay SM, Vass K. A longitudinal analysis of the association between menopause and depression. Results from the Massachusetts Women's Health Study. Ann Epidemiol. 1994;4(3):214–20.

30. Freeman EW, Sammel MD, Liu L, Gracia CR, Nelson DB, Hollander L. Hormones and menopausal status as predictors of depression in women in transition to menopause. Arch Gen Psychiatry. 2004;61(1):62–70.

31. Morrison MF, Freeman EW, Lin H, Sammel MD. Higher DHEA-S (dehydroepiandrosterone sulfate) levels are associated with depressive symptoms during the menopausal transition: results from the PENN Ovarian Aging Study. Arch Womens Ment Health. 2011;14(5):375–82.

32. Maartens LW, Knottnerus JA, Pop VJ. Menopausal transition and increased depressive symptomatology: a community based prospective study. Maturitas. 2002;42(3):195–200.

33. Freeman EW, Sammel MD, Rinaudo PJ, Sheng L. Premenstrual syndrome as a predictor of menopausal symptoms. Obstet Gynecol. 2004;103(5 Pt 1):960–6.

34. Kravitz HM, Schott LL, Joffe H, Cyranowski JM, Bromberger JT. Do anxiety symptoms predict major depressive disorder in midlife women? The Study of Women's Health Across the Nation (SWAN) Mental Health Study (MHS). Psychol Med. 2014;44(12):2593–602.

35. Freeman EW, Sammel MD, Boorman DW, Zhang R. Longitudinal pattern of depressive symptoms around natural menopause. JAMA Psychiatry. 2014;71(1):36–43.

36. Dennerstein L, Guthrie JR, Clark M, Lehert P, Henderson VW. A population-based study of depressed mood in middle-aged, Australian-born women. Menopause. 2004;11(5):563–8.

37. Payne JL, Palmer JT, Joffe H. A reproductive subtype of depression: conceptualizing models and moving toward etiology. Harv Rev Psychiatry. 2009;17(2):72–86.

38. Worsley R, Bell R, Kulkarni J, Davis SR. The association between vasomotor symptoms and depression during perimenopause: a systematic review. Maturitas. 2014;77(2):111–7.

39. Soares CN, Taylor V. Effects and management of the menopausal transition in women with depression and bipolar disorder. J Clin Psychiatry. 2007;68(Suppl 9):16–21.

40. Miller LA, A-BO G, Carusi D, Joffe H. Depression in medical illness. New York: McGraw-Hill; 2017.

41. Baune BT, Stuart M, Gilmour A, Wersching H, Arolt V, Berger K. Moderators of the relationship between depression and cardiovascular disorders: a systematic review. Gen Hosp Psychiatry. 2012;34(5):478–92.

42. Soares CN. Mood disorders in midlife women: understanding the critical window and its clinical implications. Menopause. 2014;21(2):198–206.

43. Greendale GA, Huang MH, Wight RG, Seeman T, Luetters C, Avis NE, et al. Effects of the menopause transition and hormone use on cognitive performance in midlife women. Neurology. 2009;72(21):1850–7.

44. Greendale GA, Wight RG, Huang MH, Avis N, Gold EB, Joffe H, et al. Menopause-associated symptoms and cognitive performance: results from the study of women's health across the nation. Am J Epidemiol. 2010;171(11):1214–24.

45. Zakzanis KK, Leach L, Kaplan E. On the nature and pattern of neurocognitive function in major depressive disorder. Neuropsychiatry Neuropsychol Behav Neurol. 1998;11(3):111–9.

46. Joffe H, Soares CN, Thurston RC, White DP, Cohen LS, Hall JE. Depression is associated with worse objectively and subjectively measured sleep, but not more frequent awakenings, in women with vasomotor symptoms. Menopause. 2009;16(4):671–9.

47. Portman DJ, Gass ML, Panel VATCC. Genitourinary syndrome of menopause: new terminology for vulvovaginal atrophy from the International Society for the Study of Women's Sexual Health and the North American Menopause Society. J Sex Med. 2014;11(12):2865–72.

48. Derogatis LR, Burnett AL. The epidemiology of sexual dysfunctions. J Sex Med. 2008;5(2):289–300.

49. Prairie BA, Wisniewski SR, Luther J, Hess R, Thurston RC, Wisner KL, et al. Symptoms of depressed mood, disturbed sleep, and sexual problems in midlife women: cross-sectional data from the Study of Women's Health Across the Nation. J Women's Health (Larchmt). 2015;24(2):119–26.

50. Joffe H, Petrillo LF, Koukopoulos A, Viguera AC, Hirschberg A, Nonacs R, et al. Increased estradiol and improved sleep, but not hot flashes, predict enhanced mood during the menopausal transition. J Clin Endocrinol Metab. 2011;96(7):E1044–54.

51. Worsley R, Bell RJ, Gartoulla P, Robinson PJ, Davis SR. Moderate-severe vasomotor symptoms are associated with moderate-severe depressive symptoms. J Women's Health (Larchmt). 2017;26(7):712–8.

52. Kraepelin E. Psychiatrie: ein Lehrbuch fuer Studierende und Aerzte. Leipzig: Barth; 1909.

53. Harkins EB. Effects of empty nest transition on self-report of psychological and physical well-being. J Marriage Fam. 1978;40(3):549–56.

54. Dennerstein L, Dudley E, Guthrie J. Empty nest or revolving door? A prospective study of women's quality of life in midlife during the phase of children leaving and re-entering the home. Psychol Med. 2002;32(3):545–50.

55. Freeman EW, Sammel MD, Lin H, Gracia CR, Kapoor S. Symptoms in the menopausal transition: hormone and behavioral correlates. Obstet Gynecol. 2008;111(1):127–36.

56. Gilbody S, Richards D, Barkham M. Diagnosing depression in primary care using self-completed instruments: UK validation of PHQ-9 and CORE-OM. Br J Gen Pract. 2007;57(541):650–2.

57. Heinemann LA, Potthoff P, Schneider HP. International versions of the menopause rating scale (MRS). Health Qual Life Outcomes. 2003;1:28.

58. Hilditch JR, Lewis J, Peter A, van Maris B, Ross A, Franssen E, et al. A menopause-specific quality of life questionnaire: development and psychometric properties. Maturitas. 2008;61(1–2):107–21.

59. Lynch D, Laws KR, McKenna PJ. Cognitive behavioural therapy for major psychiatric disorder: does it really work? A meta-analytical review of well-controlled trials. Psychol Med. 2010;40(1):9–24.

60. Brandon AR, Minhajuddin A, Thase ME, Jarrett RB. Impact of reproductive status and age on response of depressed women to cognitive therapy. J Women's Health (Larchmt). 2013;22(1):58–66.

61. Cuijpers P, Geraedts AS, van Oppen P, Andersson G, Markowitz JC, van Straten A. Interpersonal psychotherapy for depression: a meta-analysis. Am J Psychiatry. 2011;168(6):581–92.

62. Kornstein SG, Clayton AH, Bao W, Guico-Pabia CJ. A pooled analysis of the efficacy of desvenlafaxine for the treatment of major depressive disorder in perimenopausal and postmenopausal women. J Women's Health (Larchmt). 2015;24(4):281–90.

63. Joffe H, Groninger H, Soares CN, Nonacs R, Cohen LS, Soares C. An open trial of mirtazapine in menopausal women with depression unresponsive to estrogen replacement therapy. J Womens Health Gend Based Med. 2001;10(10):999–1004.

64. Ladd CO, Newport DJ, Ragan KA, Loughhead A, Stowe ZN. Venlafaxine in the treatment of depressive and vasomotor symptoms in women with perimenopausal depression. Depress Anxiety. 2005;22(2):94–7.

65. Pae CU, Mandelli L, Kim TS, Han C, Masand PS, Marks DM, et al. Effectiveness of antidepressant treatments in pre-menopausal versus post-menopausal women: a pilot study on differential effects of sex hormones on antidepressant effects. Biomed Pharmacother. 2009;63(3):228–35.

66. Pinto-Meza A, Usall J, Serrano-Blanco A, Suárez D, Haro JM. Gender differences in response to antidepressant treatment prescribed in primary care. Does menopause make a difference? J Affect Disord. 2006;93(1–3):53–60.

67. Kornstein SG, Toups M, Rush AJ, Wisniewski SR, Thase ME, Luther J, et al. Do menopausal status and use of hormone therapy affect antidepressant treatment response? Findings from the Sequenced Treatment Alternatives to Relieve Depression (STAR*D) study. J Women's Health (Larchmt). 2013;22(2):121–31.

68. Eker SS, Kirli S, Akkaya C, Cangur S, Sarandol A. Are there differences between serotonergic, noradrenergic and dual acting antidepressants in the treatment of depressed women? World J Biol Psychiatry. 2009;10(4 Pt 2):400–8.

69. Rossouw JE, Anderson GL, Prentice RL, LaCroix AZ, Kooperberg C, Stefanick ML, et al. Risks and benefits of estrogen plus progestin in healthy postmenopausal women: principal results From the Women's Health Initiative randomized controlled trial. JAMA. 2002;288(3):321–33.

70. Morrison MF, Kallan MJ, Ten Have T, Katz I, Tweedy K, Battistini M. Lack of efficacy of estradiol for depression in postmenopausal women: a randomized, controlled trial. Biol Psychiatry. 2004;55(4):406–12.

71. Soares CN, Almeida OP, Joffe H, Cohen LS. Efficacy of estradiol for the treatment of depressive disorders in perimenopausal women: a double-blind, randomized, placebo-controlled trial. Arch Gen Psychiatry. 2001;58(6):529–34.

72. Schmidt PJ, Nieman L, Danaceau MA, Tobin MB, Roca CA, Murphy JH, et al. Estrogen replacement in perimenopause-related depression: a preliminary report. Am J Obstet Gynecol. 2000;183(2):414–20.

73. Gordon JL, Rubinow DR, Eisenlohr-Moul TA, Xia K, Schmidt PJ, Girdler SS. Efficacy of transdermal estradiol and micronized progesterone in the prevention of depressive symptoms in the menopause transition: a randomized clinical trial. JAMA Psychiat. 2018;75(2):149–57.

74. Simon NM. Treating complicated grief. JAMA. 2013;310(4):416–23.

75. Brakemeier EL, Frase L. Interpersonal psychotherapy (IPT) in major depressive disorder. Eur Arch Psychiatry Clin Neurosci. 2012;262(Suppl 2):S117–21.

76. Jakobsen JC, Hansen JL, Simonsen S, Simonsen E, Gluud C. Effects of cognitive therapy versus interpersonal psychotherapy in patients with major depressive disorder: a systematic review of randomized clinical trials with meta-analyses and trial sequential analyses. Psychol Med. 2012;42(7):1343–57.

77. Avis NE, Ory M, Matthews KA, Schocken M, Bromberger J, Colvin A. Health-related quality of life in a multiethnic sample of middle-aged women: Study of Women's Health Across the Nation (SWAN). Med Care. 2003;41(11):1262–76.

78. Kravitz HM, Ganz PA, Bromberger J, Powell LH, Sutton-Tyrrell K, Meyer PM. Sleep difficulty in women at midlife: a community survey of sleep and the menopausal transition. Menopause. 2003;10(1):19–28.

79. Bromberger JT, Assmann SF, Avis NE, Schocken M, Kravitz HM, Cordal A. Persistent mood symptoms in a multiethnic community cohort of pre- and perimenopausal women. Am J Epidemiol. 2003;158(4):347–56.

80. Williams RE, Kalilani L, DiBenedetti DB, Zhou X, Fehnel SE, Clark RV. Healthcare seeking and treatment for menopausal symptoms in the United States. Maturitas. 2007;58(4):348–58.

81. Dennerstein L, Dudley EC, Hopper JL, Guthrie JR, Burger HG. A prospective population-based study of menopausal symptoms. Obstet Gynecol. 2000;96(3):351–8.

82. Gold EB, Colvin A, Avis N, Bromberger J, Greendale GA, Powell L, et al. Longitudinal analysis of the association between vasomotor symptoms and race/ethnicity across the menopausal transition: study of women's health across the nation. Am J Public Health. 2006;96(7):1226–35.

83. Reed SD, Lampe JW, Qu C, Copeland WK, Gundersen G, Fuller S, et al. Premenopausal vasomotor symptoms in an ethnically diverse population. Menopause. 2014;21(2):153–8.

84. Col NF, Guthrie JR, Politi M, Dennerstein L. Duration of vasomotor symptoms in middle-aged women: a longitudinal study. Menopause. 2009;16(3):453–7.

85. Tepper PG, Brooks MM, Randolph JF, Crawford SL, El Khoudary SR, Gold EB, et al. Characterizing the trajectories of vasomotor symptoms across the menopausal transition. Menopause. 2016;23(10):1067–74.

86. Politi MC, Schleinitz MD, Col NF. Revisiting the duration of vasomotor symptoms of menopause: a meta-analysis. J Gen Intern Med. 2008;23(9):1507–13.

87. Freeman EW, Sammel MD, Sanders RJ. Risk of long-term hot flashes after natural menopause: evidence from the Penn Ovarian Aging Study cohort. Menopause. 2014;21(9):924–32.

88. Avis NE, Crawford SL, Greendale G, Bromberger JT, Everson-Rose SA, Gold EB, et al. Duration of menopausal vasomotor symptoms over the menopause transition. JAMA Intern Med. 2015;175(4):531–9.

89. Randolph JF, Sowers M, Bondarenko I, Gold EB, Greendale GA, Bromberger JT, et al. The relationship of longitudinal change in reproductive hormones and vasomotor symptoms during the menopausal transition. J Clin Endocrinol Metab. 2005;90(11):6106–12.

90. Freeman EW, Sammel MD, Lin H, Liu Z, Gracia CR. Duration of menopausal hot flushes and associated risk factors. Obstet Gynecol. 2011;117(5):1095–104.

91. Kershaw EE, Flier JS. Adipose tissue as an endocrine organ. J Clin Endocrinol Metab. 2004;89(6):2548–56.

92. Thurston RC, Sowers MR, Chang Y, Sternfeld B, Gold EB, Johnston JM, et al. Adiposity and reporting of vasomotor symptoms among midlife women: the study of women's health across the nation. Am J Epidemiol. 2008;167(1):78–85.

93. Anderson GS. Human morphology and temperature regulation. Int J Biometeorol. 1999;43(3):99–109.

94. Whiteman MK, Staropoli CA, Langenberg PW, McCarter RJ, Kjerulff KH, Flaws JA. Smoking, body mass, and hot flashes in midlife women. Obstet Gynecol. 2003;101(2):264–72.

95. Michnovicz JJ, Hershcopf RJ, Naganuma H, Bradlow HL, Fishman J. Increased 2-hydroxylation of estradiol as a possible mechanism for the anti-estrogenic effect of cigarette smoking. N Engl J Med. 1986;315(21):1305–9.

96. McKinlay SM, Bifano NL, McKinlay JB. Smoking and age at menopause in women. Ann Intern Med. 1985;103(3):350–6.

97. Freeman EW, Sammel MD, Lin H, Gracia CR, Kapoor S, Ferdousi T. The role of anxiety and hormonal changes in menopausal hot flashes. Menopause. 2005;12(3):258–66.

98. Mitchell ES, Woods NF. Hot flush severity during the menopausal transition and early postmenopause: beyond hormones. Climacteric. 2015;18(4):536–44.

99. Faubion SS, Sood R, Thielen JM, Shuster LT. Caffeine and menopausal symptoms: what is the association? Menopause. 2015;22(2):155–8.

100. Thurston RC, Bromberger J, Chang Y, Goldbacher E, Brown C, Cyranowski JM, et al. Childhood abuse or neglect is associated with increased vasomotor symptom reporting among midlife women. Menopause. 2008;15(1):16–22.

101. Thurston RC, Sutton-Tyrrell K, Everson-Rose SA, Hess R, Matthews KA. Hot flashes and subclinical cardiovascular disease: findings from the Study of Women's Health Across the Nation Heart Study. Circulation. 2008;118(12):1234–40.

102. Thurston RC, Christie IC, Matthews KA. Hot flashes and cardiac vagal control: a link to cardiovascular risk? Menopause. 2010;17(3):456–61.

103. Crandall CJ, Tseng CH, Crawford SL, Thurston RC, Gold EB, Johnston JM, et al. Association of menopausal vasomotor symp-

toms with increased bone turnover during the menopausal transition. J Bone Miner Res. 2011;26(4):840–9.

104. Carpenter JS. The hot flash related daily interference scale: a tool for assessing the impact of hot flashes on quality of life following breast cancer. J Pain Symptom Manag. 2001;22(6):979–89.

105. Carpenter JS, Bakoyannis G, Otte JL, Chen CX, Rand KL, Woods N, et al. Validity, cut-points, and minimally important differences for two hot flash-related daily interference scales. Menopause. 2017;24(8):877–85.

106. Sternfeld B, Guthrie KA, Ensrud KE, LaCroix AZ, Larson JC, Dunn AL, et al. Efficacy of exercise for menopausal symptoms: a randomized controlled trial. Menopause. 2014;21(4):330–8.

107. Stefanopoulou E, Grunfeld EA. Mind-body interventions for vasomotor symptoms in healthy menopausal women and breast cancer survivors. A systematic review. J Psychosom Obstet Gynaecol. 2017;38(3):210–25.

108. Garcia MK, Graham-Getty L, Haddad R, Li Y, McQuade J, Lee RT, et al. Systematic review of acupuncture to control hot flashes in cancer patients. Cancer. 2015;121(22):3948–58.

109. Hunter MS, Mann E. A cognitive model of menopausal hot flushes and night sweats. J Psychosom Res. 2010;69(5):491–501.

110. Ayers B, Smith M, Hellier J, Mann E, Hunter MS. Effectiveness of group and self-help cognitive behavior therapy in reducing problematic menopausal hot flushes and night sweats (MENOS 2): a randomized controlled trial. Menopause. 2012;19(7):749–59.

111. McCurry SM, Guthrie KA, Morin CM, Woods NF, Landis CA, Ensrud KE, et al. Telephone-based cognitive behavioral therapy for insomnia in perimenopausal and postmenopausal women with vasomotor symptoms: a MsFLASH randomized clinical trial. JAMA Intern Med. 2016;176(7):913–20.

112. Prentice RL. Postmenopausal hormone therapy and the risks of coronary heart disease, breast cancer, and stroke. Semin Reprod Med. 2014;32(6):419–25.

113. Grady D, Gebretsadik T, Kerlikowske K, Ernster V, Petitti D. Hormone replacement therapy and endometrial cancer risk: a meta-analysis. Obstet Gynecol. 1995;85(2):304–13.

114. Suvanto-Luukkonen E, Koivunen R, Sundström H, Bloigu R, Karjalainen E, Häivä-Mällinen L, et al. Citalopram and fluoxetine in the treatment of postmenopausal symptoms: a prospective, randomized, 9-month, placebo-controlled, double-blind study. Menopause. 2005;12(1):18–26.

115. Freeman EW, Guthrie KA, Caan B, Sternfeld B, Cohen LS, Joffe H, et al. Efficacy of escitalopram for hot flashes in healthy menopausal women: a randomized controlled trial. JAMA. 2011;305(3):267–74.

116. Carroll DG, Lisenby KM, Carter TL. Critical appraisal of paroxetine for the treatment of vasomotor symptoms. Int J Womens Health. 2015;7:615–24.

117. Joffe H, Guthrie KA, LaCroix AZ, Reed SD, Ensrud KE, Manson JE, et al. Low-dose estradiol and the serotonin-norepinephrine reuptake inhibitor venlafaxine for vasomotor symptoms: a randomized clinical trial. JAMA Intern Med. 2014;174(7):1058–66.

118. Pinkerton JV, Kagan R, Portman D, Sathyanarayana R, Sweeney M, Investigators B. Phase 3 randomized controlled study of gastroretentive gabapentin for the treatment of moderate-to-severe hot flashes in menopause. Menopause. 2014;21(6):567–73.

119. Pinkerton JV. Does addition of gabapentin to antidepressant therapy improve control of hot flashes? Nat Clin Pract Endocrinol Metab. 2007;3(8):566–7.

120. Maki DG. Review: in menopause (intact uterus), estrogen + progestogen, isoflavones, and black cohosh reduce hot flashes. Ann Intern Med. 2017;167(6):JC26.

121. Kravitz HM, Zhao X, Bromberger JT, Gold EB, Hall MH, Matthews KA, et al. Sleep disturbance during the menopausal transition in a multi-ethnic community sample of women. Sleep. 2008;31(7):979–90.

122. de Zambotti M, Colrain IM, Javitz HS, Baker FC. Magnitude of the impact of hot flashes on sleep in perimenopausal women. Fertil Steril. 2014;102(6):1708–15.el.

123. Ensrud KE, Stone KL, Blackwell TL, Sawaya GF, Tagliaferri M, Diem SJ, et al. Frequency and severity of hot flashes and sleep disturbance in postmenopausal women with hot flashes. Menopause. 2009;16(2):286–92.

124. Timur S, Sahin NH. Effects of sleep disturbance on the quality of life of Turkish menopausal women: a population-based study. Maturitas. 2009;64(3):177–81.

125. Joffe H, Massler A, Sharkey KM. Evaluation and management of sleep disturbance during the menopause transition. Semin Reprod Med. 2010;28(5):404–21.

126. Woods NF, Mitchell ES. Sleep symptoms during the menopausal transition and early postmenopause: observations from the Seattle Midlife Women's Health Study. Sleep. 2010;33(4):539–49.

127. Naufel MF, Frange C, Anderen ML, Girao MJBC, Tufik S, Beraldi Ribeiro E, Hachul H. Association between obesity and sleep disorders in postmenopausal women. Menopause. 2018;25(2):139–44.

128. Mirer AG, Young T, Palta M, Benca RM, Rasmuson A, Peppard PE. Sleep-disordered breathing and the menopausal transition among participants in the Sleep in Midlife Women Study. Menopause. 2017;24(2):157–62.

129. Lampio L, Polo-Kantola P, Polo O, Kauko T, Aittokallio J, Saaresranta T. Sleep in midlife women: effects of menopause, vasomotor symptoms, and depressive symptoms. Menopause. 2014;21(11):1217–24.

130. Lampio L, Saaresranta T, Engblom J, Polo O, Polo-Kantola P. Predictors of sleep disturbance in menopausal transition. Maturitas. 2016;94:137–42.

131. Joffe H, Crawford S, Economou N, Kim S, Regan S, Hall JE, et al. A gonadotropin-releasing hormone agonist model demonstrates that nocturnal hot flashes interrupt objective sleep. Sleep. 2013;36(12):1977–85.

132. Thurston RC, Joffe H. Vasomotor symptoms and menopause: findings from the Study of Women's Health across the Nation. Obstet Gynecol Clin N Am. 38. United States2011:489–501.

133. Hall MH, Matthews KA, Kravitz HM, Gold EB, Buysse DJ, Bromberger JT, et al. Race and financial strain are independent correlates of sleep in midlife women: the SWAN sleep study. Sleep. 2009;32(1):73–82.

134. Durrence HH, Lichstein KL. The sleep of African Americans: a comparative review. Behav Sleep Med. 2006;4(1):29–44.

135. Steinberg EM, Rubinow DR, Bartko JJ, Fortinsky PM, Haq N, Thompson K, et al. A cross-sectional evaluation of perimenopausal depression. J Clin Psychiatry. 2008;69(6):973–80.

136. Woods NF, Hohensee C, Carpenter JS, Cohen L, Ensrud K, Freeman EW, et al. Symptom clusters among MsFLASH clinical trial participants. Menopause. 2016;23(2):158–65.

137. Bastien CH, Vallières A, Morin CM. Validation of the insomnia severity index as an outcome measure for insomnia research. Sleep Med. 2001;2(4):297–307.

138. Buysse DJ, Reynolds CF, Monk TH, Berman SR, Kupfer DJ. The Pittsburgh sleep quality index: a new instrument for psychiatric practice and research. Psychiatry Res. 1989;28(2):193–213.

139. Stepanski EJ, Wyatt JK. Use of sleep hygiene in the treatment of insomnia. Sleep Med Rev. 2003;7(3):215–25.

140. Guthrie KA, Larson JC, Ensrud KE, Anderson GL, Carpenter JS, Freeman EW, et al. Effects of pharmacologic and nonpharmaco-

logic interventions on insomnia symptoms and subjective sleep quality in women with hot flashes: a pooled analysis of individual participant data from 4 MsFLASH trials. Sleep. 2017.

141. Dorsey CM, Lee KA, Scharf MB. Effect of zolpidem on sleep in women with perimenopausal and postmenopausal insomnia: a 4-week, randomized, multicenter, double-blind, placebo-controlled study. Clin Ther. 2004;26(10):1578–86.

142. Joffe H, Petrillo L, Viguera A, Koukopoulos A, Silver-Heilman K, Farrell A, et al. Eszopiclone improves insomnia and depressive and anxious symptoms in perimenopausal and postmenopausal women with hot flashes: a randomized, double-blinded, placebo-controlled crossover trial. Am J Obstet Gynecol. 2010;202(2):171. e1–e11.

143. Campbell S, Whitehead M. Oestrogen therapy and the menopausal syndrome. Clin Obstet Gynaecol. 1977;4(1):31–47.

144. Burleson MH, Todd M, Trevathan WR. Daily vasomotor symptoms, sleep problems, and mood: using daily data to evaluate the domino hypothesis in middle-aged women. Menopause. 2010;17(1):87–95.

Stroke Risk Factors in Women

Emer R. McGrath and Kathryn M. Rexrode

Introduction

Stroke is the leading cause of acquired adult disability worldwide and the second leading cause of death worldwide [1]. In the US, stroke is the fifth leading cause of death in men, but the fourth leading cause of death in women [2, 3]. The lifetime risk of stroke for individuals aged 55–75 years is higher in women (20%) compared to men (17%), in part due to the longer life expectancy of women [4]. The majority (60%) of stroke deaths occur in women, partially due to the fact that women tend to be older when they experience a stroke [5, 6]. Women are more likely than men to experience stroke as their first manifestation of cardiovascular disease (CVD), and stroke comprises a greater percentage of their cardiovascular events [7]. In the recent Greater Cincinnati/Northern Kentucky Stroke Study of over 1.3 million people, the incidence of stroke was shown to have decreased between 2005 and 2010 in men but not women, largely driven by a reduction in ischemic stroke in men [8]. The decline in stroke incidence rates in men but not women may be explained by sex differences in the distribution and/or treatment of risk factors, as well as lower rates of risk factor optimization in women [9].

In this chapter we provide an overview of stroke risk factors in women, focusing primarily on ischemic stroke, and provide an in-depth discussion of the differential effect of traditional stroke risk factors in women compared to men, as well as those stroke risk factors which are unique to women.

Risk Factors

Women have a number of unique risk factors for stroke, including menarche and menopause, pregnancy and its related complications, use of oral contraceptive medication and postmenopausal hormone therapy. In addition, the prevalence of traditional stroke risk factors and the strength of their association, varies between men and women (Table 1). Women who experience stroke more commonly have atrial fibrillation and hypertension while men who present with

Table 1 Risk factors for stroke in women

	Sex specific risk factors	Risk factors stronger/more prevalent in women	Risk factors similar between men and women
Pregnancy	X		
Preeclampsia/eclampsia	X		
Gestational diabetes	X		
Oral contraceptive use	X		
Postmenopausal hormone use	X		
Migraine with aura		X	
Atrial fibrillation		X	
Diabetes mellitus		X	
Hypertension		X	
Depression		X	
Psychosocial stress		X	
Age			X
Physical inactivity			X
Obesity			X
Diet			X
Smoking			X
Metabolic syndrome			X
Prior cardiovascular disease			X

Adapted from Bushnell et al. [12] with permission from Wolters Kluwer Health, Inc.

E. R. McGrath (✉)
Department of Neurology, Brigham and Women's Hospital and Harvard Medical School, Boston, MA, USA
e-mail: emcgrath2@bwh.harvard.edu

K. M. Rexrode
Division of Women's Health, Department of Medicine, Brigham and Women's Hospital and Harvard Medical School, Boston, MA, USA
e-mail: krexrode@bwh.harvard.edu

© Springer Nature Switzerland AG 2019
M. A. O'Neal (ed.), *Neurology and Psychiatry of Women*, https://doi.org/10.1007/978-3-030-04245-5_23

stroke are more likely to have coronary artery disease and peripheral vascular disease [10].

Risk Factors Unique to Women

Pregnancy

The absolute incidence of stroke in young women is low, however the incidence increases during pregnancy and puerperium, with the highest risk occurring in the third trimester and the early postpartum period [11, 12]. The risk of stroke in pregnancy and the puerperium is further increased in association with migraine, gestational diabetes and preeclampsia or eclampsia [13, 14] as well as in the presence of more traditional vascular risk factors, including hypertension, pre-existing CVD and non-gestational diabetes mellitus. Advanced maternal age (≥35 years), African American race, systemic lupus erythematosus, thrombophilic disorders and sickle cell disease are also associated with an increased risk [15]. Furthermore, complications of pregnancy including preeclampsia, gestational diabetes and pregnancy induced hypertension, are now known to be associated with an elevated risk of stroke and CVD, beyond the childbearing years [12, 16]. Please refer to chapter "Stroke in Pregnancy" for a detailed discussion of stroke in pregnancy.

Pre-eclampsia

Pregnancy related hypertension is the most important risk factor for stroke in pregnancy [12]. Preeclampsia is one of the pregnancy hypertensive disorders, affecting 8–12% of all pregnancies and causing cerebrovascular complications, including stroke, in up to 1% [17]. Women with preeclampsia-eclampsia have a significantly higher risk of stroke during pregnancy and in the first postpartum year, with an almost eightfold increased risk of antenatal stroke (OR 7.7, 95% CI 1.3–55.7) [13]. Multiple studies have now shown that a history of preeclampsia increases the risk of stroke and other CVD beyond the childbearing years [18, 19]. In a meta-analysis of 4 studies of over 64,000 women with preeclampsia, women with a history of preeclampsia had twice the lifetime risk of stroke compared to a woman with an uncomplicated pregnancy history (OR 2.16; 95% CI 1.86–2.52) [20], with similar results for stroke risk reported in a more recent meta-analysis of all-cause CVD (OR 1.76; 95% CI 1.43–2.21) [21]. In addition, preeclampsia is associated with a more than fourfold increased risk of hypertension after pregnancy, [20] with even higher risk among women with overweight or obesity [22]. Potential mechanisms responsible for the association between preeclampsia and risk of subsequent stroke include shared risk factors for preeclampsia/eclampsia and stroke (including hypertension and dyslipidemia), endothelial dysfunction, underlying genetic factors and induction of cerebrovascular abnormalities in pregnancy that persist postpartum [23].

Gestational Diabetes Mellitus

Data on the risk of stroke associated with gestational diabetes is limited to a few observational studies. In one population-based cohort and nested case-control study, gestational diabetes was associated with an increased risk of antenatal stroke, with a RR of 26.8, 95% CI 3.2-∝ [13]. In the Nurses' Health Study II, a history of gestational diabetes mellitus was associated with an increased risk of future CVD including stroke (HR 1.43, 95% CI 1.12–1.81), although this association was not observed for the outcome of stroke alone after full adjustment (HR 1.10, 95% CI 0.75–1.61) [24]. Similarly, in a Swedish study, women with a history of gestational diabetes had an odds ratio of 1.51 (95% CI 1.07–2.14) for CVD, although analyses were not adjusted for intercurrent diabetes. No data specific to stroke were presented [25]. Up to one in every two women with gestational diabetes mellitus will develop type 2 diabetes mellitus (an independent risk factor for stroke) within 5–10 years of their pregnancy, which will affect long-term stroke risk [12].

Other Pregnancy Complications

A history of miscarriage or stillbirth, [26] as well as a history of preterm delivery particularly before 32 weeks, [27] have also been associated with an increased risk of CVD in later life.

Menarche and Menopause

Duration of reproductive years in women has also been associated with risk of stroke and CVD [26, 28], with a shorter duration of reproductive lifespan associated with a higher risk of stroke in the Nurses' Health Study, mostly due to an earlier age of onset (<40 years) of menopause (RR 1.27; 95% CI, 1.06–1.52). Early age at menopause (<45 years) has been consistently associated with increased risk of stroke, whether from natural or surgical causes [28]. Additionally, an extremely early age of onset (≤10 years) of menarche has also been associated with a higher stroke risk (RR 1.25; 95% CI, 1.07–1.46) [28].

Hormonal Contraceptive Use

Estrogen-containing oral contraceptives (OC) have consistently been associated with an increased risk of stroke. In a large population-based cohort of over 1.6 million women, the incidence of ischemic stroke in contraceptive users was reported to be 21.4 per 100,000 person-years [29]. However, it is important to note that the risk of stroke associated with OC appears to be lower than that associated with pregnancy [15]. Based on five prior meta-analyses, the risk of stroke associated with current use of combined low dose OC ranges from an OR of 1.9 to 2.75 [30–34]. The risk appears dose dependent: the adjusted RR for ethinyl-estradiol doses of 30–40 μg ranges from 1.40 (95% CI, 0.97–2.03) to 2.20 (1.79–2.69), whereas the RR for the 20-μg dose ranges from 0.88 (0.22–3.53) to 1.53 (1.26–1.87) [29]. It is unclear if third generation OCs (desogestrel or gestodene) are associated with a higher risk of ischemic stroke compared to second generation OCs (levonorgestrel) [35]. In studies to date, progestin-only OC have not been associated with an increased stroke risk [29, 34]. Fewer data are available for non-oral hormonal contraceptives. The vaginal contraceptive ring is associated with a 2.5-fold increased risk, while the transdermal contraceptive patch is associated with a nonsignificant trend towards an increased stroke risk [29].

In healthy young women, the absolute risk of stroke associated with OC is low, [29] although the risk is increased in the presence of other stroke risk factors, including smoking, hypertension, dyslipidemia, obesity, migraine with aura and a history of thromboembolic disease. In the RATIO Study, the risk of stroke with OC use was even greater in those who also had a history of hypertension or current smoking [35]. The risk of stroke with OC use is also increased in those with a genetic predisposition to thrombosis, including the Factor V Leiden mutation and the methylenetetrahydrofolate 677T mutation [36]. A history of migraine with aura also appears to result in a greater risk of stroke among OC users (see section below on migraine).

Postmenopausal Hormone Therapy

Previous observational studies and clinical trials have consistently demonstrated an association between postmenopausal hormone therapy, estrogen alone or combined estrogen and progesterone use, and risk of stroke [37–40]. In the Women's Health Initiative of over 27,000 postmenopausal women, women randomized to estrogen therapy or combined estrogen and progestogen therapy had a 40% increase in risk of ischemic stroke compared with placebo [39, 41]. Whether there is a lower risk of stroke with transdermal preparations has not been clearly proven. In a large case-cohort study of postmenopausal women, transdermal estrogen use was not associated with an increased stroke risk, while increased risk was observed for oral use [42]. Timing of hormone initiation does not appear to influence the association for stroke [43]. In the Nurses' Health Study, an increased risk of stroke was noted among women initiating hormone therapy at young ages or close to menopause as well as at older ages or more than 10 years post-menopause, in contrast to results observed for coronary heart disease. There is also clear evidence of a dose-response relationship between higher doses of conjugated estrogens and risk of stroke (P for trend, <.001) [37]. For those with established cerebrovascular or CVD, hormones have been clearly associated with risk [44, 45].

Risk Factors with a Differential Effect in Women Compared to Men

Migraine with Aura

The prevalence of migraine in the population is approximately 18.5%, and is 4.4% for migraine with aura [46]. Migraine has a marked female predominance, with a three to fourfold higher prevalence in women compared to men [46, 47]. Studies have consistently found an association between migraine and stroke across different populations [48–51]. In the Nurses' Health Study II a history of migraine was associated with a 60% increased risk of stroke (HR 1.62, 95% CI 1.37–1.92) [52]. Data suggest that the risk of stroke associated with migraine is higher in women (RR 2.08, 95% CI 1.13–3.84) compared to men (RR 1.37, 95% CI 0.89–2.11) and in those who have a history of migraine with aura compared to those with migraine without aura [53–55].

The combination of migraine with aura and use of hormonal contraceptives is associated with a sixfold increased risk of stroke compared to neither risk factor, while migraine with aura alone is associated with a 2.7 fold increased risk and migraine without aura alone is associated with a 2.2 fold increased risk [48]. In addition, cigarette smoking in individuals with migraine is associated with an even greater stroke risk [53].

Hypertension

Hypertension is the most important modifiable risk factor for stroke. In the INTERSTROKE study, approximately 35% of all stroke cases could be attributed to hypertension (OR 2.64) [56]. Hypertension predisposes to ischemic stroke by causing endothelial damage and predisposing to thrombus formation. It also accelerates intracranial and extracranial atherosclerosis and contributes to cardiac conditions like atrial fibrillation and, that can lead to cardioembolic strokes [57]. In the US, the prevalence of hypertension (systolic blood pressure ≥140 mmHg and/or diastolic blood pressure ≥90 mmHg) in women aged 18 years or above is 28% [58]. In individuals aged over 65 years, the prevalence of hypertension is higher in women compared to men, with the highest age-adjusted prevalence of hypertension noted in black women aged over 75 years (prevalence of over 70%) [59]. Women over 65 years are more likely to have uncontrolled hypertension compared to men of the same age (44.5% vs. 38.2%), with the difference even greater at over 75 years (61.5% vs 46.5%) [60]. This may partly be explained by differences in care delivery in older women or a higher prevalence of resistant hypertension in women, due to older age and a higher rates of obesity [61]. The higher prevalence of hypertension noted in older women, along with poorer control, together contribute to the increased stroke risk attributable to hypertension observed in older women [62]. In addition, pregnancy-related hypertensive disorders may have chronic effects on cardiovascular health in women, which could contribute to an elevated stroke risk later in life [63]. In a meta-analysis of observational studies, the risk of ischemic stroke per each incremental increase in systolic blood pressure has been found to be similar between the sexes [64].

Atrial Fibrillation

Atrial fibrillation (AF) is the most common cardiac arrhythmia and is a significant risk factor for stroke, associated with a fivefold increase in risk [65]. Irregular contractions of the atria lead to stasis of blood and an increased risk of thrombus formation, particularly in the left atrial appendage. This in turn predisposes to intracardiac thrombosis and, subsequently, ischemic stroke. In high-income countries, about 25% of all ischemic strokes and 36% of strokes in patients >80 years are due to AF [66]. The incidence rates of atrial fibrillation have remained stable; however due to the aging of the population the overall prevalence is rising. The prevalence of AF increases in a stepwise fashion with increasing age, from 1.9% in those aged 40 years or younger, to 46.0% in those aged 90 years or older [67]. Women have a 1.5 to twofold lower risk of developing AF compared to men, however due to a longer life expectancy in women, a higher absolute number of older women have AF compared to men [68]. Approximately 60% of patients with AF aged over 75 years are women [69]. Women with AF have a higher risk of stroke compared to men with AF [70, 71]. For this reason, commonly used stroke risk scoring systems for AF, most notable the CHA_2DS_2-VASc score [Cardiac Failure, Hypertension, Age 75, Diabetes Mellitus, Stroke, Vascular Disease, Age 65–74 and Sex Category (female)]), incorporate female sex as an independent risk factor for stroke [72, 73]. Women with AF, compared to men, tend to have more severe strokes [74] and also have a greater risk of recurrent stroke and post-stroke dependency, even after accounting for comorbidities, stroke subtype and stroke severity [75]. The higher post-stroke mortality in women compared to men has been attributed primarily to advanced age, in addition to increased stroke severity, greater pre-stroke disability and the increased prevalence of AF in older women [76]. Women with AF are less likely than men to be treated appropriately with oral anticoagulant therapy or antiplatelet therapy [77–80]. A recent population based study reported a greater likelihood of women been prescribed a lower dose of dabigatran compared to men (higher dose is considered to be more efficacious), even after accounting for age and comorbidities [81].

Diabetes Mellitus

Diabetes mellitus is a potent risk factor for stroke in both men and women, with an overall twofold increased risk of ischemic stroke [82]. Diabetes mellitus contributes to an increased risk of atherosclerosis and subsequently ischemic stroke. Among ischemic strokes, the risk of lacunar stroke may be particularly increased [83, 84]. The prevalence of diabetes among men and women with stroke is similar; [85] however, diabetes is a stronger risk factor for stroke in women compared to men, with women with diabetes having a 27% higher risk of stroke compared to men with diabetes [86]. Furthermore, women with diabetes have a twofold higher risk of fatal stroke compared to men with diabetes, even after controlling for other stroke risk factors and severity of diabetes [87]. Women with diabetes have a risk of fatal stroke which is comparable to that observed in women who have had a prior stroke, indicating that diabetes mellitus is a stroke risk equivalent [88]. The increasing incidence rates of diabetes and obesity, and their associated higher risk in women compared to men, have been suggested as one explanation for the slower decline in stroke incidence rates in women compared to men in recent decades.

Depression

Depression is an important risk factor for stroke and depression is twice as common in women than men. In a meta-analysis of prospective studies, depression was associated with a 45% increased risk of total stroke, and 55% increased risk of fatal stroke [89]. In the prospective Nurses' Health Study, women with a history of depression had a 30% increased risk of total stroke, compared to with women without a history of depression [90]. Specific tests for effect modification of the association by sex have not been done. The association between depression and stroke is believed to be multifactorial, including increased prevalence of cardiovascular comorbidities; subclinical small vessel cerebrovascular disease predisposing to vascular depression; poor health behaviors including unhealthy diet, reduced physical activity and reduced compliance with medications; and potential biological effects including greater inflammation and increased sympathetic tone [91, 92].

Psychosocial Stress

Chronic stress at home or in the workplace, social isolation, and anxiety are all now thought to be associated with an increased stroke risk [93]. In the INTERSTROKE study, the presence of psychosocial stress, defined as general stress at home and in the workplace (permanent or several periods of stress versus no or some periods of stress in the past year) was associated with a 30% increased risk of stroke (OR 1.30, 99% CI) [56]. Major life events have also been associated with an increased risk of stroke [94]. Women are more likely to have a history of sexual abuse or assault. In the Nurses' Health Study II, 9% of women reported a history of severe physical abuse and 11% reported sexual abuse, and such abuse was associated and 80% increased risk of stroke. Women with a history of abuse were noted to have worse adult health behaviors including higher BMI in adulthood and higher rates of depression and smoking. A history of severe childhood physical abuse and sexual abuse were associated with an increased risk of stroke, partially but not completely mediated by adult health behaviors and medical risk factors [95].

It is important to note that several risk factors appear to have relatively equal associations for stroke risk among both women and men, but should not be ignored for their impact in women. These risk factors include smoking, physical activity, diet, obesity and prior cardiovascular disease.

Future Directions

Whether stroke prevention should look the same in women in men is not clear. Testing and development of sex-specific risk prediction models incorporating risk factors unique to and differentially associated with stroke in women may improve risk classification and stroke prevention in women.

Conclusion

- Stroke is the leading cause of acquired adult disability worldwide and the fourth leading cause of death in women in developed countries, with 60% of stroke deaths occurring in women.
- Women have a number of unique risk factors for stroke, including pregnancy, preeclampsia, gestational diabetes, duration of reproductive life, use of oral contraceptives and post-menopausal hormone therapy.
- Some risk factors are more prevalent or have a stronger association with stroke in women compared to men, including migraine with aura, atrial fibrillation, diabetes mellitus, hypertension, depression and psychosocial stress
- Sex-specific risk prediction models incorporating risk factors unique to and differentially associated with women may improve risk classification and stroke prevention in women.

References

1. World Health Organization. The top 10 causes of death worldwide 2017. Available from: http://www.who.int/mediacentre/factsheets/fs310/en/.
2. Leading causes of death in females. In: Centers for Disease Control and Prevention Website [online]. Available at: cdc.gov/women/lcod/index.htm. Accessed 28 Jan 2018.
3. Leading causes of death in males: United States. In: Centers for Disease Control and Prevention Website [online]. Available at: cdc.gov/men/lcod/2013/index.htm. Accessed 20 Apr 2017.
4. Seshadri S, Beiser A, Kelly-Hayes M, Kase CS, Au R, Kannel WB, et al. The lifetime risk of stroke: estimates from the Framingham Study. Stroke. 2006;37(2):345–50.
5. Benjamin EJ, Blaha MJ, Chiuve SE, Cushman M, Das SR, Deo R, et al. Heart disease and stroke statistics-2017 update: a report from the American Heart Association. Circulation. 2017;135(10):e146–603.
6. Reeves MJ, Bushnell CD, Howard G, Gargano JW, Duncan PW, Lynch G, et al. Sex differences in stroke: epidemiology, clinical presentation, medical care, and outcomes. Lancet Neurol. 2008;7(10):915–26.
7. Leening MJ, Ferket BS, Steyerberg EW, Kavousi M, Deckers JW, Nieboer D, et al. Sex differences in lifetime risk and first manifestation of cardiovascular disease: prospective population based cohort study. BMJ. 2014;349:g5992.
8. Madsen TE, Khoury J, Alwell K, Moomaw CJ, Rademacher E, Flaherty ML, et al. Sex-specific stroke incidence over time in the Greater Cincinnati/Northern Kentucky Stroke Study. Neurology. 2017;89(10):990–6.
9. Koton S, Rexrode KM. Trends in stroke incidence in the United States. Will women overtake men? Neurology. 2017;89(10):982–3.
10. Koton S, Telman G, Kimiagar I, Tanne D. Gender differences in characteristics, management and outcome at discharge and three months after stroke in a national acute stroke registry. Int J Cardiol. 2013;168(4):4081–4.
11. Kittner SJ, Stern BJ, Feeser BR, Hebel R, Nagey DA, Buchholz DW, et al. Pregnancy and the risk of stroke. N Engl J Med. 1996;335(11):768–74.
12. Bushnell C, McCullough LD, Awad IA, Chireau MV, Fedder WN, Furie KL, et al. Guidelines for the prevention of stroke in women: a statement for healthcare professionals from the American Heart Association/American Stroke Association. Stroke. 2014;45(5):1545–88.
13. Scott CA, Bewley S, Rudd A, Spark P, Kurinczuk JJ, Brocklehurst P, et al. Incidence, risk factors, management, and outcomes of stroke in pregnancy. Obstet Gynecol. 2012;120(2 Pt 1):318–24.
14. Bushnell CD, Jamison M, James AH. Migraines during pregnancy linked to stroke and vascular diseases: US population based case-control study. BMJ. 2009;338:b664.
15. James AH, Bushnell CD, Jamison MG, Myers ER. Incidence and risk factors for stroke in pregnancy and the puerperium. Obstet Gynecol. 2005;106(3):509–16.
16. Berends AL, de Groot CJ, Sijbrands EJ, Sie MP, Benneheij SH, Pal R, et al. Shared constitutional risks for maternal vascular-related pregnancy complications and future cardiovascular disease. Hypertension. 2008;51(4):1034–41.
17. Steegers EA, von Dadelszen P, Duvekot JJ, Pijnenborg R. Pre-eclampsia. Lancet. 2010;376(9741):631–44.
18. Smith GN, Pudwell J, Walker M, Wen SW. Ten-year, thirty-year, and lifetime cardiovascular disease risk estimates following a pregnancy complicated by preeclampsia. Can: JOGC = J Obstet Gynecol Can: JOGC. 2012;34(9):830–5.
19. McDonald SD, Malinowski A, Zhou Q, Yusuf S, Devereaux PJ. Cardiovascular sequelae of preeclampsia/eclampsia: a systematic review and meta-analyses. Am Heart J. 2008;156(5):918–30.
20. Bellamy L, Casas JP, Hingorani AD, Williams DJ. Pre-eclampsia and risk of cardiovascular disease and cancer in later life: systematic review and meta-analysis. BMJ. 2007;335(7627):974.
21. Brown MC, Best KE, Pearce MS, Waugh J, Robson SC, Bell R. Cardiovascular disease risk in women with pre-eclampsia: systematic review and meta-analysis. Eur J Epidemiol. 2013;28(1):1–19.
22. Timpka S, Stuart JJ, Tanz LJ, Rimm EB, Franks PW, Rich-Edwards JW. Lifestyle in progression from hypertensive disorders of pregnancy to chronic hypertension in Nurses' Health Study II: observational cohort study. BMJ. 2017;358:j3024.

23. Romundstad PR, Magnussen EB, Smith GD, Vatten LJ. Hypertension in pregnancy and later cardiovascular risk: common antecedents? Circulation. 2010;122(6):579–84.

24. Tobias DK, Stuart JJ, Li S, Chavarro J, Rimm EB, Rich-Edwards J, et al. Association of history of gestational diabetes with long-term cardiovascular disease risk in a large prospective cohort of US women. JAMA Intern Med. 2017;177(12):1735–42.

25. Fadl H, Magnuson A, Ostlund I, Montgomery S, Hanson U, Schwarcz E. Gestational diabetes mellitus and later cardiovascular disease: a Swedish population based case-control study. BJOG: Int J Obstet Gynaecol. 2014;121(12):1530–6.

26. Peters SA, Woodward M. Women's reproductive factors and incident cardiovascular disease in the UK Biobank. Heart. 2018;104:1069–75.

27. Tanz LJ, Stuart JJ, Williams PL, Rimm EB, Missmer SA, Rexrode KM, et al. Preterm delivery and maternal cardiovascular disease in young and middle-aged adult women. Circulation. 2017;135(6):578–89.

28. Ley SH, Li Y, Tobias DK, Manson JE, Rosner B, Hu FB, et al. Duration of reproductive life span, age at menarche, and age at menopause are associated with risk of cardiovascular disease in women. J Am Heart Assoc. 2017;6(11):e006713.

29. Lidegaard O, Lokkegaard E, Jensen A, Skovlund CW, Keiding N. Thrombotic stroke and myocardial infarction with hormonal contraception. N Engl J Med. 2012;366(24):2257–66.

30. Gillum LA, Mamidipudi SK, Johnston SC. Ischemic stroke risk with oral contraceptives: a meta-analysis. JAMA. 2000;284(1):72–8.

31. Chan WS, Ray J, Wai EK, Ginsburg S, Hannah ME, Corey PN, et al. Risk of stroke in women exposed to low-dose oral contraceptives: a critical evaluation of the evidence. Arch Intern Med. 2004;164(7):741–7.

32. Peragallo Urrutia R, Coeytaux RR, McBroom AJ, Gierisch JM, Havrilesky LJ, Moorman PG, et al. Risk of acute thromboembolic events with oral contraceptive use: a systematic review and meta-analysis. Obstet Gynecol. 2013;122(2 Pt 1):380–9.

33. Baillargeon JP, McClish DK, Essah PA, Nestler JE. Association between the current use of low-dose oral contraceptives and cardiovascular arterial disease: a meta-analysis. J Clin Endocrinol Metab. 2005;90(7):3863–70.

34. Chakhtoura Z, Canonico M, Gompel A, Thalabard JC, Scarabin PY, Plu-Bureau G. Progestogen-only contraceptives and the risk of stroke: a meta-analysis. Stroke. 2009;40(4):1059–62.

35. Kemmeren JM, Tanis BC, van den Bosch MA, Bollen EL, Helmerhorst FM, van der Graaf Y, et al. Risk of arterial thrombosis in relation to oral contraceptives (RATIO) study: oral contraceptives and the risk of ischemic stroke. Stroke. 2002;33(5):1202–8.

36. Slooter AJ, Rosendaal FR, Tanis BC, Kemmeren JM, van der Graaf Y, Algra A. Prothrombotic conditions, oral contraceptives, and the risk of ischemic stroke. J Thromb Haemost. 2005;3(6):1213–7.

37. Grodstein F, Manson JE, Stampfer MJ, Rexrode K. Postmenopausal hormone therapy and stroke: role of time since menopause and age at initiation of hormone therapy. Arch Intern Med. 2008;168(8):861–6.

38. Grodstein F, Manson JE, Colditz GA, Willett WC, Speizer FE, Stampfer MJ. A prospective, observational study of postmenopausal hormone therapy and primary prevention of cardiovascular disease. Ann Intern Med. 2000;133(12):933–41.

39. Anderson GL, Limacher M, Assaf AR, Bassford T, Beresford SA, Black H, et al. Effects of conjugated equine estrogen in postmenopausal women with hysterectomy: the women's health initiative randomized controlled trial. JAMA. 2004;291(14):1701–12.

40. Hendrix SL, Wassertheil-Smoller S, Johnson KC, Howard BV, Kooperberg C, Rossouw JE, et al. Effects of conjugated equine estrogen on stroke in the Women's Health Initiative. Circulation. 2006;113(20):2425–34.

41. Rossouw JE, Anderson GL, Prentice RL, LaCroix AZ, Kooperberg C, Stefanick ML, et al. Risks and benefits of estrogen plus progestin in healthy postmenopausal women: principal results from the Women's Health Initiative randomized controlled trial. JAMA. 2002;288(3):321–33.

42. Renoux C, Dell'aniello S, Garbe E, Suissa S. Transdermal and oral hormone replacement therapy and the risk of stroke: a nested case-control study. BMJ. 2010;340:c2519.

43. Rossouw JE, Prentice RL, Manson JE, Wu L, Barad D, Barnabei VM, et al. Postmenopausal hormone therapy and risk of cardiovascular disease by age and years since menopause. JAMA. 2007;297(13):1465–77.

44. Viscoli CM, Brass LM, Kernan WN, Sarrel PM, Suissa S, Horwitz RI. A clinical trial of estrogen-replacement therapy after ischemic stroke. N Engl J Med. 2001;345(17):1243–9.

45. Clarke SC, Kelleher J, Lloyd-Jones H, Slack M, Schofiel PM. A study of hormone replacement therapy in postmenopausal women with ischaemic heart disease: the Papworth HRT atherosclerosis study. BJOG: Int J Obstet Gynaecol. 2002;109(9):1056–62.

46. Merikangas KR. Contributions of epidemiology to our understanding of migraine. Headache. 2013;53(2):230–46.

47. Vetvik KG, MacGregor EA. Sex differences in the epidemiology, clinical features, and pathophysiology of migraine. Lancet Neurol. 2017;16(1):76–87.

48. Champaloux SW, Tepper NK, Monsour M, Curtis KM, Whiteman MK, Marchbanks PA, et al. Use of combined hormonal contraceptives among women with migraines and risk of ischemic stroke. Am J Obstet Gynecol. 2017;216(5):489.e1–7.

49. Li H, Yu Y. Association between ischemic stroke and migraine in elderly Chinese: a case-control study. BMC Geriatr. 2013;13:126.

50. Li L, Schulz UG, Kuker W, Rothwell PM, Oxford Vascular S. Age-specific association of migraine with cryptogenic TIA and stroke: population-based study. Neurology. 2015;85(17):1444–51.

51. Rambarat CA, Elgendy IY, Johnson BD, Reis SE, Thompson DV, Sharaf BL, et al. Migraine headache and long-term cardiovascular outcomes: an extended follow-up of the women's ischemia syndrome evaluation. Am J Med. 2017;130(6):738–43.

52. Kurth T, Winter AC, Eliassen AH, Dushkes R, Mukamal KJ, Rimm EB, et al. Migraine and risk of cardiovascular disease in women: prospective cohort study. BMJ. 2016;353:i2610.

53. Schurks M, Rist PM, Bigal ME, Buring JE, Lipton RB, Kurth T. Migraine and cardiovascular disease: systematic review and meta-analysis. BMJ. 2009;339:b3914.

54. Abanoz Y, Gulen Abanoz Y, Gunduz A, Uluduz D, Ince B, Yavuz B, et al. Migraine as a risk factor for young patients with ischemic stroke: a case-control study. Neurol Sci. 2017;38(4):611–7.

55. Peng KP, Chen YT, Fuh JL, Tang CH, Wang SJ. Migraine and incidence of ischemic stroke: a nationwide population-based study. Cephalalgia. 2017;37(4):327–35.

56. O'Donnell MJ, Xavier D, Liu L, Zhang H, Chin SL, Rao-Melacini P, et al. Risk factors for ischaemic and intracerebral haemorrhagic stroke in 22 countries (the INTERSTROKE study): a case-control study. Lancet. 2010;376(9735):112–23.

57. Johansson BB. Hypertension mechanisms causing stroke. Clin Exp Pharmacol Physiol. 1999;26(7):563–5.

58. Yoon SS, Carroll MD, Fryar CD. Hypertension prevalence and control among adults: United States, 2011-2014. NCHS Data Brief. 2015(220):1–8.

59. Ong KL, Cheung BM, Man YB, Lau CP, Lam KS. Prevalence, awareness, treatment, and control of hypertension among United States adults 1999-2004. Hypertension. 2007;49(1):69–75.

60. 2016. Available from: https://www.cdc.gov/nchs/data/hus/2016/.

61. Muntner P, Davis BR, Cushman WC, Bangalore S, Calhoun DA, Pressel SL, et al. Treatment-resistant hypertension and the incidence of cardiovascular disease and end-stage renal disease: results from

the Antihypertensive and Lipid-Lowering Treatment to Prevent Heart Attack Trial (ALLHAT). Hypertension. 2014;64(5):1012–21.

62. Wenger NK, Ferdinand KC, Bairey Merz CN, Walsh MN, Gulati M, Pepine CJ. Women, hypertension, and the systolic blood pressure intervention trial. Am J Med. 2016;129(10):1030–6.

63. Appelman Y, van Rijn BB, Ten Haaf ME, Boersma E, Peters SA. Sex differences in cardiovascular risk factors and disease prevention. Atherosclerosis. 2015;241(1):211–8.

64. Peters SA, Huxley RR, Woodward M. Comparison of the sex-specific associations between systolic blood pressure and the risk of cardiovascular disease: a systematic review and meta-analysis of 124 cohort studies, including 1.2 million individuals. Stroke. 2013;44(9):2394–401.

65. Wolf P, Abbott R, Kannel W. Atrial fibrillation as an independent risk factor for stroke: the Framingham Study. Stroke. 1991;22(8):983–8.

66. Wolf PA, Abbott RD, Kannel WB. Atrial fibrillation: a major contributor to stroke in the elderly. The Framingham Study. Arch Intern Med. 1987;147(9):1561–4.

67. McGrath ER, Kapral MK, Fang J, Eikelboom JW, O'Conghaile A, Canavan M, et al. Association of atrial fibrillation with mortality and disability after ischemic stroke. Neurology. 2013;81(9):825–32.

68. Ko D, Rahman F, Schnabel RB, Yin X, Benjamin EJ, Christophersen IE. Atrial fibrillation in women: epidemiology, pathophysiology, presentation, and prognosis. Nat Rev Cardiol. 2016;13(6):321–32.

69. Feinberg WM, Blackshear JL, Laupacis A, Kronmal R, Hart RG. Prevalence, age distribution, and gender of patients with atrial fibrillation. Analysis and implications. Arch Intern Med. 1995;155(5):469–73.

70. Shroff GR, Solid CA, Herzog CA. Atrial fibrillation, stroke, and anticoagulation in Medicare beneficiaries: trends by age, sex, and race, 1992-2010. J Am Heart Assoc. 2014;3(3):e000756.

71. Emdin CA, Wong CX, Hsiao AJ, Altman DG, Peters SA, Woodward M, et al. Atrial fibrillation as risk factor for cardiovascular disease and death in women compared with men: systematic review and meta-analysis of cohort studies. BMJ. 2016;532:h7013.

72. Lip GY, Nieuwlaat R, Pisters R, Lane DA, Crijns HJ. Refining clinical risk stratification for predicting stroke and thromboembolism in atrial fibrillation using a novel risk factor-based approach: the euro heart survey on atrial fibrillation. Chest. 2010;137(2):263–72.

73. Gage BF, Waterman AD, Shannon W, Boechler M, Rich MW, Radford MJ. Validation of clinical classification schemes for predicting stroke: results from the National Registry of Atrial Fibrillation. JAMA. 2001;285(22):2864–70.

74. Wagstaff AJ, Overvad TF, Lip GY, Lane DA. Is female sex a risk factor for stroke and thromboembolism in patients with atrial fibrillation? A systematic review and meta-analysis. QJM. 2014;107(12):955–67.

75. Hong Y, Yang X, Zhao W, Zhang X, Zhao J, Yang Y, et al. Sex differences in outcomes among stroke survivors with non-valvular atrial fibrillation in China. Front Neurol. 2017;8:166.

76. Phan HT, Blizzard CL, Reeves MJ, Thrift AG, Cadilhac D, Sturm J, et al. Sex differences in long-term mortality after stroke in the INSTRUCT (INternational STRoke oUtComes sTudy): a meta-analysis of individual participant data. Circ Cardiovasc Qual Outcomes. 2017;10(2):e003436. https://doi.org/10.1161/CIRCOUTCOMES.116.003436.

77. Thompson LE, Maddox TM, Lei L, Grunwald GK, Bradley SM, Peterson PN, et al. Sex differences in the use of oral anticoagulants for atrial fibrillation: a report from the National Cardiovascular Data Registry (NCDR(R)) PINNACLE Registry. J Am Heart Assoc. 2017;6(7):e005801. https://doi.org/10.1161/JAHA.117.005801.

78. Humphries KH, Kerr CR, Connolly SJ, Klein G, Boone JA, Green M, et al. New-onset atrial fibrillation: sex differences in presentation, treatment, and outcome. Circulation. 2001;103(19):2365–70.

79. Singer DE, Chang Y, Fang MC, Borowsky LH, Pomernacki NK, Udaltsova N, et al. The net clinical benefit of warfarin anticoagulation in atrial fibrillation. Ann Intern Med. 2009;151(5):297–305.

80. McGrath ER, Kapral MK, Fang J, Eikelboom JW, Conghaile AO, Canavan M, et al. Antithrombotic therapy after acute ischemic stroke in patients with atrial fibrillation. Stroke. 2014;45(12):3637–42.

81. Avgil Tsadok M, Jackevicius CA, Rahme E, Humphries KH, Pilote L. Sex differences in dabigatran use, safety, and effectiveness in a population-based cohort of patients with atrial fibrillation. Circ Cardiovasc Qual Outcomes. 2015;8(6):593–9.

82. Emerging Risk Factors C, Sarwar N, Gao P, Seshasai SR, Gobin R, Kaptoge S, et al. Diabetes mellitus, fasting blood glucose concentration, and risk of vascular disease: a collaborative meta-analysis of 102 prospective studies. Lancet. 2010;375(9733):2215–22.

83. Iso H, Rexrode K, Hennekens CH, Manson JE. Application of computer tomography-oriented criteria for stroke subtype classification in a prospective study. Ann Epidemiol. 2000;10(2):81–7.

84. Ohira T, Shahar E, Chambless LE, Rosamond WD, Mosley TH Jr, Folsom AR. Risk factors for ischemic stroke subtypes: the Atherosclerosis Risk in Communities study. Stroke. 2006;37(10):2493–8.

85. Madsen TE, Khoury JC, Alwell KA, Moomaw CJ, Demel SL, Flaherty ML, et al. Sex differences in cardiovascular risk profiles of ischemic stroke patients with diabetes in the Greater Cincinnati/Northern Kentucky Stroke Study. J Diabetes. 2017;10:496–501.

86. Peters SA, Huxley RR, Woodward M. Diabetes as a risk factor for stroke in women compared with men: a systematic review and meta-analysis of 64 cohorts, including 775 385 individuals and 12 539 strokes. Lancet. 2014;383:1973–80.

87. Stevens RJ, Coleman RL, Adler AI, Stratton IM, Matthews DR, Holman RR. Risk factors for myocardial infarction case fatality and stroke case fatality in type 2 diabetes: UKPDS 66. Diabetes Care. 2004;27(1):201–7.

88. Ho JE, Paultre F, Mosca L. Is diabetes mellitus a cardiovascular disease risk equivalent for fatal stroke in women? Data from the women's pooling project. Stroke. 2003;34(12):2812–6.

89. Pan A, Sun Q, Okereke OI, Rexrode KM, Hu FB. Depression and risk of stroke morbidity and mortality: a meta-analysis and systematic review. JAMA. 2011;306(11):1241–9.

90. Pan A, Okereke OI, Sun Q, Logroscino G, Manson JE, Willett WC, et al. Depression and incident stroke in women. Stroke. 2011;42(10):2770–5.

91. Wassertheil-Smoller S, Shumaker S, Ockene J, Talavera GA, Greenland P, Cochrane B, et al. Depression and cardiovascular sequelae in postmenopausal women. The Women's Health Initiative (WHI). Arch Intern Med. 2004;164(3):289–98.

92. Smoller JW, Allison M, Cochrane BB, Curb JD, Perlis RH, Robinson JG, et al. Antidepressant use and risk of incident cardiovascular morbidity and mortality among postmenopausal women in the Women's Health Initiative study. Arch Intern Med. 2009;169(22):2128–39.

93. Mackay J, Mensah G. The atlas of heart disease and stroke. Geneva: World Health Organization; 2004.

94. House A, Dennis M, Mogridge L, Hawton K, Warlow C. Life events and difficulties preceding stroke. J Neurol Neurosurg Psychiatry. 1990;53(12):1024–8.

95. Rich-Edwards JW, Mason S, Rexrode K, Spiegelman D, Hibert E, Kawachi I, et al. Physical and sexual abuse in childhood as predictors of early-onset cardiovascular events in women. Circulation. 2012;126(8):920–7.

Gender Differences in Parkinson's Disease

Michael T. Hayes

Parkinson's disease is a fairly common, progressive degenerative disease which affects motor systems (rigidity, bradykinesia, tremor, balance, speech and swallowing) and nonmotor systems (anxiety, depression, insomnia, cognitive function, bowel function and autonomic function). It afflicts one million people in United States and at least four million people worldwide. It's estimated that the disease effects 0.3% of people with in the developed world and 4% of individuals over the age of 80 [1]. The onset, clinical manifestations and, perhaps, responsiveness to medications varies between males in females.

Multiple studies [2–4] demonstrate that the onset of Parkinson's disease occurs about 2 years earlier, on average, in men than women and that approximately twice as many men as women will develop the disease. Some studies [2, 5, 6] suggest that women tend to present with a "milder" phenotype characterized by tremor, depression and medication associated dyskinesias while men tend to present with a form characterized by rigidity, eye movement abnormalities, daytime somnolence, sialorrhea and bradykinesia. Obviously, these clinical subtypes are not specific to males or females but merely tendencies.

Genetic Factors

As to the mechanism, environmental factors, genetic differences and, of course, the effect of sex hormones on development and function of the brain have been implicated in some way. From an environmental standpoint, factors like exposure to herbicides (like paraquat) [7] and head trauma [8] have been implicated in higher rates of Parkinson's disease.

M. T. Hayes (✉)
Department of Neurology, Brigham and Women's Hospital, Boston, MA, USA

South Shore Hospital, Weymouth, MA, USA

Harvard Medical School, Boston, MA, USA
e-mail: mthayes@bwh.harvard.edu

Traditionally, men have been more involved in agricultural jobs and professions and sports that have a higher risk of head trauma associated with them. However, while a correlation has been established, no clear cause and effect has been established related to these factors.

Understandably, the genetics of Parkinson's disease has been an active area of investigation. A growing number of genes have been associated with Parkinson's disease including the LRRK2, PARK7, PINK, PRKN and SCNA genes. The genes associated with Parkinson's disease are, however, only associated with about 2–3% of the cases of Parkinson's disease and thus cannot be a significant factor in explaining the differences in prevalence between males in females.

A specific gene on the Y chromosome, the SRY gene, is important in sex determination insofar as it has a roll in testicular development. More recent investigations show that its expression during adulthood has now been identified and a number of male nonreproductive tissues including the brain (humans, rats and mice). In postmortem and immunologic studies [9], SRY was found to co-localize to neurons of the superchiasmatic nucleus (SCN) that express tyrosine hydrogenous which controls the rate limiting step of dopamine synthesis. This finding suggests that the SRY gene may have a role in regulating the nigrostriatal dopamine system. It was also shown that SRY positively regulated expression of enzymes involved in dopamine synthesis including tyrosine hydroxylase, DOPA decarboxylase in dopamine beta hydroxylase. It has not been clearly determined, however, whether SRY has a roll in midbrain dopamine related disorders that show a sex bias as Parkinson's disease does.

The Effect of Estrogen

All sex hormones are critically important in the structure and functional development of the brain and are uniquely important in determining sex differences and susceptibility to disease. Estrogen is the most abundant and arguably the most active hormone that is likely to convey protection against degenerative diseases that show lower incidences in women than men. There are a number of studies (although mostly retrospective) that show a neuroprotective effect of estrogen. Estrogen replacement therapy can help with Parkinson's disease symptoms early in the disease course and can decrease the risk of developing Parkinson's disease. Bilateral oophorectomy before menopause increases the risks of Parkinson's disease. Parkinson's disease symptoms may increase during menses (when estrogen levels are at their lowest) [10–13]. In patients with early Parkinson's disease, symptoms may deteriorate with the cessation of estrogen therapy [14]. Once the patient has the established disease, however, estrogen does not seem to slow down the progression in females relative to males.

Estrogen has, therefore, been implicated as a hormone that may modify the effects of Parkinson's disease. It is not clear how that occurs. It also does not account for the entire difference in the way that males in females are affected by Parkinson's as the decreased incidence of Parkinson's disease in women continues beyond menopause.

Animal studies have suggested some mechanisms. These models look at the effect of neurotoxins (usually 6 hydroxy-dopamine or 1-methyl-4 phenyl tetrahydropyridine) on the striatum and how that toxicity is modulated by other factors. Sexual dimorphism in the development of the male and female brain may be a factor. Certain anti-apoptotic and anti-oxidant molecules had higher expression in the striatum of female vs. male mice [15]. In the toxin induced models of Parkinson's disease, males suffer greater losses of dopaminergic neurons than females [16, 17]. Furthermore, in this animal model, ovariectomy resulted in larger losses of dopaminergic neurons in females while gonadectomy might males had less severe lesions in the dopaminergic system than gonad intact males.

Clinical observations show gender differences in the onset and course of Parkinson's disease. Some studies have demonstrated earlier onset of Parkinson's disease after ovariectomy or hysterectomy [10, 13]. Haaxma et al. [2] studied 253 Parkinson's disease patients (62% men) with disease duration of less than 10 years, who had yet to be placed on dopaminergic medication. The age of onset was 2.1 years later in females that males. Effects of estrogen were also demonstrated in this study. The more children that a female had, the later the onset of the disease (estimated at 2.7 years/child). The duration of fertile lifespan also positively affected the age of onset. The earlier a woman experienced menopause, the earlier the onset of Parkinson's disease.

This group of patients also underwent single photon emission computed tomography (SPECT) imaging using the tracer [^{123}I] FR-CIT to quantify the amount of nigrostriatal dopamine uptake binding. Women had a 16% higher striatal binding at the onset of disease suggesting a less severe lesion at the time of diagnosis. The rate of decline of tracer binding

(3.1%/year) did not vary between men and women suggesting that progression of the disease (at least by this measure) was about the same. This finding correlates with animal data (very well reviewed by Gillies et al. [20]) which showed a protective effect of estrogen in smaller lesions in the neurotoxic animal model of Parkinson's disease. Once a lesion was greater than 60–70% of the striatal dopaminergic neurons, the protective effect was lost [18, 19]. It is estimated that patients do not become symptomatic until approximately 80% of the dopaminergic neurons are lost. This fits with the clinical finding that, while the onset of Parkinson's disease may be delayed by estrogen (or another factor that correlates with estrogen levels), progression of the disease after it is established is about the same between males in females.

Motor Symptoms

A number of studies have looked at gender differences in the motor manifestations of Parkinson's disease [21–24]. As noted previously, Haaxma et al. found that women tend to present with tremor (which correlated with a slower progression as measured by the Unified Parkinson's Disease Rating Scale (UPDRS III) scores over time) while men presented with bradykinesia and rigidity. Studies noted that women had more difficulty with dyskinesias. Zappia and Accolla [23, 24] both commented that body weight was not taken into account when dosing levodopa and that the levodopa/kilogram ratio tended to be higher in women. However, in clinical practice, levodopa is titrated by clinical response and unwanted side effects. Response to specific doses of levodopa varies widely between individuals. It is also not clear that body weight has any correlation with CNS utilization of levodopa.

Two studies looked at the gender differences in clinical response to functional neurosurgical treatment of Parkinson's disease. Hariz look at the effective pallidotomy, thalamotomy and deep brain stimulation related to gender. He found that women had their surgeries later in the disease course and had lower ADLs scores prior to surgery than men who came to surgery. While the ADLs scores for women were lower prior to surgery, they were similar to the postop scores of men (thus women had a more ADL score improvement than men. It is not clear, from this study, why women presented later in the disease course. It is possible that the women in this group tolerated their symptoms for longer periods of time before considering surgery or treating physicians may have had an element of bias about referring female patients to surgery.

Accolla et al. evaluated patient's before and after deep brain stimulation to the subthalamic nuclei. In this study, no preoperative differences were noted between men and women in terms of duration of disease nor in severity of disease in regards to tremor, rigidity or the ability to perform ADLs. However, women were noted to be more dyskinetic and less responsive to dopaminergic medication for the treatment of bradykinesia (it is, of course, possible that the use of dopaminergic medication was limited by dyskinesias). A year after surgery, both groups were improved but women were still more bradykinetic than men. Women did to do better on performing ADLs but that measure did not reach statistical significance.

Cognition and Other Nonmotor Symptoms

Cognitive decline, anxiety, depression, sleep disturbances and other nonmotor symptoms of Parkinson's disease can, in some cases, be as debilitating as the motor aspects of the disease. Some differences in nonmotor symptoms related to gender, have been found. Picillo et al. [25] studied the prevalence of a number of nonmotor symptoms of Parkinson's disease and found that women suffered more with anxiety, mood changes, and pain than their male counterparts. Interestingly, in the cohort that they studied, there was no difference in the prescribing of dopaminergic or antidepressant/antianxiety medications suggesting that the symptoms were underrecognized or undertreated.

Parkinson's disease patients also developed difficulties in cognition primarily affecting executive function which affects ADLs, verbal recall, visuospatial recognition and attention. Locascio et al. [26] the longitudinal study of males in females with Parkinson's disease over 10 years. As the disease progressed males performed better in the roadmap test direction which requires mental rotation of a map. Women performed better at the letter fluency test. Men's performance deteriorated more quickly for category fluency.

Davidsdottir et al. [27] evaluated visual and spatial abilities in female and male patient with Parkinson's disease. Interestingly, gender and side of onset both played roles. Parkinson's disease is usually an asymmetric process. Men with left-sided onset (right-sided symptoms) had more difficulty estimating spatial relations than the women with left-sided onset. No differences were noted between the sexes who had right-sided onset.

Clark et al. [28] found that male patients with Parkinson's disease had more difficulty recognizing facial emotion (particularly anger and surprise). In the Parkinson's disease group, men had specific difficulties recognizing fearful facial expressions while in the control group, the opposite was noted. Women in the Parkinson's group also reported more difficulty with self assertive and over accommodating behavior.

A study by Nicoletti et al. [29] also looked at non-motor symptoms and found that depression was significantly more frequent in females as were urinary disturbances but that

men had more difficulty with cognitive impairment, hallucinations and sleep disorders. Furthermore, Perrin et al. [30] found that depression tended to be manifested differently relative to gender, with women having more melancholy and men having more apathy and loss of libido.

Cereda and Cilia [31] looked at the onset of dementia by DSM-IV criteria in 6599 patients and found that age and disease duration were independently associated with dementia. Male gender was also an independent risk factor and higher rates of dementia were found in males between the age of 60 and 80. The prevalence of dementia in females also increased after the age of 65 but did not catch up with the male prevalence until after age 80. Fernandez et al. [32] focused on Parkinson's disease patients in nursing homes diagnosed with dementia. They found that men showed more wandering, verbal and physical abusiveness and inappropriate behavior while women exhibited more depression (as seen in other studies). Another interesting finding in this study was that men were more likely to be treated with antipsychotic medication while women were treated with antidepressant medication regardless of the behavioral symptoms.

Pregnancy

Because Parkinson's disease is a disease with typical onset after the age of 50, pregnancies are fairly rare. Parkinson's disease presents before the age of 40 in only about 5% of cases. Still, pregnancies do occur. The literature (understandably) consists mainly of reports of small numbers of patients with varying findings, some reporting worsening of Parkinson's disease during pregnancies and other suggesting stabilization or even improvement. Two large studies, Golbe [33] in 1987 and a review by Hagell et al. [34] in 1998, looked at larger numbers of patients. In the Golbe study, 65% (11 patients) reported worsening of their parkinsonian symptoms and 10 of the 11 patients felt that they did not return to baseline after the pregnancy. Five of those patients did not receive any medication for the treatment of Parkinson's disease during her pregnancy. In the Hagell review (26 women with a total of 35 pregnancies), 46% of patients reported worsening of the symptoms. A quarter of those patients did not receive medication for Parkinson's disease during pregnancies.

Sier and Hiller [35] reviewed the aggregate data of 28 studies done between 1985 and 2016 is reported births to Parkinson's disease. Seventy-four births were recorded. Forty-eight percent reported worsening symptoms during pregnancy. Fifty-two percent had no change or improved symptoms. Treatment regimens were so disperate that conclusions about optimal treatment were difficult to make. In this group, however, 83% received medications for Parkinson's disease of which 63% felt that they were unchanged or improved through their pregnancies. In the patients not treated with antiparkinsonian medications, only 33% felt that there was no change or that there was improvement. Based on that data alone, it would seem advisable to treat Parkinson's disease during pregnancy.

The authors suggest that it is counterintuitive for symptoms to be worse in pregnancy when estrogen levels are high as estrogen is felt to be protective. However, as noted earlier here, the protective action of estrogen ceases to be a factor once the disease is established.

Potential reasons for worsening of Parkinson's disease include the progression of a degenerative neurologic disorder, physiologic changes during pregnancy, for instance increased plasma volume and changes in volume distribution and metabolic state and physical and psychological stress area.

The review of the literature by Seier and Hiller found no problems with fertility or conception, no increased Cesarian-section rate, no bleeding issues beyond a single placental abruption and no increased rate of spontaneous abortions. It also detailed 46 levodopa exposed pregnancies. Eight complications were noted which included a case of placental abruption (with concurrent use of cabergoline), preeclampsia (concurrent use of amantadine), seizure in the infant 1 h after birth (concurrent use of high-dose bromocriptine), a ventricular septal defect (concurrent use of entacapone and selegiline), osteomalacia and transient hypotonia. All of these children were subsequently reported to be healthy with normal development.

There is little human data on the effects of medication for Parkinson's disease in terms of teratogenicity except for some data on amantadine [36–38]. Amantadine should not be considered as a treatment for Parkinson's disease during pregnancy.

Report by Scelzo et al. [39] included three cases of women implanted with deep brain stimulators for Parkinson's disease which resulted in reduced motor fluctuations and dyskinesias as well as reductions in medication which allowed for them to have successful pregnancies.

Pregnancies can occur during Parkinson's disease and can be brought to full term with successful births. It appears advisable to treat the patient's symptomatically during the pregnancies, primarily with carbidopa levodopa as opposed to other medications. Whether the pregnancy itself has any negative impact on the progression of the disease is unclear at present.

References

1. Dexter DT, Jenner P. Parkinson's disease from pathology to molecular disease mechanisms. Free Radic Biol Med. 2013;62:132–44.

2. Haaxma CA, Bloem BR, Borm GT, et al. Gender differences in Parkinson's disease. J Neurol Neurosurg Psychiatry. 2007;78:819–24.

3. Wooten GF, Currie LJ, Boubjerg VE, et al. Are men at greater risk for Parkinson's disease than women? J Neurol Neurosurg Psychiatry. 2004;75:637–9.

4. Van Den Eeden SK, Tanner CM, Bernstein AL, et al. Incidence of Parkinson's disease: variations by age, gender and race/ethnicity. Am J Epidemiol. 2003;157:1015–22.

5. Shulman LM, Bhat V. Gender disparities in Parkinson's disease. Expert Rev Neurother. 2006;6:407–16.

6. Martinez-Martin P, Falup P, Odin P, et al. Gender-related differences in the burden of nonmotor symptoms in Parkinson's disease. J Neurol. 2012;259:1639–47.

7. Semchuk KM, Love EJ, Lee RG. Parkinson's disease and exposure to agricultural work and pesticide chemicals. Neurology. 1992;42:1328–35.

8. Bruns J, Hauser WA. The epidemiology of traumatic brain injury: a review. Epilepsia. 2003;44(suppl.10):2–10.

9. Czech DP, Lee J, et al. The human testis-determining factor SRY localizes in midbrain dopamine neurons and regulates multiple components of catecholamine synthesis and metabolism. J Neurochem. 2012;122:260–71.

10. Benedetti MD, Maraganore DM, et al. Hysterectomy, menopause and estrogen use preceding Parkinson's disease: an exploratory case control study. Mov Disord. 2001;16:830–7.

11. Currie LJ, Harrison MB, et al. Postmenopausal estrogen use affects risk for Parkinson's disease. Arch Neurol. 2004;61:886–8.

12. Liu B, Dluzen DE, et al. Oestrogen and nigrostriatal dopaminergic neurodegeneration: animal models and clinical reports of Parkinson's disease. Clin Exp Pharmacol Physiol. 2007;34:555–65.

13. Rocca WA, Bower JH, et al. Increased risk of parkinsonism in women who underwent oophorectomy before menopause. Neurology. 2008;70:200–9.

14. Sandyk R. Estrogens and the pathophysiology of Parkinson's disease. Int J Neurosci. 1989;45:119–22.

15. Rodriguez-Navarro JA, Solano RM, et al. Gender differences and estrogen effects and parkin null mice. J Neurochem. 2008;106:2143–57.

16. Gillies GE, Murray HE, et al. Sex dimorphisms in the neuroprotective effects of estrogen in an animal model of Parkinson's disease. Pharmacol Biochem Behav. 2004;78:513–22.

17. McArthur S, Murray HE, et al. Striatal susceptibility to a dopaminergic neurotoxin is independent of sex hormone effects on cell survival and DAT expression but is exacerbated by central aromatase inhibition. Neuropsychopharmacology. 2007;32:1462–76.

18. Dluzen D. Estrogen decreases corpus striatal neurotoxicity in response to 6-hydroxydopamine. Brain Res. 1997;767:340–4.

19. Ferraz AC, Matheussi F, et al. Evaluation of estrogen neuroprotective effect on nigrostriatal dopaminergic neurons following 6-hydroxydopamine injection into the substantia nigra pars compacta or the medial forebrain bundle. Neurochem Res. 2008;33:1238–46.

20. Gillies GE, Pienaar IS, et al. Sex differences in Parkinson's disease. Front Neuroendocrinol. 2014;35:370–84.

21. Hariz GM, Lindberg M, et al. Gender differences in disability and health-related quality of life in patients with Parkinson's disease treated with stereotactic surgery. Acta Neurol Scand. 2003;108:28–37.

22. Baba Y, Putzke JD, et al. Gender and Parkinson's disease phenotype. J Neurol. 2005;252:1201–5.

23. Accolla E, Caputo E, et al. Gender differences in patients with Parkinson's disease treated with subthalamic deep brain stimulation. Mov Disord. 2007;22:1150–6.

24. Zappia M, Crescibene L, et al. Body weight influences pharmacokinetics of levodopa in Parkinson's disease. Neurol Sci. 2002;23(Suppl 2):S53–4.

25. Picillo M, Palladino R, et al. Gender and non-motor fluctuations and Parkinson's disease: a prospective study. Parkinsonism Relat Disord. 2016;27:89–92.

26. Locascio JJ, Corkin S, et al. Relation between clinical characteristics of Parkinson's disease and cognitive decline. J Clin Exp Neuropsychol. 2003;25(1):94–109.

27. Davidsdottir S, Cronin-Golomb A, Lee A. Visual and facial symptoms in Parkinson's disease. Vis Res. 2005;45(10):1285–96.

28. Clark US, Neargardner S, Cronin-Golomb A. A visual exploration of emotional facial expressions in Parkinson's disease. Neurophychologia. 2010;48(7):1901–13.

29. Nicolletti A, Vaste R. Gender effect on nonmotor symptoms of Parkinson's disease. Parkinsonism Relat Disord. 2016;35:69–74.

30. Perrin AJ, Nosova E, et al. Gender differences in Parkinson's disease depression. Parkinsonism Relat Disord. 2017;36:93–7.

31. Cereda E, Cilia R, et al. Dementia in Parkinson's disease: is male gender a risk factor? Parkinsonism Relat Disord. 2016;26:67–72.

32. Fernandez HH, Lapane KL, et al. Gender differences in the frequency and treatment of behavior problems in Parkinson's disease. SAGE Study Group. Systemic assessment and geriatric drug use the a epidemiology. Mov Disord. 2000;15(3):490–6.

33. Golbe LI. Parkinson's disease and pregnancy. Neurology. 1987;37:1245–9.

34. Hagell P, Odin P, Vinge E. Pregnancy in Parkinson's disease: a review of the literature and a case report. Mov Disord. 1998;13:34–8.

35. Seier M, Hiller A. Parkinson's disease and pregnancy: an updated review. Parkinsonism Relat Disord. 2017;40:11–7.

36. Rosa F. Amantadine pregnancy experience. Reprod Toxicol. 1994;8:531.

37. Nora JJ, Nora AH, Way GL. Cardiovascular maldevelopment associated with maternal exposure to amantadine. Lancet. 1975;2:607.

38. Pandit PB, Chitayat D, Jefferie AL, Qamar IU, Koren G. Tibial hemimelia and tetralogy of Fallot associated with first trimester exposure to amantadine. Reprod Toxicol. 1994;8:89–92.

39. Scelzo E, Mehrkens JH, Botzel K, Krack P, Mendes A, Chabardes S, et al. Deep brain stimulation during pregnancy and delivery: experience from a series of "DBS babies". Front Neurol. 2015;6:191.

Sex-Related Differences in Alzheimer's Disease

Diler Acar and Carolyn Jane King

Alzheimer's disease (AD) is a progressive neurodegenerative disease leading to cognitive deficits, functional impairment as well as behavioral changes. The pathophysiology of AD involves the accumulation of neurotoxic amyloid beta protein (Aβ), in early phases, inducing inflammatory and microglial cascades, mitochondrial dysfunction and oxidative stress. These processes then lead to hyperphosphorylation of the microtubule stabilizing protein tau and formation of neurofibrillary tangles. These changes cause synaptic and neuronal dysfunction by disruption of intracellular signaling and widespread cortical dysfunction. Accumulation of amyloid plaques and neurofibrillary tangles further disrupt synaptic integrity and result in neuronal cell death. Despite these well-defined neuropathological hallmarks, human and animal models demonstrate that amyloid plaque burden and distribution do not correlate with cognitive deficit. Neurofibrillary tangles can exist without neuronal impairment, and it is the synaptic loss and network dysfunction that are thought to be related to cognitive deficit [1–4].

AD is the most common cause of dementia, affecting 5.5 million Americans. In 2014, AD was recorded to be the sixth leading cause of death in the United States and the fifth leading cause of death in among those 65 years of age and older. Between 2000 and 2014, the number of deaths from AD increased 89%, whereas deaths resulting from stroke and heart disease decreased by 21% and 14% [5], respectively.

In the United States, two-thirds of patients with AD are women with 3.3 million women carrying the diagnosis. In age 71 and older, 16% of women have AD or other dementias compared to 11% of men [5]. Hormones exert significant effects on brain function and there are multiple complexities of their action on the pathogenesis of AD. Due to these complexities, there is limited research exploring sex differences in AD.

Higher prevalence of AD among women is not well understood. The sex-related disparity may be partially due to greater female lifespan as older age is the strongest risk factor for AD [6–8]. The Framingham heart study reported that men who survive beyond age 65 might have lower cardiovascular risk factors – "survival bias" – which may explain the lower risk of dementia in men compared to women after age 80 [9]. While men have a higher prevalence of Mild Cognitive Impairment (MCI) preceding AD, women tend to transition from normal cognition to AD at a later age but more precipitously [10–14]. Also, AD has a less aggressive course in women compared to men [8, 15, 16]. Although most studies in the United States report no significant difference in incidence between men in women, multiple European studies and the Cache County study showed a higher incidence of AD in women compared to men after age 80 [17–23]. Furthermore, women tend to have a higher rate of conversion from MCI to AD after age 80 [13].

Potential Risk Factors for Women

Sex-specific neuroanatomical, neurochemical and psychosocial differences may be pertinent for the development of AD pathology. The male brain is 10% larger than female brain [24]. Gray and white matter volumes also vary by sex [25, 26]. When compared for intracranial volume, height and weight, women have a higher percentage of gray matter, whereas men have a higher percentage of white matter and cerebrospinal fluid (CSF) [27]. Studies show consistently higher gray/white matter ratio in frontal, temporal, parietal, and occipital lobes, cingulate gyrus, and insula in women versus men [25, 27–30] as well as thicker gray matter in the parietal cortex in women [25, 31, 32]. Men have larger amygdala and hypothalamus; women have larger caudate and hippocampus [33].

Sex-related differences in the human brain are of increasing interest, with studies exploring differences in cognitive abilities, namely better verbal skills in women

D. Acar (✉) · C. J. King
Brigham and Women's Hospital, Boston, MA, USA
e-mail: dacar@bwh.harvard.edu

© Springer Nature Switzerland AG 2019
M. A. O'Neal (ed.), *Neurology and Psychiatry of Women*, https://doi.org/10.1007/978-3-030-04245-5_25

and better spatial abilities in men. In men, IQ score correlates with gray matter volume in the frontal and parietal lobes; whereas in women, it correlates mainly with gray matter volume in the frontal lobe [30]. There is accumulating data suggesting that the adult male brain is asymmetrically organized compared to women [34]. In adult men, volume loss in the whole brain, frontal and temporal lobes increases with age, whereas in women, volume loss in the hippocampus and parietal lobes increases with age [35]. Global grey matter volume decreases linearly with age with a steeper decline in men [36, 37], a finding that has been confirmed postmortem [38]. In individuals with MCI or AD, brain volume declines faster in women than men [39]. Studies of sex differences in cognitive change over time also indicated resilience in women compared with men [40]. The reasons for these differences are thought to be related to the female sex steroids. There are, however, no studies on the effects of female sex steroids in the living human brain.

Some studies showed that women have higher global cerebral blood flow compared to men during rest [41, 42] and cognitive activity [42–46]. The cerebral metabolic rate of glucose utilization tends to be higher in women compared to men [47], particularly in the orbitofrontal area [48], although this finding has not been replicated consistently [49–51]. Regional glucose utilization also varies with the phases of menstrual cycle, emphasizing the hormonal effects on the brain glucose metabolism [52].

Presence of APOE ε4 allele significantly increases the risk of AD and lowers the age of onset [53–55]. Earlier studies suggested that women who carry one or two copies of APOE ε4 have a higher risk of AD and are significantly more likely to convert from MCI to AD than men [55, 56]. In a recent meta-analysis of 27 studies, while women and men between ages 55 and 85 years with one copy of ApoE ε4 showed no difference in AD risk, women who were between ages 55 and 70 years had increased risk of MCI [55].

There are some studies suggesting that sex can modify the expression of ApoE ε4 in the human brain. Female ε4 carriers showed reduced functional connectivity in the precuneus, a major hub of default-mode network [57] and smaller hippocampal volume [56]. Female ε4 carriers with a diagnosis of MCI had significantly higher CSF levels of total tau, indicative of neuronal injury [56]. Sex-related differences on the effect of ApoE genotype raises the possibility of gene-hormone interactions, which may have both diagnostic and therapeutic implications.

DNA telomere length is linked with normal cellular aging and shortening of it has been shown in neurodegeneration, particularly in AD [58]. Estrogen depletion has been shown to cause telomer shortening in healthy, postmenopausal women with ApoE ε4 genotype, which was reversed by hormonal therapy [59].

Hormones and AD

Animals studies have identified neuroprotective actions of sex hormones by means of increasing neuronal plasticity, improving their functioning, counteracting AD pathogenesis. In the aging brain, depletion of sex gonadal steroids increases the susceptibility to AD, but the mechanism of such effect is unclear. The hormonal loss due to menopause is quite abrupt in women but more gradual in aging men. There are studies indicating that AD pathology may cause negative feedback on hormonal levels by inhibiting neurosteroidogenesis, thus reducing their neuroprotection. Sex hormones have been implicated in regulation and clearance of Aβ by promoting amyloid precursor protein processing (APP), stimulating microglial phagocytosis [60] and increasing the expression of Aβ degrading enzymes [61–64].

There are studies indicating estradiol's role in synaptic plasticity and hippocampal-dependent learning and memory as well as increased excitability [65–67] in normal brain. Similar effects of estradiol have not been consistently observed in the diseased brain.

Estradiol suppresses β secretase enzyme which initiates Aβ accumulation [68] and increases the beta-amyloid catabolizing insulin degrading enzyme [69]. There are multiple studies indicating that hormone replacement therapy (HRT) can decrease Aβ levels and plaques [68–75] but increased levels of Aβ do not seem to improve cognition. Neurological symptoms that appear during perimenopause are mostly due to disruption in estrogen-dependent systems (including thermoregulation, sleep, circadian rhythms) which can affect multiple domains of cognition [76]. Women in the first year of post-menopause performed significantly worse than women in the late menopausal transition stages on measures of verbal learning, verbal memory, and motor function [77], most likely indicating the effects of hormonal changes on cognition.

Most studies found that HRT does not provide any benefit for the treatment of AD, and the preventative trials showed inconsistent results. Other studies suggested that postmenopausal women treated with HRT are less likely to develop AD, and the risk may be negatively associated with dose and duration. The Cache County study showed that the greatest reduction of risk was achieved when HRT was used more than 10 years [78]. The Women's Health Initiative Memory study showed an increased risk of dementia with HRT, particularly in the estrogen plus progesterone treated group [79–81]. These results were attributed to late start of HRT.

HRT regimens, as well as formulations have also been studied to understand these discrepant findings [82]. The start age of HRT may be the key factor in explaining the potential protective effect of HRT ("window of opportunity hypothesis"). The Cache County study found that HRT within 5 years of menopause was protective. Recent studies paying attention to this observation revealed that HRT during the critical window resulted in reduced Aβ accumulation [83] but no benefit on cognition [84–86]. A recent prospective cohort study of 8195 women-concluded that there was no strong evidence for a protective effect of postmenopausal HRT although risk of AD was reduced among those with long-term (more than 10 years) self-reported use [87].

The KEEPS study compared the effects of conjugated equine estrogen plus progesterone and transdermal estradiol to placebo [84]. On average participants were 52.6-years-old with 1.4 year past their last menstrual period. HRT did not make any improvement in cognition, but oral conjugated equine estrogen improved affective symptoms (anxiety and depression).

Education

Education is a key factor for cognitive reserve which affects the onset of AD. There is a well-known discrepancy between women and men in educational achievement in United States population older than 65 years, putting women at risk. Low education is a risk factor for dementia [88–93], which may explain the higher risk of dementia in women especially born in the first half of 20 the century [94]. Low education results in low-skilled jobs and less occupational engagement which can directly affect cognitive reserve. Even though women, in general, are more engaged in social cognitive activities, low education has greater impact on cognitive reserve.

Cardiovascular and Metabolic Factors

There is a strong correlation between cardiovascular disease and a higher incidence of dementia. Obesity is a well-known precursor to many disorders, including type 2 diabetes, metabolic syndrome, cardiovascular disease, hypertension (HTN) and hyperlipidemia [95, 96]. Obesity-related comorbidities increase the risk of AD [97]. Insulin resistance and dysregulation of insulin increase risk of dementia [98]. Metabolic syndrome, as well as type 2 diabetes have been associated with increased risk of AD [99–101]. Type 2 diabetes has been also shown to accelerate the age-related cognitive decline [102]. Some studies suggest that dementia risk is adversely affected by central obesity rather than body mass index [103]. Obesity and high-fat diet induce the release of inflammatory cytokines that are detrimental to the brain [104]. Menopause and aging increase central obesity and inflammation both of which are implicated in the initiation and progression of AD [105].

Although mid-adulthood HTN is more common in men, HTN was associated with higher risk of dementia in women [106]. The Framingham Heart Study also showed that women develop cardiovascular disease a decade later than men and men have higher mortality from cardiovascular diseases between the ages of 45 and 65 which might partly explain the higher prevalence of dementia in women compared to men in older ages [9].

Depression, Stress, and Insomnia

Depression is considered a risk factor and prodromal state for AD [107], MCI and for progression from MCI to AD [108]. Women are more likely to suffer from depression [109–111] and anxiety, and thus are found to be more at risk for MCI and AD [112, 113]. However, one study showed that depression was a risk factor for men, not for women [114]. Another study reported that female APOE e4 carriers with more than 10 years of depression was at risk for dementia [115].

Variations in serotonin 5-HT function may explain the known sex-related difference (higher levels in women than men) in the prevalence of depression [109]. There is some evidence that treatment with selective serotonin reuptake inhibitors reduces accumulation of Aβ plaques in animal brains and decreases levels of Aβ in CSF in humans [116].

Insomnia is also a risk factor for dementia [117] which is more commonly seen in women [118]. Poor sleep quality was found to be associated with a higher amyloid burden and decreased connectivity in the default mode network [119].

There is limited data on the sex-specific efficacy and safety of cholinesterase inhibitors and memantine. A systematic review of 48 studies showed that only two studies examined the potential effects of sex on treatment efficacy and did not show any sex-related differences [120].

Role as a Caregiver

In 2016, more than 15 million family members and other unpaid caregivers provided an estimated about 18 billion hours of care to people with AD or other dementias [5]. Sex-related differences in caregiving are particularly relevant for dementia care. Approximately two-thirds of the caregivers are women [121, 122], one-third are daughters [123–126] In general, it is more common for wives to be the care givers for their husbands [127]. Women spent more time, take more responsibility, have more endurance than men as caregivers [128] thus, they are more likely to experience stress-related physical and mental health problems. Women lose income due to the reduction in the number of work hours or early exit from the workforce. For those who remain in the workforce, the responsibility of being a caregiver can increase absenteeism, stress-related health plan spending as well as disability claims.

We need an expansion of neuroscience research to study sex-related susceptibility to neurodegenerative diseases. There is much to study on sex-related differences in dementia and AD as the incidence, prevalence, morbidity, and mortality disparities are well known facts. Further studies should also explore the contribution of sex chromosomes, use approaches to address sex as a biological variable, and must include sex-specific data analyses.

References

1. Palop JJ, Chin J, Mucke L. A network dysfunction perspective on neurodegenerative diseases. Nature. 2006;443(7113):768–73.
2. DeKosky ST, Scheff SW. Synapse loss in frontal cortex biopsies in Alzheimer's disease: correlation with cognitive severity. Ann Neurol. 1990;27(5):457–64.
3. Pievani M, de Haan W, Wu T, Seeley WW, Frisoni GB. Functional network disruption in the degenerative dementias. Lancet Neurol. 2011;10(9):829–43.
4. Palop JJ, Mucke L. Amyloid-beta-induced neuronal dysfunction in Alzheimer's disease: from synapses toward neural networks. Nat Neurosci. 2010;13(7):812–8.
5. Association As. 2017 Alzheimer's disease facts and figures. Alzheimers Dement. 2017;13(4):325–73.
6. Seshadri S, Wolf PA, Beiser A, Au R, McNulty K, White R, et al. Lifetime risk of dementia and Alzheimer's disease. The impact of mortality on risk estimates in the Framingham Study. Neurology. 1997;49(6):1498–504.
7. Hebert LE, Scherr PA, McCann JJ, Beckett LA, Evans DA. Is the risk of developing Alzheimer's disease greater for women than for men? Am J Epidemiol. 2001;153(2):132–6.
8. Larson EB, Shadlen MF, Wang L, McCormick WC, Bowen JD, Teri L, et al. Survival after initial diagnosis of Alzheimer disease. Ann Intern Med. 2004;140(7):501–9.
9. Chêne G, Beiser A, Au R, Preis SR, Wolf PA, Dufouil C, et al. Gender and incidence of dementia in the Framingham Heart Study from mid-adult life. Alzheimers Dement. 2015;11(3):310–20.
10. Petersen RC, Roberts RO, Knopman DS, Geda YE, Cha RH, Pankratz VS, et al. Prevalence of mild cognitive impairment is higher in men. The Mayo Clinic Study of Aging. Neurology. 2010;75(10):889–97.
11. Ganguli M, Dodge HH, Shen C, DeKosky ST. Mild cognitive impairment, amnestic type: an epidemiologic study. Neurology. 2004;63(1):115–21.
12. Koivisto K, Reinikainen KJ, Hänninen T, Vanhanen M, Helkala EL, Mykkänen L, et al. Prevalence of age-associated memory impairment in a randomly selected population from eastern Finland. Neurology. 1995;45(4):741–7.
13. Roberts RO, Geda YE, Knopman DS, Cha RH, Pankratz VS, Boeve BF, et al. The incidence of MCI differs by subtype and is higher in men: the Mayo Clinic Study of Aging. Neurology. 2012;78(5):342–51.
14. Caracciolo B, Palmer K, Monastero R, Winblad B, Bäckman L, Fratiglioni L. Occurrence of cognitive impairment and dementia in the community: a 9-year-long prospective study. Neurology. 2008;70(19 Pt 2):1778–85.
15. Fitzpatrick AL, Kuller LH, Lopez OL, Kawas CH, Jagust W. Survival following dementia onset: Alzheimer's disease and vascular dementia. J Neurol Sci. 2005;229-230:43–9.
16. Ganguli M, Dodge HH, Shen C, Pandav RS, DeKosky ST. Alzheimer disease and mortality: a 15-year epidemiological study. Arch Neurol. 2005;62(5):779–84.
17. Knopman DS, Roberts RO, Pankratz VS, Cha RH, Rocca WA, Mielke MM, et al. Incidence of dementia among participants and nonparticipants in a longitudinal study of cognitive aging. Am J Epidemiol. 2014;180(4):414–23.
18. Bachman DL, Wolf PA, Linn RT, Knoefel JE, Cobb JL, Belanger AJ, et al. Incidence of dementia and probable Alzheimer's disease in a general population: the Framingham Study. Neurology. 1993;43(3 Pt 1):515–9.
19. Miech RA, Breitner JC, Zandi PP, Khachaturian AS, Anthony JC, Mayer L. Incidence of AD may decline in the early 90s for men, later for women: The Cache County study. Neurology. 2002;58(2):209–18.
20. Letenneur L, Gilleron V, Commenges D, Helmer C, Orgogozo JM, Dartigues JF. Are sex and educational level independent predictors of dementia and Alzheimer's disease? Incidence data from the PAQUID project. J Neurol Neurosurg Psychiatry. 1999;66(2):177–83.
21. Ott A, Breteler MM, van Harskamp F, Stijnen T, Hofman A. Incidence and risk of dementia. The Rotterdam Study. Am J Epidemiol. 1998;147(6):574–80.
22. Fratiglioni L, Viitanen M, von Strauss E, Tontodonati V, Herlitz A, Winblad B. Very old women at highest risk of dementia and Alzheimer's disease: incidence data from the Kungsholmen Project, Stockholm. Neurology. 1997;48(1):132–8.
23. Brayne C, Gill C, Huppert FA, Barkley C, Gehlhaar E, Girling DM, et al. Incidence of clinically diagnosed subtypes of dementia in an elderly population. Cambridge Project for Later Life. Br J Psychiatry. 1995;167(2):255–62.
24. Giedd JN, Raznahan A, Mills KL, Lenroot RK. Review: magnetic resonance imaging of male/female differences in human adolescent brain anatomy. Biol Sex Differ. 2012;3(1):19.
25. Allen JS, Damasio H, Grabowski TJ, Bruss J, Zhang W. Sexual dimorphism and asymmetries in the gray-white composition of the human cerebrum. NeuroImage. 2003;18(4):880–94.
26. Paus T, Otaky N, Caramanos Z, MacDonald D, Zijdenbos A, D'Avirro D, et al. In vivo morphometry of the intrasulcal gray matter in the human cingulate, paracingulate, and superior-rostral sulci: hemispheric asymmetries, gender differences and probability maps. J Comp Neurol. 1996;376(4):664–73.
27. Gur RC, Turetsky BI, Matsui M, Yan M, Bilker W, Hughett P, et al. Sex differences in brain gray and white matter in healthy young adults: correlations with cognitive performance. J Neurosci. 1999;19(10):4065–72.
28. Peters M, Jäncke L, Staiger JF, Schlaug G, Huang Y, Steinmetz H. Unsolved problems in comparing brain sizes in Homo sapiens. Brain Cogn. 1998;37(2):254–85.
29. Goldstein JM, Seidman LJ, Horton NJ, Makris N, Kennedy DN, Caviness VS, et al. Normal sexual dimorphism of the adult human brain assessed by in vivo magnetic resonance imaging. Cereb Cortex. 2001;11(6):490–7.
30. Haier RJ, Jung RE, Yeo RA, Head K, Alkire MT. The neuroanatomy of general intelligence: sex matters. NeuroImage. 2005;25(1):320–7.
31. Nopoulos P, Flaum M, O'Leary D, Andreasen NC. Sexual dimorphism in the human brain: evaluation of tissue volume, tissue composition and surface anatomy using magnetic resonance imaging. Psychiatry Res. 2000;98(1):1–13.
32. Carne RP, Vogrin S, Litewka L, Cook MJ. Cerebral cortex: an MRI-based study of volume and variance with age and sex. J Clin Neurosci. 2006;13(1):60–72.
33. Cosgrove KP, Mazure CM, Staley JK. Evolving knowledge of sex differences in brain structure, function, and chemistry. Biol Psychiatry. 2007;62(8):847–55.
34. Mcglone J. Sex differences in human brain asymmetry: a critical survey. Behav Brain Sci. 1980;3(2):215–27.

35. Murphy DG, DeCarli C, McIntosh AR, Daly E, Mentis MJ, Pietrini P, et al. Sex differences in human brain morphometry and metabolism: an in vivo quantitative magnetic resonance imaging and positron emission tomography study on the effect of aging. Arch Gen Psychiatry. 1996;53(7):585–94.

36. Blatter DD, Bigler ED, Gale SD, Johnson SC, Anderson CV, Burnett BM, et al. Quantitative volumetric analysis of brain MR: normative database spanning 5 decades of life. AJNR Am J Neuroradiol. 1995;16(2):241–51.

37. Good CD, Johnsrude IS, Ashburner J, Henson RN, Friston KJ, Frackowiak RS. A voxel-based morphometric study of ageing in 465 normal adult human brains. NeuroImage. 2001;14(1 Pt 1):21–36.

38. Witelson SF, Beresh H, Kigar DL. Intelligence and brain size in 100 postmortem brains: sex, lateralization and age factors. Brain. 2006;129(Pt 2):386–98.

39. Skup M, Zhu H, Wang Y, Giovanello KS, Lin JA, Shen D, et al. Sex differences in grey matter atrophy patterns among AD and aMCI patients: results from ADNI. NeuroImage. 2011;56(3):890–906.

40. McCarrey AC, An Y, Kitner-Triolo MH, Ferrucci L, Resnick SM. Sex differences in cognitive trajectories in clinically normal older adults. Psychol Aging. 2016;31(2):166–75.

41. Devous MD, Stokely EM, Chehabi HH, Bonte FJ. Normal distribution of regional cerebral blood flow measured by dynamic single-photon emission tomography. J Cereb Blood Flow Metab. 1986;6(1):95–104.

42. Gur RC, Gur RE, Obrist WD, Hungerbuhler JP, Younkin D, Rosen AD, et al. Sex and handedness differences in cerebral blood flow during rest and cognitive activity. Science. 1982;217(4560):659–61.

43. Jones K, Johnson KA, Becker JA, Spiers PA, Albert MS, Holman BL. Use of singular value decomposition to characterize age and gender differences in SPECT cerebral perfusion. J Nucl Med. 1998;39(6):965–73.

44. Slosman DO, Chicherio C, Ludwig C, Genton L, de Ribaupierre S, Hans D, et al. (133) Xe SPECT cerebral blood flow study in a healthy population: determination of T-scores. J Nucl Med. 2001;42(6):864–70.

45. Esposito G, Van Horn JD, Weinberger DR, Berman KF. Gender differences in cerebral blood flow as a function of cognitive state with PET. J Nucl Med. 1996;37(4):559–64.

46. Podreka I, Baumgartner C, Suess E, Müller C, Brücke T, Lang W, et al. Quantification of regional cerebral blood flow with IMP-SPECT. Reproducibility and clinical relevance of flow values. Stroke. 1989;20(2):183–91.

47. Baxter LR, Mazziotta JC, Phelps ME, Selin CE, Guze BH, Fairbanks L. Cerebral glucose metabolic rates in normal human females versus normal males. Psychiatry Res. 1987;21(3):237–45.

48. Andreason PJ, Zametkin AJ, Guo AC, Baldwin P, Cohen RM. Gender-related differences in regional cerebral glucose metabolism in normal volunteers. Psychiatry Res. 1994;51(2):175–83.

49. Hatazawa J, Brooks RA, Di Chiro G, Campbell G. Global cerebral glucose utilization is independent of brain size: a PET Study. J Comput Assist Tomogr. 1987;11(4):571–6.

50. Azari NP, Rapoport SI, Grady CL, DeCarli C, Haxby JV, Schapiro MB, et al. Gender differences in correlations of cerebral glucose metabolic rates in young normal adults. Brain Res. 1992;574(1–2):198–208.

51. Kuhl DE, Metter EJ, Riege WH, Phelps ME. Effects of human aging on patterns of local cerebral glucose utilization determined by the [18F]fluorodeoxyglucose method. J Cereb Blood Flow Metab. 1982;2(2):163–71.

52. Reiman EM, Armstrong SM, Matt KS, Mattox JH. The application of positron emission tomography to the study of the normal menstrual cycle. Hum Reprod. 1996;11(12):2799–805.

53. Corder EH, Saunders AM, Strittmatter WJ, Schmechel DE, Gaskell PC, Small GW, et al. Gene dose of apolipoprotein E type 4 allele and the risk of Alzheimer's disease in late onset families. Science. 1993;261(5123):921–3.

54. Liu CC, Kanekiyo T, Xu H, Bu G. Apolipoprotein E and Alzheimer disease: risk, mechanisms and therapy. Nat Rev Neurol. 2013;9(2):106–18.

55. Neu SC, Pa J, Kukull W, Beekly D, Kuzma A, Gangadharan P, et al. Apolipoprotein E genotype and sex risk factors for Alzheimer disease: a meta-analysis. JAMA Neurol. 2017;74(10):1178–89.

56. Altmann A, Tian L, Henderson VW, Greicius MD, Investigators ADNI. Sex modifies the APOE-related risk of developing Alzheimer disease. Ann Neurol. 2014;75(4):563–73.

57. Damoiseaux JS, Seeley WW, Zhou J, Shirer WR, Coppola G, Karydas A, et al. Gender modulates the APOE ε4 effect in healthy older adults: convergent evidence from functional brain connectivity and spinal fluid tau levels. J Neurosci. 2012;32(24):8254–62.

58. Panossian LA, Porter VR, Valenzuela HF, Zhu X, Reback E, Masterman D, et al. Telomere shortening in T cells correlates with Alzheimer's disease status. Neurobiol Aging. 2003;24(1):77–84.

59. Jacobs EG, Kroenke C, Lin J, Epel ES, Kenna HA, Blackburn EH, et al. Accelerated cell aging in female APOE-ε4 carriers: implications for hormone therapy use. PLoS One. 2013;8(2):e54713.

60. Li R, Shen Y, Yang LB, Lue LF, Finch C, Rogers J. Estrogen enhances uptake of amyloid beta-protein by microglia derived from the human cortex. J Neurochem. 2000;75(4):1447–54.

61. Tang YP, Haslam SZ, Conrad SE, Sisk CL. Estrogen increases brain expression of the mRNA encoding transthyretin, an amyloid beta scavenger protein. J Alzheimers Dis. 2004;6(4):413–20; discussion 43-9

62. Quintela T, Gonçalves I, Baltazar G, Alves CH, Saraiva MJ, Santos CR. 17beta-estradiol induces transthyretin expression in murine choroid plexus via an oestrogen receptor dependent pathway. Cell Mol Neurobiol. 2009;29(4):475–83.

63. Murphy GM, Zhao F, Yang L, Cordell B. Expression of macrophage colony-stimulating factor receptor is increased in the AbetaPP(V717F) transgenic mouse model of Alzheimer's disease. Am J Pathol 200;157 (3):895–904.

64. Huang J, Guan H, Booze RM, Eckman CB, Hersh LB. Estrogen regulates neprilysin activity in rat brain. Neurosci Lett. 2004;367(1):85–7.

65. Woolley CS. Acute effects of estrogen on neuronal physiology. Annu Rev Pharmacol Toxicol. 2007;47:657–80.

66. Spencer JL, Waters EM, Romeo RD, Wood GE, Milner TA, McEwen BS. Uncovering the mechanisms of estrogen effects on hippocampal function. Front Neuroendocrinol. 2008;29(2):219–37.

67. Foy MR, Baudry M, Diaz Brinton R, Thompson RF. Estrogen and hippocampal plasticity in rodent models. J Alzheimers Dis. 2008;15(4):589–603.

68. Amtul Z, Wang L, Westaway D, Rozmahel RF. Neuroprotective mechanism conferred by 17beta-estradiol on the biochemical basis of Alzheimer's disease. Neuroscience. 2010;169(2):781–6.

69. Zhao L, Yao J, Mao Z, Chen S, Wang Y, Brinton RD. 17β-Estradiol regulates insulin-degrading enzyme expression via an ERβ/PI3-K pathway in hippocampus: relevance to Alzheimer's prevention. Neurobiol Aging. 2011;32(11):1949–63.

70. Levin-Allerhand JA, Lominska CE, Wang J, Smith JD. 17Alpha-estradiol and 17beta-estradiol treatments are effective in lowering cerebral amyloid-beta levels in AbetaPPSWE transgenic mice. J Alzheimers Dis. 2002;4(6):449–57.

71. Carroll JC, Pike CJ. Selective estrogen receptor modulators differentially regulate Alzheimer-like changes in female 3xTg-AD mice. Endocrinology. 2008;149(5):2607–11.

72. Carroll JC, Rosario ER, Chang L, Stanczyk FZ, Oddo S, LaFerla FM, et al. Progesterone and estrogen regulate Alzheimer-like neuropathology in female 3xTg-AD mice. J Neurosci. 2007;27(48):13357–65.

73. Carroll JC, Rosario ER, Villamagna A, Pike CJ. Continuous and cyclic progesterone differentially interact with estradiol in the regulation of Alzheimer-like pathology in female 3xTransgenic-Alzheimer's disease mice. Endocrinology. 2010;151(6):2713–22.

74. Xu H, Wang R, Zhang YW, Zhang X. Estrogen, beta-amyloid metabolism/trafficking, and Alzheimer's disease. Ann N Y Acad Sci. 2006;1089:324–42.

75. Zheng H, Xu H, Uljon SN, Gross R, Hardy K, Gaynor J, et al. Modulation of A(beta) peptides by estrogen in mouse models. J Neurochem. 2002;80(1):191–6.

76. Brinton RD, Yao J, Yin F, Mack WJ, Cadenas E. Perimenopause as a neurological transition state. Nat Rev Endocrinol. 2015;11(7):393–405.

77. Weber MT, Rubin LH, Maki PM. Cognition in perimenopause: the effect of transition stage. Menopause. 2013;20(5):511–7.

78. Zandi PP, Carlson MC, Plassman BL, Welsh-Bohmer KA, Mayer LS, Steffens DC, et al. Hormone replacement therapy and incidence of Alzheimer disease in older women: the Cache County Study. JAMA. 2002;288(17):2123–9.

79. Espeland MA, Rapp SR, Shumaker SA, Brunner R, Manson JE, Sherwin BB, et al. Conjugated equine estrogens and global cognitive function in postmenopausal women: Women's Health Initiative Memory Study. JAMA. 2004;291(24):2959–68.

80. Shumaker SA, Legault C, Kuller L, Rapp SR, Thal L, Lane DS, et al. Conjugated equine estrogens and incidence of probable dementia and mild cognitive impairment in postmenopausal women: Women's Health Initiative Memory Study. JAMA. 2004;291(24):2947–58.

81. Shumaker SA, Legault C, Rapp SR, Thal L, Wallace RB, Ockene JK, et al. Estrogen plus progestin and the incidence of dementia and mild cognitive impairment in postmenopausal women: the Women's Health Initiative Memory Study: a randomized controlled trial. JAMA. 2003;289(20):2651–62.

82. Henderson VW. Estrogen-containing hormone therapy and Alzheimer's disease risk: understanding discrepant inferences from observational and experimental research. Neuroscience. 2006;138(3):1031–9.

83. Kantarci K, Lowe VJ, Lesnick TG, Tosakulwong N, Bailey KR, Fields JA, et al. Early postmenopausal transdermal 17β-estradiol therapy and amyloid-β deposition. J Alzheimers Dis. 2016;53(2):547–56.

84. Gleason CE, Dowling NM, Wharton W, Manson JE, Miller VM, Atwood CS, et al. Effects of hormone therapy on cognition and mood in recently postmenopausal women: findings from the randomized, controlled KEEPS-cognitive and affective study. PLoS Med. 2015;12(6):e1001833; discussion e

85. Henderson VW, St John JA, Hodis HN, McCleary CA, Stanczyk FZ, Shoupe D, et al. Cognitive effects of estradiol after menopause: a randomized trial of the timing hypothesis. Neurology. 2016;87(7):699–708.

86. Espeland MA, Shumaker SA, Leng I, Manson JE, Brown CM, LeBlanc ES, et al. Long-term effects on cognitive function of postmenopausal hormone therapy prescribed to women aged 50 to 55 years. JAMA Intern Med. 2013;173(15):1429–36.

87. Imtiaz B, Tuppurainen M, Rikkonen T, Kivipelto M, Soininen H, Kröger H, et al. Postmenopausal hormone therapy and Alzheimer disease: a prospective cohort study. Neurology. 2017;88(11):1062–8.

88. Stern Y. Cognitive reserve in ageing and Alzheimer's disease. Lancet Neurol. 2012;11(11):1006–12.

89. Sando SB, Melquist S, Cannon A, Hutton M, Sletvold O, Saltvedt I, et al. Risk-reducing effect of education in Alzheimer's disease. Int J Geriatr Psychiatry. 2008;23(11):1156–62.

90. Roe CM, Xiong C, Miller JP, Morris JC. Education and Alzheimer disease without dementia: support for the cognitive reserve hypothesis. Neurology. 2007;68(3):223–8.

91. Stern Y. Cognitive reserve and Alzheimer disease. Alzheimer Dis Assoc Disord. 2006;20(3 Suppl 2):S69–74.

92. McDowell I, Xi G, Lindsay J, Tierney M. Mapping the connections between education and dementia. J Clin Exp Neuropsychol. 2007;29(2):127–41.

93. Tom SE, Hubbard RA, Crane PK, Haneuse SJ, Bowen J, McCormick WC, et al. Characterization of dementia and Alzheimer's disease in an older population: updated incidence and life expectancy with and without dementia. Am J Public Health. 2015;105(2):408–13.

94. Rocca WA, Mielke MM, Vemuri P, Miller VM. Sex and gender differences in the causes of dementia: a narrative review. Maturitas. 2014;79(2):196–201.

95. Bonomini F, Rodella LF, Rezzani R. Metabolic syndrome, aging and involvement of oxidative stress. Aging Dis. 2015;6(2):109–20.

96. Kim B, Feldman EL. Insulin resistance as a key link for the increased risk of cognitive impairment in the metabolic syndrome. Exp Mol Med. 2015;47:e149.

97. Jayaraman A, Pike CJ. Alzheimer's disease and type 2 diabetes: multiple mechanisms contribute to interactions. Curr Diab Rep. 2014;14(4):476.

98. Yaffe K, Blackwell T, Kanaya AM, Davidowitz N, Barrett-Connor E, Krueger K. Diabetes, impaired fasting glucose, and development of cognitive impairment in older women. Neurology. 2004;63(4):658–63.

99. Cigolle CT, Lee PG, Langa KM, Lee YY, Tian Z, Blaum CS. Geriatric conditions develop in middle-aged adults with diabetes. J Gen Intern Med. 2011;26(3):272–9.

100. Whitmer RA, Gustafson DR, Barrett-Connor E, Haan MN, Gunderson EP, Yaffe K. Central obesity and increased risk of dementia more than three decades later. Neurology. 2008;71(14):1057–64.

101. Thaler JP, Guyenet SJ, Dorfman MD, Wisse BE, Schwartz MW. Hypothalamic inflammation: marker or mechanism of obesity pathogenesis? Diabetes. 2013;62(8):2629–34.

102. Christensen A, Pike CJ. Menopause, obesity and inflammation: interactive risk factors for Alzheimer's disease. Front Aging Neurosci. 2015;7:130.

103. Carr MC. The emergence of the metabolic syndrome with menopause. J Clin Endocrinol Metab. 2003;88(6):2404–11.

104. Luchsinger JA, Tang MX, Shea S, Mayeux R. Hyperinsulinemia and risk of Alzheimer disease. Neurology. 2004;63(7):1187–92.

105. Profenno LA, Porsteinsson AP, Faraone SV. Meta-analysis of Alzheimer's disease risk with obesity, diabetes, and related disorders. Biol Psychiatry. 2010;67(6):505–12.

106. Gilsanz P, Mayeda ER, Glymour MM, Quesenberry CP, Mungas DM, DeCarli C, et al. Female sex, early-onset hypertension, and risk of dementia. Neurology. 2017;89(18):1886–93.

107. Diniz BS, Butters MA, Albert SM, Dew MA, Reynolds CF. Late-life depression and risk of vascular dementia and Alzheimer's disease: systematic review and meta-analysis of community-based cohort studies. Br J Psychiatry. 2013;202(5):329–35.

108. Richard E, Reitz C, Honig LH, Schupf N, Tang MX, Manly JJ, et al. Late-life depression, mild cognitive impairment, and dementia. JAMA Neurol. 2013;70(3):374–82.

109. Kessler RC, McGonagle KA, Swartz M, Blazer DG, Nelson CB. Sex and depression in the National Comorbidity Survey. I: lifetime prevalence, chronicity and recurrence. J Affect Disord. 1993;29(2–3):85–96.

110. Steiner M, Dunn E, Born L. Hormones and mood: from menarche to menopause and beyond. J Affect Disord. 2003;74(1):67–83.

111. Piccinelli M, Wilkinson G. Gender differences in depression. Critical review. Br J Psychiatry. 2000;177:486–92.

112. Goveas JS, Espeland MA, Woods NF, Wassertheil-Smoller S, Kotchen JM. Depressive symptoms and incidence of mild cognitive impairment and probable dementia in elderly women: the Women's Health Initiative Memory Study. J Am Geriatr Soc. 2011;59(1):57–66.

113. Yaffe K, Blackwell T, Gore R, Sands L, Reus V, Browner WS. Depressive symptoms and cognitive decline in nondemented elderly women: a prospective study. Arch Gen Psychiatry. 1999;56(5):425–30.

114. Dal Forno G, Palermo MT, Donohue JE, Karagiozis H, Zonderman AB, Kawas CH. Depressive symptoms, sex, and risk for Alzheimer's disease. Ann Neurol. 2005;57(3):381–7.

115. Karlsson IK, Bennet AM, Ploner A, Andersson TM, Reynolds CA, Gatz M, et al. Apolipoprotein E ε4 genotype and the temporal relationship between depression and dementia. Neurobiol Aging. 2015;36(4):1751–6.

116. Sheline YI, West T, Yarasheski K, Swarm R, Jasielec MS, Fisher JR, et al. An antidepressant decreases CSF Aβ production in healthy individuals and in transgenic AD mice. Sci Transl Med. 2014;6(236):236re4.

117. Osorio RS, Pirraglia E, Agüera-Ortiz LF, During EH, Sacks H, Ayappa I, et al. Greater risk of Alzheimer's disease in older adults with insomnia. J Am Geriatr Soc. 2011;59(3):559–62.

118. Phillips BA, Collop NA, Drake C, Consens F, Vgontzas AN, Weaver TE. Sleep disorders and medical conditions in women. Proceedings of the Women & Sleep Workshop, National Sleep Foundation, Washington, DC, March 5–6, 2007. J Womens Health (Larchmt). 2008;17(7):1191–9.

119. Scullin MK. Do older adults need sleep? A review of neuroimaging, sleep, and aging studies. Curr Sleep Med Rep. 2017;3(3):204–14.

120. Canevelli M, Quarata F, Remiddi F, Lucchini F, Lacorte E, Vanacore N, et al. Sex and gender differences in the treatment of Alzheimer's disease: a systematic review of randomized controlled trials. Pharmacol Res. 2017;115:218–23.

121. Kasper JD, Freedman VA, Spillman BC. Disability and care needs of older Americans by dementia status: An analysis of the 2011 national health and aging trends study. Washington, DC: U.S. Department of Health and Human Services; 2014.

122. Bouldin ED, Andresen E. Caregiving across the United States: caregivers of persons with Alzheimer's disease or dementia in 8 states and the District of Columbia. 2009.

123. Friedman EM, Shih RA, Langa KM, Hurd MD. US prevalence and predictors of informal caregiving for dementia. Health Aff (Millwood). 2015;34(10):1637–41.

124. Wolff JL, Spillman BC, Freedman VA, Kasper JD. A national profile of family and unpaid caregivers who assist older adults with health care activities. JAMA Intern Med. 2016;176(3):372–9.

125. Hurd MD, Martorell P, Langa KM. Monetary costs of dementia in the United States. N Engl J Med. 2013;369(5):489–90.

126. Kasper JD, Freedman VA, Spillman BC, Wolff JL. The disproportionate impact of dementia on family and unpaid caregiving to older adults. Health Aff (Millwood). 2015;34(10):1642–9.

127. AARP NAfCa. Caregiving in the U.S.: unpublished data analyzed under contract for the Alzheimer's Association. 2009.

128. Association As. 2014 Alzheimer's disease facts and figures. Spec Rep Women Alzheimer's Dis. 2014;

Successful Aging

Marie Pasinski

Successful Aging

Maintaining a healthy, vibrant brain is the key to successful aging. Achieving a healthy brain encompasses actively preventing brain disease and maximizing brain function across the lifespan. Unlike any other organ, the brain has a remarkable capacity to change. It is continually evolving, molded and influenced by the way we use our brain, our experiences and the lifestyle choices we make every day. As you will see in the sections below, an exciting growing body of research suggests that there are numerous modifiable lifestyle choices we can make to optimize our chances of maintaining a healthy brain.

Alzheimer's Disease

Developing dementia is one of our greatest fears of aging. Alzheimer's disease, the most common type of dementia, disproportionately affects women. Alzheimer's is two to three times more common in women than men and this is not fully explained by woman's longer life expectancy. At age 65, healthy women have a greater than 1 in 6 chance of developing Alzheimer's disease in the future, compared with a 1 in 11 chance for men. In addition, women shoulder the burden of caring for those with dementia. There are 2.5 times as many women as men providing 24-h care for someone with dementia.

It's unclear why women have a higher risk of Alzheimer's compared to men. Although advancing age is the biggest risk factor for Alzheimer's and women have a longer life expectancy, on average living 3 years longer than men, this does not fully account for the increased burden of Alzheimer's in women. Genetic, hormonal, environmental and lifestyle factors may contribute to this greater vulnerability.

The apolipoprotien E4 genotype (APOE4) is the most potent known genetic risk factor for late-onset Alzheimer's in both sexes. In the brain, APOE transports cholesterol to neurons and it occurs in three alleles, E2, E3 and E4. Having one E4 allele increases the risk of developing Alzheimer's threefold compared those without an E4 allele, while those homozygous for E4 have up to 20 times the risk of developing Alzheimer's. Previous studies suggested that having the APOE4 allele conferred a greater risk of developing Alzheimer's in females compared to their male counterparts with the same genotype. More recently, a meta- analysis by Neu et al. of 27 independent studies with 58,000 participants did not show a difference in the risk of Alzheimer's disease between men and women with one copy of the apolipoprotein E4 allele from age 55 to 85 years. However, in a subgroup analysis, women were at an increased risk compared to men between the ages 65 and 75 [1].

Although the decline in estrogen associated with menopause is thought to underlie multiple negative brain changes, including reduced glucose metabolism, decreased synaptic formation and increased deposition of beta-amyloid plaques, a hallmark of Alzheimer's pathology, currently there is no role for hormonal replacement to prevent or treat Alzheimer's. The Women's Health Initiative Memory Study (WHIMS) a large, randomized, double blind, controlled trial in 2003, showed that estrogen with or without medroxyprogesterone, significantly increased the risk of Alzheimer's disease and other forms of dementia [2]. However, women in the WHIMS were over age 65 which raised the question that perhaps the timing of hormonal replacement was critical. An observational study by Shao et al. in 2012 found that women who used hormone replacement therapy within 5 years of menopause had a 30% lower risk of Alzheimer's disease [3]. However, these results have not been supported by a recent randomized trial comparing initiation of hormonal therapy within 6 years versus more than 10 years after menopause. This trial showed that hormone therapy neither benefited or impaired cognitive function regardless of the timing post menopause [4].

M. Pasinski (✉)
Harvard Medical School, Nahant, MA, USA
e-mail: mpasinski@mgh.harvard.edu

© Springer Nature Switzerland AG 2019
M. A. O'Neal (ed.), *Neurology and Psychiatry of Women*, https://doi.org/10.1007/978-3-030-04245-5_26

Mixed Dementia

Dementia is not a single disease; it includes an array of disorders that produce abnormal changes in the brain that in turn cause a decline in cognitive skills and behavioral changes severe enough to impair daily life and independent function. Although Alzheimer's is the most common clinical diagnosis of dementia, "mixed dementia" is the most common pathologic diagnosis of dementia.

Mixed dementia is diagnosed when abnormalities characteristic of more than one type of dementia occur simultaneously in the brain. The Rush Memory and Aging Project showed that 54% of participants whose brains met pathological criteria for Alzheimer's also had pathologic evidence of one or more coexisting dementias such as vascular, Lewy body and others.

In fact, there are many other factors that negatively influence brain function some of which are not easily quantifiable or readily diagnosed pathologically such as traumatic brain injuries, concussions, substance abuse, nutritional deficiencies, toxins, infections, chemotherapy and radiation. That is why when we think about brain health we must consider all the factors that influence brain function.

The most common form of mixed dementia is the coexistence of Alzheimer's and vascular pathology [5]. This may explain why studies show a significant overlap between the major risk factors for vascular disease and the more recently identified risk factors for Alzheimer's disease. Barnes et al. performed a meta-analysis of all major studies on risk factor reduction for Alzheimer's disease and determined that one third of Alzheimer's cases are attributable to seven modifiable risk factors including diabetes, hypertension, obesity, smoking, physical inactivity, depression and cognitive inactivity [6]. It is notable that five of these seven risk factors are vascular risk factors and that physical inactivity was shown to be the most significant modifiable risk factor for Alzheimer's disease in the United States.

Preventing vascular disease is therefore vital to brain health. Addressing vascular risk factors and optimizing blood flow to the brain not only reduces the risk of stroke and dementia, but it also assures the proper delivery of nutrients and oxygen to brain tissue for optimal function.

Gender Risk Factor Disparities

For women, addressing modifiable lifestyle risk factors may be especially important, as women have a higher prevalence of multiple dementia risk factors compared to men. For example, women have higher rates of obesity, they are less physically active and inherently have a greater risk for concussion and brain injury. In addition, women have more mental health disorders, higher rates of insomnia, lower levels of educational attainment and have less mentally challenging occupations. These striking gender disparities are further detailed individually in the section below.

Fortunately, it is never too late to modify lifestyle risk factors. Two major scientific breakthroughs underlie our new understanding that the lifestyle choices we make every day directly influence brain structure and function. First is the concept of neuroplasticity, the realization that the brain is incredibly dynamic and constantly evolving. It has the ability to form new synapses and create new neurons throughout our lives. Secondly, the emerging field of epigenetics which studies how gene expression is directly influenced by environment and lifestyle, provides a mechanism for how lifestyle choices can induce phenotypic change. In other words, while we cannot change our genes, we can make healthy lifestyle choices that directly alter gene expression, which in turn, benefit our brain.

Modifiable Brain Health Risk Factors

General Health

Every organ system supports brain function. Consequently, diseases of all organ systems can impair brain homeostasis. For example, pulmonary, cardiac, respiratory, gastrointestinal, hepatic, renal, immune and endocrine disorders can negatively affect cognition both in the short term and in the long run. Maintaining general health and optimally treating any medical disorders is the first step in maintaining a healthy brain. A typical initial work up for cognitive decline includes the following: complete blood count (CBC), comprehensive metabolic profile (CMP), thyroid screening panel, vitamin B12, folate, syphilis antibody (RPR), human immunodeficiency virus (HIV) testing and neuroimaging.

Blood Pressure

Hypertension is a significant risk factor for stroke, and dementia, including Alzheimer's disease. However, it is woefully underdiagnosed and undertreated. Approximately 47% of American adults have hypertension, and this increases significantly with age. Hypertension is present in 76% of adults age 65–74 years and 82% of adults age 75 years or older. According to a national survey, hypertension was under good control in less than 50% of adults. Although men are more likely to develop hypertension through early middle age, women are more likely to have high blood pressure after age 65, especially systolic hypertension which is more damaging to the brain. Regular blood pressure checks and aggressive treatment of hypertension is one of the pillars of brain health.

Diabetes

Nearly 70% of those with type 2 diabetes mellitus ultimately develop Alzheimer's disease. Although hyperinsulinemia and insulin resistance, the hallmarks of type 2 diabetes have been shown to cause memory impairment and that diabetics are more likely to develop cortical atrophy and the pathologic hallmarks of Alzheimer's disease, ongoing research has yet to explain a shared pathophysiology. It is staggering to consider that approximately 25 million Americans have diabetes, and an estimated 54 million U.S. adults have prediabetes, most of whom will develop type 2 diabetes within 10 years. Educating patients about the cognitive risks of diabetes, counseling them on diet and weight control and performing HgA1C testing could significantly decrease the burden of Alzheimer's disease.

Weight

Midlife obesity is a recognize risk factor for Alzheimer's disease. In particular, increased central adiposity as measured by waist circumference is correlated with an increased risk of dementia. Visceral fat produces inflammatory cytokines leading to chronic inflammation. A growing body of research suggests that chronic inflammation, as measured by high levels of CRP and IL-6 may weaken the blood brain barrier, triggering inflammation within the brain and the development of Alzheimer's related pathology. According to a CDC report in 2014, the prevalence of mid- life obesity among women ages 40–59 is 42%, compared to 38% for middle-aged men. Across all adult age groups, 38% of women are obese compared to 34% of men. This disparity is even greater for women of color. The obesity rate among African-American women it is 57% and 46% among Hispanic women.

Diet

A Mediterranean style diet is supported by countless observational studies as the best diet to maintain a healthy brain. It is associated with a decreased risk of dementia, Alzheimer's disease, and stroke, as well as improved cognitive performance. The mainstays of a Mediterranean style diet include: vegetables, legumes, whole grains, fruits, nuts, seeds, fish, seafood, herbs, spices and olive oil. Poultry, eggs, cheese and yogurt should be eaten in moderation while red meat, processed foods and sweets should be limited to special occasions.

This diet has a naturally low glycemic index which prevents pro-inflammatory blood glucose and insulin spikes. Elevated blood glucose and insulin levels promote abdominal fat deposition, which in turn, increase the risk of multiple other Alzheimer's risk factors including: obesity, diabetes and hypertension as well as producing inflammatory mediators that cause chronic inflammation throughout the body including the brain.

The MIND diet (Mediterranean- DASH Intervention for Neurodegenerative Delay) study showed that participants who followed this diet for an average of 4 years had a 54% decreased risk of Alzheimer's disease when the diet was followed rigorously and a 35% decreased risk of Alzheimer's when followed moderately [7]. The MIND diet is a combination of the Mediterranean diet and the DASH diet (Dietary Approaches to Stop Hypertension). The DASH diet which is naturally low in sodium and high in potassium has been shown lower blood pressure.

Physical Activity

Exercise is key to maintaining a healthy brain. According to the previously mentioned study by Norton et al., physical inactivity is the number one modifiable risk factor for Alzheimer's disease in the United States. Physical activity triggers the release of brain derived neurotrophic factor (BDNF) which promotes synaptic plasticity and neurogenesis. In addition, numerous studies have shown that regular aerobic exercise increases brain volume on magnetic resonance imaging volumetric brain imaging. The hippocampus, the area of the brain important for memory consolidation and spatial navigation has been shown to become more robust with aerobic training. Studies also show a strong correlation between physical fitness and improved cognitive functioning. The general recommendation for brain health is 150 min per week of moderate exercise or 75 min per week of vigorous exercise. According to the US Department of Health and Human Services only 14.7% of women meet the recommendation for adequate physical activity, compared to 21.1% of men and these percentages decrease with age.

Mental Health

Depression and anxiety are linked to an increased risk of Alzheimer's. Although this association does not establish a causal link, both depression and anxiety trigger increased levels of cortisol which have been shown to be toxic to hippocampal neurons. Additionally, both conditions are also associated with lower levels of BDNF and decreased rates of hippocampal neurogenesis. From the time of puberty, females are twice as likely to have an anxiety disorder and have a 1.7-fold greater incidence of depression compared to men. Screening for these conditions and appropriate treatment can improve quality of life and may in turn, decrease the risk of dementia.

Socialization

Maintaining an active social life appears to preserve brain health, while social isolation is a recognized risk factor for cognitive decline in elderly. The protective effect of socialization extends to all types of social interactions including family, friends and community contacts. A Harvard School of Public Health Study showed that individuals who engaged in frequent social activity in their 50s and 60s had the slowest rate of memory decline [8]. In fact, those subjects who had the highest social integration scores had less than half the rate of memory loss compared to those who were the least socially active. In general, women have larger, more diverse social networks than men as well as more people they consider as close contacts. However, during midlife, women's socialization may be reduced by the demands of parenting and caring for elderly family members. Encouraging socialization and participation in caretaker support groups can be beneficial.

Head Trauma

Over recent years there's been a growing body of research on the long-term effects of concussions on cognition. It appears that even minor head injuries may compromise the blood brain barrier and lead to inflammation in the brain. Data suggests that in sports with similar rules, female athletes sustain more concussions than males. In addition, female athletes experience more severe symptoms and require longer recovery than their male counterparts. The reason for this is unclear and is likely multifactorial. Anatomical differences including weaker neck musculature and decreased neck girth in women result in less shock absorption with impact and increase acceleration forces on the brain. Interesting research also suggests that female hormones may influence brain vulnerability to injury. While progesterone appears to have a protective effect, higher estrogen levels may increase the degree of injury. Work by Wunderle et al. suggests that women injured during the follicular phase, the first 2 weeks of the menstrual cycle have better outcomes after mild traumatic brain injury compared to those injured during the luteal phase [9]. Additionally, recent research by Dolle et al. found that female axons were smaller, had fewer microtubules and were more vulnerable to simulated traumatic brain injury in vitro compared to male axons [10]. While it is impossible to quantify the degree to which cumulative head trauma contributes to cognitive loss over time, it is prudent to protect the brain from trauma by wearing seatbelts, using appropriate head protective wear/helmets for sports and avoiding falls.

Sleep

Sleep disorders and sleep deprivation are recognized risk factors for Alzheimer's disease. Sleep disordered breathing for example, is associated with twice the odds of developing dementia. Although this does not determine causality, it has been shown that neurogenesis and neuroplastic changes required for memory formation and learning new skills occur during sleep. It has also been shown that beta-amyloid, which forms the pathological amyloid plaques in Alzheimer's disease, is cleared from the brain during sleep and that adequate amounts of deep slow wave and rapid eye movement sleep are required for optimal brain homeostasis.

According to the US Center of Disease Control and Prevention, 30% of Americans are sleep deprived, sleeping less than 6 h per night. Insomnia is the most common type of sleep disorder. A 2002 National Sleep Foundation poll showed that 63% of women report insomnia several times per week compared to 54% of men.

In light of the fact that sleep deprivation can increase the risk of other dementia risk factors including, hypertension, diabetes, stroke, obesity and depression, making sleep a priority and instructing patients on proper sleep hygiene is extremely important. When proper sleep hygiene does not correct insomnia or when fragmented sleep persists, a sleep study or referral to a sleep specialist is recommended.

Toxins, Substance Use and Medications

Alcohol-related dementia is an umbrella term for dementia caused by long-term, excessive consumption of alcohol causing neurologic damage and impaired cognitive function. Alcohol is toxic to neurons which directly damages the brain. It can also cause malnutrition, in particular, a loss of thiamine (vitamin B1) resulting in Korsakoff's syndrome causing profound short term memory loss. Diagnosing alcohol-related dementia is difficult due to the wide range of symptoms and lack of specific brain pathology. It is unknown to what degree even moderate alcohol consumption may contribute to a diagnosis of dementia in any given individual. An observational cohort study measuring weekly alcohol intake and cognitive performance measures repeatedly over 30 years concluded that alcohol consumption even at moderate levels is associated with adverse brain outcomes including hippocampal atrophy [11]. The current thinking is that less is more when it comes to alcohol consumption and brain health. For women, intake should be limited to no more than one standard alcoholic beverage per day. For those with pre-existing memory difficulties, abstinence is recommended.

Smoking is a significant risk factor for Alzheimer's and should be discouraged. Similarly, all forms of substance abuse alter brain physiology and are believed to negatively impact brain function and structure over time.

It is important to realize that medications, particularly those that are psychoactive and those that cross the blood brain barrier can impair memory and cognition. Depending on the duration of treatment and disruption of brain physiology and structure, these effects may be present in both the short term and in the long run. For example, chemotherapeutic agents have been shown to decrease neurogenesis, while radiation may result in irreversible changes in brain structure. There is growing concern that chronic use of some prescription medications may predispose individuals to dementia. For example, chronic use of benzodiazepines and anti-cholinergics such as diphenhydramine (commonly used in over the counter sleeping aids) have been associated with an increased risk of dementia. Reviewing patients' medication lists regularly and discontinuing unnecessary psychoactive medications is recommended.

Cognitive Stimulation

Higher educational attainment and engagement in mentally challenging activities throughout life are associated with improved cognitive function and lower risk of dementia. Globally, low educational attainment is considered the number one modifiable risk factor for Alzheimer's disease [12]. Mental challenge has been shown to induce neuroplastic changes and stimulate the release of brain growth factors including BDNF that promote neurogenesis and fortify neural synapses. Neurogenesis and synaptic remodeling have been shown to be active processes throughout life.

Traditionally, women are at a significant disadvantage due to lower levels of educational attainment and less mentally stimulating occupations compared to men. In addition, many women sacrifice educational goals and cognitively challenging careers to raise children and care for ailing family members. Encouraging women to pursue an education, strive for mentally stimulating occupations and stay mentally active by engaging in new experiences and new learning throughout their lives is key to maintaining a healthy brain.

Conclusion

Preserving cognition is imperative for successful aging. Women are disproportionately at risk for dementia and have a higher prevalence of multiple modifiable dementia risk factors compared to men. Encouraging our patients to make brain healthy lifestyle choices can be life changing and is the key to maintaining a healthy brain.

References

1. Neu S, Pa J, et al. Apolipoprotein E genotype and sex risk factors for Alzheimer disease, a meta-analysis. JAMA. 2017;74(10):1178–89.
2. Shumaker SA, Legault C, et al. Estrogen progestin and the incidence of dementia and mild cognitive impairment in postmenopausal women: the Women's Health Initiative Memory Study: a randomized controlled trial. JAMA. 2003;289:2651–62.
3. Shao H, Breitner JCS, et al. Hormone therapy and Alzheimer's disease dementia: new findings from the Cache County Study. Neurology. 2012;79(18):1846–52.
4. Henderson VW, St John JA, et al. Cognitive effects of estradiol after menopause: a randomized trial of the timing hypothesis. Neurology. 2016;87(7):699–708.
5. Rahimi J, Kovacs G. Prevalence of mixed pathology in the aging brain. Alzheimers Res Ther. 2014;6:82.
6. Norton S, Matthews F, et al. Potential for primary prevention of Alzheimer's disease: an analysis of population–based data. Lancet Neurol. 2014;13(8):788–94.
7. Morris MC, Tangey CC, Wang Y, et al. MIND diet associated with reduced incidence of Alzheimer's disease. Alzheimers Dement. 2015;11(9):1007–14.
8. Ertel K, Glymour MM. Effects of social integration on preserving memory function in a nationally representative US elderly population. Am J Public Health. 2008;98(7):1215–20.
9. Wunderle K, Hoeger KM, et al. Menstrual phase as predictor of outcome after mild traumatic brain injury in women. Am J Public Health. 2014;29(5):1–8.
10. Dolle JP, Stewart AJ, et al. New found sex differences in axonal structure underlie differential outcomes from in vitro traumatic axonal injury. Exp Neurol. 2018;300:121–34.
11. Topiwala A, Allan CL, et al. Moderate alcohol consumption as risk factor for adverse brain outcomes and cognitive decline: longitudinal cohort study. BMJ. 2017;357:2353–62.
12. Barnes DE, Yaffe K. The projected impact of risk factor reduction on Alzheimer's disease prevalence. Lancet Neurol. 2011;10(9):819–28.

Index

A

Acceptance and Commitment Therapy (ACT), 50
Acetazolamide, 91, 93, 134
Acetylcholine receptor (AChR) antibodies, 177, 181
Achilles reflex, 175
ACTH deficiency, 41
Acupuncture, 166
Acute adrenal insufficiency, 42
Acute disseminated encephalomyelitis (ADEM), 78
Adaptive immunity, 8, 78, 79
Adjustment disorder, 194
    treatment, 195
Adrenal insufficiency, 41
Aging
    Alzheimer's disease, 227
    gender risk factor disparities, 228
    mixed dementia, 228
    modifiable brain health risk factors
        blood pressure, 228
        cognitive stimulation, 231
        diabetes, 229
        diet, 229
        general health, 228
        head trauma, 230
        mental health, 229
        physical activity, 229
        sleep disorder, 230
        socialization, 230
        toxins, substance use and medications, 230–231
        weight, 229
Agoraphobia, 70
Alcohol-related dementia, 230
Alemtuzumab, 81, 150
Alexithymia, 48
Allopregnanolone, 69, 91
Alzheimer's disease (AD)
    aging, 227
    diabetes, 229
    diet, 229
    hypertension, 228
    obesity, 229
    pathophysiology of, 219
    physical activity, 229
    prevalence of, 219
    sex-related differences
        cardiovascular and metabolic factors, 221
        caregivers, role as, 221, 222
        depression, 221
        education, 221
        hormones, 220, 221
        insomnia, 221
        risk factors for women, 219, 220
    sleep disorder and deprivation, 230
    in United States, 219
Amantadine, 216
Amyloid plaque, 219
Amyloid precursor protein processing (APP), 220
Androgen deprivation therapy, 79
Aneurysmal- related hemorrhage, 122
Anterior spinal artery syndrome, 176
Anticoagulation, 142, 175
Antidepressants, 39, 163–165, 167, 194, 196, 198
Anti-epileptic drugs (AEDs), 30
    best and worst choices for, 126–127
        CBZ, 126
        LTG and LEV, 126
        OXC, 127
        TPM, 126
        VPA, 126, 127
    breastfeeding, 128
    epilepsy management, 128
    seizure control, 125
Antinuclear antibody (ANA), 8
Antiplatelet agents, 142, 175
Antiprogesterone therapy, 96
Antipsychotics, 165, 166
Antithrombotic therapy, 142
Anxiety, 40, 48, 49, 158, 196, 197, 229
    GAD, 71
    gynecological pain
        bladder pain syndrome, 73
        chronic pelvic pain, 73
        pelvic organ prolapse, 74
        urinary incontinence, 74
        vulvar pain, 73
    hormonal influence, 69
    OSD, 71, 72
    panic disorder, 71
    pregnanacy
        and postpartaum, 70, 71
        loss (*see* Pregnancy loss)
    PTSD, 71
    specific differences in
        GAD, 70
        obsessive compulsive disorder, 70
        panic disorder, 70
        phobias, 70
        PTSD, 70
    in women, 69
Apolipoprotien E4 genotype (APOE4), 220, 227
Arterial ischemic strokes, 142
Arteriovenous malformation (AVM), 122, 183
Arthrogryposis multiplex congenita (AMC), 181
Artificial reproductive therapies, 73

M. A. O'Neal (ed.), *Neurology and Psychiatry of Women*, https://doi.org/10.1007/978-3-030-04245-5

Assisted reproductive technology (ART), 146
Atrial fibrillation (AF), 208
Aubagio, 149
Autoimmune diseases, 7, 77–79
Autoimmune hepatitis, 79
Autoimmunity, 7
Axonal injuries, 173
Azathioprine, 80, 81, 153, 178, 179, 181

B
Baby blues, 157
Barbiturates, 180
B-cell activating factor (BAFF), 77
B-cell depleting therapies, 150
Bem's gender role theory, 69
Benzodiazepines, 72, 91, 180
Bereavement, 194
Bilateral femoral neuropathy, 174
Bilateral oophorectomy, 95, 214
Bipolar disorder
    clinical course, 159, 160
    epidemiology, 159
    risk factors, 159
Bladder pain syndrome (BPS), 73
Blood pressure, 228
Bodily preoccupation, 49
Bone health risk, 196
Brachial plexopathies, 99
Brain and leptomeningeal metastases, 98
Brain derived neurotrophic factor (BDNF), 229
Breast cancers, 98
Breastfeeding, 151, 152, 162
    antidepressants, 165
    antipsychotics, 166
    mood stabilizers, 165, 166
Bromocriptine, 39, 216

C
Cabergoline, 39, 40, 216
Caffeine, 137, 196, 198
Carbamazepine (CBZ), 73, 126, 127, 164, 166
Cardiomyopathy, 140
Cardiovascular disease, 196, 221
Catamenial epilepsy
    definition, 85
    epidemiology, 85
    management, 89, 90
        alternative strategies, 91–93
        hormonal treatment, 90, 91
    pathophysiology
        antiepileptic medication clearance changes, 88
        hypothalamic-pituitary-ovarian axis, 85
        menstrual cycle, neurological and non-neurological disorders,
            88–89
        sex hormones and epileptogenesis, 85–88
    patterns of, 86
Catheter-based angiography, FMD, 12
CDC USMEC categories of medical eligibility for contraceptive use,
    27
CDC USMEC recommendations for hormonal contraceptive use, 29
Centers for Disease Control (CDC), 27
Central Brain Tumor Registry of the United States (CBTRUS), 95
Cerebral infarctions, 122
Cerebral vasculitis, 9
Cerebral venous and sinus vasculature, 122

Cerebral venous thrombosis (CVT), 122, 141
    clinical manifestations, 136
    epidemiology, 136
    pathophysiology, 136
    treatment, 136
Cervical cancer, 80, 96
Chemoradiation therapy, 100
Chemotherapy
    conception, 99
    into semen/other body fluids, 99
Cholinesterase inhibitors, 180
Chronic pelvic pain (CPP), 73
Chronic vulvar pain, 73
Citalopram, 165, 196
Clobazam, 93
Clomipramine, 164
Clonazepam (CLO), 126
Clozapine, 166
Cognitive behavioral therapy (CBT), 49, 50, 52
    FND, 18
    hot flashes, 196
    major depression, 194
    mood disorder, 163
    sleep disturbances, 198
Cognitive impairment, 9, 40
Combined hormonal contraception (CHC), 27, 28
Computed tomography (CT), 119, 175
    deterministic effects, 117
    direct exposure, 117
    dose units, 117
    effects of radiation, 117
    gestational age of fetus, 117
    headache, 131
    indirect exposure, 117
    radiology reports and radiation dosimetry, 118
    rate of absorption, 117
    stochastic effects, 117
Computed tomography angiography (CTA), 118
Congenital myasthenic syndromes, 181
Connective tissue disorders
    with autoimmune etiologies, 7
    fascia, 7
    genetic and autoimmune causes, 7
Contraception, neurologic and psychiatric disorders
    copper and levonorgestrel IUDs, 27
    hormonal and non-hormonal options, 27
    and method selection, 27
    teratogenic medications, 27
Contraceptive counseling, 33
Conus medullaris injury, 175
Conversion disorder (CD), 53
    clinical manifestation, 56
    cognitive symptoms, 51
    definition of, 50
    diagnosis, 51
    epidemiology, 52
    functional neurologic symptoms, 51
    motor manifestations, 50
    neuropsychologic characteristics, 51, 52
    organic neurologic symptoms, 51
    psychogenic movement disorders rating scale, 55
    symptoms, 51
    treatment, 52, 53
Copaxone, 148
Copper IUD, 30
Corticosteroids, 177, 179, 181
Corticotrophic tumors, 40

Corticotropin-releasing hormone (CRH), 158
Cortisol level, 69
CT, *see* Computed tomography (CT)
Cushing's syndrome, 39, 40
    diagnosis, 40
    medical comorbidities, 39
    mood disorders, 40
    signs and symptoms, 39
    treatment, 40
Cyclophosphamide, 80, 81
Cyclophosphamide-induced infertility, 79
Cyclosporine, 178, 181
CYP3A4 enzyme inducing status, 30

D
Daclizumab, 81, 149
DDAVP, 41
Dementia, 219, 221, 222, 227, 230
Demyelinating disease
    multiple sclerosis (MS) (*see* Multiple sclerosis (MS))
    NMOSD (*see* Neuromyelitis optica spectrum disorders
        (NMOSD))
Denosumab, 79
Depersonalization/derealization disorder, 19–22
Depression, 40, 192, 197, 198, 208, 215, 221, 229
    adjustment disorder, treatment, 195
    assessment scales, 194
    bereavement, 195
    coinciding symptoms
        concentration, 193
        difficulty sleeping, 193
        fatigue, 193
        sexual dysfunction, 193
        weight gain, 193
    complicating symptoms and challenges
        hot flashes, 193
        psychological and daily life challenges, 193, 194
    complicating symptoms and challenges
    depressive symptoms
        definition of, 192
        demographic factors, 192
        epidemiology, 192
        lifestyle factors, 193
        medical factors, 193
        psychiatric factors, 192
        psychological factors, 193
        psychosocial factors, 193
        treatment, 195
    diagnosis, 33
    differential diagnosis, 194
    major depression
        antidepressants, 194
        CBT, 194
        definition of, 192
        demographic factors, 192
        epidemiology, 192
        hormone therapy, 194
        IPT, 194
        lifestyle factors, 193
        medical factors, 193
        psychiatric factors, 192
        psychological factors, 193
        psychosocial factors, 193
    psychological distress
        definition of, 192
        demographic risk factors, 192

        epidemiology, 192
        lifestyle risk factors, 193
        medical risk factors, 193
        psychiatric risk factors, 193
        psychosocial risk factors, 193
        treatment, 195
    SLE, 9
Depressive symptoms
    definition of, 192
    epidemiology, 192
    risk factors
        demographic factors, 192
        lifestyle factors, 193
        medical factors, 193
        psychiatric factors, 192
        psychological factors, 193
        psychosocial factors, 193
    treatment, 195
Desmopression, 41
Desogestrel, 152
Diabetes insipidus, 41
Diabetes mellitus, 208, 229
Dialectical behavioral therapy (DBT), 52
Diet, 229
Dietary Approaches to Stop Hypertension (DASH) diet, 229
Difficulty sleeping, 193
Digital subtraction angiography (DSA), 118, 119
Dimethyl fumarate (DMF), 81, 148
Diphenhydramine, 231
Disease conviction, 49
Disease fear, 49
Disease-modifying antirheumatic drugs (DMARD), 79
Disease-modifying therapies (DMTs), 79, 146, 151
    conception, changes of, 146
    gestation, 147, 148
        alemtuzumab, 150
        daclizumab, 149
        dimethyl fumarate, 148
        fingolimod, 148, 149
        natalizumab, 149, 150
        ocrelizumab, 150
        rituximab, 150
        teriflunomide, 149
    glatiramer acetate, 148
    lactation, 148
        alemtuzumab, 150
        daclizumab, 149
        dimethyl fumarate, 148
        fingolimod, 149
        glatiramer acetate, 148
        natalizumab, 150
        ocrelizumab, 150
        rituximab, 150
        teriflunomide, 149
    safety profile of drug, 147, 148
Dissociative amnesia, 21
Dissociative disorder, 19
    clinical evaluation, 21, 22
    clinical phenomenology, 19
    comorbidities, 19
    differential diagnosis, 20
    epidemiology, 19
    pharmacologic interventions, 22
    psychological theories and pathophysiology, 21
    treatment, 22
Dissociative fugue, 21
Dissociative identity disorder (DID), 19, 21

Domino theory, 198
Dopamine, 213
  agonists, 39
Dyskinesias, 213, 215, 216

E

Ebstein's anomaly, 164
Eclampsia, 134, 179
Eculizumab, 178, 179, 181
Edinburgh postnatal depression scale (EPDS), 161
Electroconvulsive therapy (ECT), 161, 166
Encephalitis, 99
Endocrinopathies, 43
End-of-life decisions, 186, 187
Endogenous ovarian hormones, 29
Entacapone, 216
Epidural anesthesia, 173–175
  and breastfeeding, 146
Epidural catheter, 174
Epidural hematoma, 175, 176
Epigenetics, 228
Epilepsy, 29, 31, 122, 123, 131
  AED choices for childbearing WWE, 126
  anti-epileptic drugs and hormonal contraception, 30
  breastfeeding in pregnancy, 128
  hormonal contraception safety, 29, 30
  management during pregnancy, 128
  prepregnancy planning, 125
  WWE
    AED choices for childbearing, 126–127
    folic acid used in, 127
Epileptogenesis, 85, 86
Escitalopram, 196
Estradiol, 220
Estriol, 152
Estrogen, 69, 79, 86, 87, 158
  effects of, 214
  supplementation, 4, 8
Estrogen-containing methods, 31
Estrogen-medroxyprogesterone hormone replacement therapy, 91
Estrogen replacement therapy, 214
Eszopiclone, 198
Ethical decisions
  AVM, 183
  end-of-life decisions, 186, 187
  ethical priority, 184
  of fetus, 184–185
  gestational age, 185–187
  gestational continuum, 185
  incapacitated, previously-competent patient, 183–184
  LST, 184–187
  substituted judgement, 183, 184
Ethinylstradiol, 152
Ethosuximide (ESM), 126
Evidence-based guidelines, 27
Exogenous hormones, 152, 153
Expanded Disability Status Scale (EDSS) score, 146
Extrapyramidal symptoms (EPS), 165

F

Factitious disorder (FD), 53
  diagnosis of, 53
  epidemiology, 54
  external motivation, 53
  FD-O, 54

  gender, 57
  treatment, 54
  women, 56
Factitious Disorder Imposed on Another (FD-O), 54
Fatigue, 193
Femoral nerve injury, 173
Femoral neuropathy, 173, 174
Fertility, 41, 95
  and pregnancy, 80
Fibromuscular dysplasia (FMD), 11–13
Fibular nerve compression, 174
Fibular neuropathy, 174
Fight/flight response, 70
Fingolimod, 81, 148, 149
First-generation antipsychotics (FGAs), 165
Fluoxetine, 50, 165
Fluvoxamine, 50
Folic acid, 127
Freeze response, 70
Functional neurological disorder (FND)
  altered voluntary motor or sensory function, 15
  and dissociative disorder
    behavioral profiles, 23
    classification, 22
    co-occurrence, 23
    somatoform and psychoform dissociation, 23
  antidepressant treatment, 18
  brain anatomy and function, 18
  clinical phenomenology, 15–17
  diagnosis, 15
  diagnostic certainty, 15
  disability and symptomatic outcomes, 15
  electromyography studies, 18
  epidemiological data, 15
  neuropsychiatric assessment, 17
  physical therapy, 18
  positive signs, 16
  psychological theories, 17, 18
  semiological differences between sexes, 17
  subtypes, 15
  treatment, 18, 19
  vulnerability traits/ neuropsychological deficits, 17
Functional Neurologic Symptom Disorder, *see* Conversion disorder (CD)

G

Gabapentin (GBP), 126, 196, 198
Gadolinium, 119, 132, 151
Gender differences in Parkinson's disease, *see* Parkinson's disease, gender differences in
Generalized anxiety disorder (GAD), 69
  PPGAD, 71
  preexisting anxiety, 71
  sex differences, 70
Gestation, 147, 148
Gestational diabetes mellitus, 206
GH deficiency, 41
GH replacement therapy, 41
Gilenya, 148–149
Glatiramer acetate (GA)
  gastation, 148
  lactation, 148
Glioblastoma (GBM), 98
Gliomas, 98, 99
Glucocorticoid-induced osteoporosis and fractures (GIOP), 79
Glucocorticoids, 81

Gonadotropin deficiency, 41
Gonadotropin releasing hormone (GnRH), 91
Gonaotrophs, 40
Granulomatosis with polyangiitis, 150
Granulomatous hypophysitis, 43
Groin puncture, 118
Gynecological pain
    bladder pain syndrome, 73
    chronic pelvic pain, 73
    pelvic organ prolapse, 74
    urinary incontinence, 74
    vulvar pain, 73

H
Head trauma, 230
Headache
    CVT
        clinical manifestations, 136
        epidemiology, 136
        pathophysiology, 136
        treatment, 136
    features, 131
    frequency of, 132
    IIH
        definition, 134
        diagnosis, 134
        epidemiology, 134
        treatment, 134
    imaging, 131–132
    migraine (*see* Migraine)
    nonsteroidal anti-inflammatory medications, 131
    PDPH
        definition, 136, 137
        epidemiology, 137
        pathophysiology, 137
        treatment, 137
    PEE
        definition, 134
        morbidity and mortality, 134
        pathophysiology, 134, 135
        treatment, 135
    RCVS
        definition, 135
        epidemiology, 135
        pathophysiology, 135
        treatment, 135
Health anxiety, 49, 50, 55
Health-related distress, 56
High-dose estrogen therapy, 153
Hippocampal atrophy, 230
Hook effect, 39
Hormonal birth control method, 28
Hormonal contraceptive method, 28, 29, 206–207
Hormonal imbalance, 37
Hormonal replacement therapy (HRT), 91,
        96, 220, 227
Hormone therapy (HT), 194, 196
    contraindications, 5
Hot flashes, 193, 198
    assessment scales, 196
    cardiovascular disease and bone health risk, 196
    epidemiology, 195
    nonpharmacological interventions
        CBT, 196
        gabapentin, 196
        HT, 196

        serotonergic agents, 196
        supportive tools, 196
    physiology, 195
    risk factors
        age and manopausal stage, 195
        anxiety, 196
        caffeine, 196
        early childhood adversity, 196
        metabolic, 195
        race, 195
        smoking, 196
    time course, 195
Hot Flash Interference Scale (HFI), 196
Hot Flash Related Daily Interference Scale (HFRDIS), 196
Hydralazine, 135, 180
Hydrocortisone, 41
Hydroxychloroquine, 80, 81
Hypercortisolemia, 39
Hypercortisolism, 40
Hyperinsulinemia, 229
Hypernatremia, 183
Hyperosmolality, 183
Hyperprolactinemia, 39, 42
Hypertension, 207, 208, 221, 228
Hypnosis, 18
    agents, 198
Hypochondriasis (HC), 49
Hypomania, 159, 160
Hypophysitis, 43
Hypopituitarism
    ACTH deficiency, 41
    causes of, 40
    diagnosis, 41
    fertility, 41
    GH deficiency, 41
    gonadotropin deficiency, 41
    pituitary apoplexy, 41, 42
    pre-menopausal woman, 41
    Sheehan syndrome, 42
    treatment, 41
    TSH deficiency, 41
Hypotension, 41
Hypothalamic-pituitary-adrenal (HPA) axis, 158
Hysteria, 15

I
ICHD 3 Beta Diagnostic Criteria for Menstrual Migraine, 4
Idiopathic Intracranial Hypertension (IIH)
    definition, 134
    diagnosis, 134
    epidemiology, 134
    treatment, 134
Illness anxiety disorder (IAD), 54
    diagnosis of, 49
    epidemiology, 49, 50
    neuropsychologic characteristics, 49
    treatment, 50
Immunomodulating therapy, 151
Immunosuppressants, 77, 79
    and non-infectious adverse effects
        breastfeeding, 80
        cervical cancer, 80
        fertility and pregnancy, 80
        GIOP, 79
Immunosuppressives (IS), 179
Individual psychotherapy, 163

Infertility, 72, 73
Innate immunity, 8
Insomnia, 221
Insomnia Severity Index (ISI), 198
Interferon β, 147
Internal carotid artery (ICA) aneurysms, 37
International Classification of Headache Disorders Third Edition Beta
        (ICHD), 3
Interpersonal psychotherapy (IPT), 163
Interpersonal therapy (IPT), 194
Interstitial cystitis, 73
Intimate Partner Violence (IPV), 70
Intracerebral pressure (ICP), 183
Intracranial hemorrhage, 122
Intrathecal chemotherapy, 98
Intravenous immunoglobulin (IVIG) therapy, 151
Intravenous labetolol, 135
Intravenous methylprednisolone, 152
Intraventricular hemorrhage (IVH)., 183
Involutional melancholia, 193
Iodinated contrast, 118, 119
Irritable bowel syndrome (IBS), 47
Ischemic stroke, 141, 196, 207, 208
IV immunoglobulin, 152

K
Ketoconazole, 40
Korsakoff's syndrome, 230

L
Lactation, 80, 148, 178, 181
        alemtuzumab, 150
        daclizumab, 149
        DMF, 148
        fingolimod, 149
        GA, 148
        mood disorder, 162
        natalizumab, 150
        ocrelizumab, 150
        rituximab, 150
        teriflunomide, 149
Lactotrope tumors secreting prolactin (prolactinomas), 38
Lactotrophs, 40, 43
Lamotrigine, 91, 92, 123, 126–128, 164, 166
Langerhans cell histiocytosis, 43
Leflunomide, 81, 149
Left parasagittal meningioma, 97
Lemtrada, 150
Levetiracetam, 91, 92, 123, 126–128, 180
Levodopa, 214
Life-sustaining therapy (LST), 184–187
Light therapy, 166
Lithium, 164, 165
Long-acting reversible contraceptives (LARC), 27
Low-dose aspirin, 142
Low-molecular-weight heparin, 142
Lumbosacral plexus injury, 175
Lymphocytic hypophysitis, 42, 43

M
Macroadenomas, 38, 39, 41
Magnesium, 135

Magnesium sulfate, 180
Magnetic resonance imaging (MRI), 118, 119
        adverse effects, 119
        cerebral venous and sinus thrombosis, 122
        fetal risk, 119
        headache, 132
        safe imaging, 119
        stroke, 141
Major congenital malformations (MCMs), 126, 127, 163
Major depression, 157, 194
        definition, 192
        epidemiology, 192
        nonpharmacological interventions
                CBT, 194
                IPT, 194
        pharmacological interventions
                antidepressants, 194
                hormone therapy, 194
        risk factors
                demographic factors, 192
                lifestylefactors, 193
                medical factors, 193
                psychiatric factors, 192
                psychological factors, 193
                psychosocial factors, 193
Major depressive disorder (MDD), 71
Maladaptive behaviors, 49
Maternal depression, 158
Maternal physiology, 121
Maternal suicide, 158
MCMs, *see* Major congenital malformations (MCMs)
Mechanical thrombectomy, 141
Medical child abuse, 54
Medication induced hypophysitis, 43
Mediterranean-DASH Intervention for Neurodegenerative Delay
        (MIND) diet, 229
Mediterranean style diet, 229
Medroxyprogesterone acetate (MPA), 91
Menarche, 206
Meningiomas, 95, 96, 98
Menopausal transition, 191–198
Menopause, 206
        definition of, 191
                menopausal transition, 191
                postmenopause, 191
                reproductive stage, 191
        depression (*see* Depression)
        hot flashes, 198
                assessment scales, 196
                cardiovascular disease and bone health risk, 196
                CBT, 196
                epidemiology, 195
                gabapentin, 196
                HT, 196
                physiology, 195
                risk factors, 195, 196
                serotonergic agents, 196
                supportive tools, 196
                time course, 195
        sleep disturbance (*see* Sleep disturbances)
Menopause Rating Scale, 194
Menopause-Specific Quality of Life Scale, 194
Menstrual cycle, 88
Menstrual cycle on neurological and non-neurological
        disorders, 88–89

Menstrually related migraine, 4
    hormonal contraceptive use, 4
    phenotype of, 4
    prophylactic medication, 4
    prostaglandins, 4
    serum estrogen, 4
    short-term prophylaxis, 4
    treatment, 4
    triptans, 4
    without aura, 4
Mental health (MH), 229
Meralgia paresthetica, 173
Metabolic syndrome, 221
Methotrexate, 80, 81, 178, 179
Methyldopa, 180
Methylprednisolone, 81, 151
MG, see Myasthenia gravis (MG)
Microadenomas, 38, 39
Microchimerism, 99
Mifeprisone, 40
Migraine, 131, 207
    attacks, 4
    definition, 132
    diagnosis, 3
    epidemiology in pregnancy and postpartum, 132
    menstrual association, 3
    treatments, 133–134
    with aura, 3
    without aura, 3
Migraine disease
    clotting factors, 28
    hormonal contraception, 28, 29
    hormonal interventions, 29
    hormonal methods, 28
    incidence/prevalence, 28
    ischemic stroke risk, 28
    levonorgestrel IUD, 28
    menstruation, 28
    national health care claims, 28
    nociceptive and anti-nociceptive etiologies, 29
    pregnancy, 28
    prevalence, 28
    risk factors, 29
    systemic hormonal contraceptives, 29
    without aura, 28
Migraine with aura, 207
    characteristics, 132
    definition, 132
Mild Cognitive Impairment (MCI), 219–221
Mild depression, 162
Mindfulness Based Cognitive Therapy (MBCT), 50
Minor depression, 157
Miscarriages, 72, 127, 150, 153
Mitoxantrone, 80, 81
Mitoxanthrone-induced infertility, 79
Mixed connective tissue disorder, see Connective tissue disorders
Mixed dementia, 228
Mood Disorder Questionnaire (MDQ), 161
Mood disorders, 40, 49
    baby blues, 157
    lactation considerations, 162
    perinatal bipolar disorder
        clinical course, 159, 160
        epidemiology, 159
        risk factors, 159

perinatal depression
    clinical features, 158
    course, 158
    epidemiology, 157
    etiology, 158
    risk factors, 157, 158
postpartum psychosis
    clinical course, 160
    epidemiology, 160
    etiology, 160
    evaluation and treatment, 161
    risk factors, 160
pregnancy and postpartum, medication and treatment in
    acupuncture, 166
    antidepressants, 163–165
    antipsychotics, 165, 166
    breastfeeding, 165, 166
    electroconvulsive therapy, 166
    individual psychotherapy, 163
    light therapy, 166
    lithium, 164
    mood stabilizers, 164–166
    omega-3 fatty acids, 166
    SNRIs, 163
    SSRIs, 163
risk-benefit analysis, treating perinatal
        patient, 161, 162
screening, pregnancy and postpartum, 161
Mood stabilizers, 164–166
Motor conversion disorders, 57
Multiple sclerosis (MS), 31, 51, 78–80, 100
    DMT (see Disease-modifying therapies (DMTs))
    evaluation and treating relapse, 151
    exogenous hormones, 152, 153
    on fertility, 145
    on gastation, 145
    general postpartum management and counseling, 151
    long-term effects, 146
    management in women planning
        ART and relapse risk, 146
        general pre-conception care and counseling, 146
    on neonatal outcomes, 145
    prevention and management of relapses
        breastfeeding, 151–152
        steroids and IVIg, 152
    short-term effects, 145, 146
Munchausen's Syndrome, 53
Muscle-specific kinase (MuSK), 177
Myasthenia gravis (MG), 78
    caused by, 177
    fetal considerations, 180, 181
    general considerations in women, 181
    hormonal effects, 177
    labor and delivery, 180
    lactation, 181
    pregnancy complications, 179, 180
    pregnancy considerations and treatment
        first-line therapies, 179
        immunosuppressive, 179
        rapid-acting therapies, 179
        thymectomy, 179
    treatment modalities, 177
Myasthenic crisis, 177
Mycophenolate, 153
Mycophenolate mofetil, 80, 81, 178, 179, 181

N
Narcotics, 180
Natalizumab, 80, 81, 149, 150
Neuraxial anesthesia, 173
Neuroendocrine disorders
    hypopituitarism
        ACTH deficiency, 41
        autoimmune hypophysitis (*see* Lymphocytic hypophysitis)
        causes of, 40
        diagnosis, 41
        fertility, 41
        GH deficiency, 41
        GH replacement therapy, 41
        gonadotropin deficiency, 41
        lymphocytic hypophysitis, 42, 43
        pituitary apoplexy, 41, 42
        pre-menopausal woman, 41
        Sheehan syndrome, 42
        treatment, 41
        TSH deficiency, 41
    pituitary adenomas (*see* Pituitary adenomas)
    symptoms, 37
Neurofibrillary tangles, 219
Neuro-inflammatory disorders
    adaptive immune responses, 78, 79
    autoimmune disease activity, 78, 79
    genetic risk and reproductive counseling, 80–82
    immunosuppressants and non-infectious adverse effects (*see* Immunosuppressants)
    sex-related differences, 77–78
Neurological impairment, SLE, 9
Neurological paraneoplastic disorders, 77
Neurologic imaging in pregnancy
    CT, 119
        deterministic effects, 117
        direct exposure, 117
        dose units, 117
        effects of radiation, 117
        gestational age of fetus, 117
        indirect exposure, 117
        radiology reports and radiation dosimetry, 118
        rate of absorption, 117
        stochastic effects, 117
    CT angiography, 118
    digital subtraction angiography, 118, 119
    gadolinium, 119
    iodinated contrast, 118, 119
    magnetic resonance imaging, 118, 119
Neurologic manifestations, SS, 10
Neuromuscular junction, 180, 181
Neuromyelitis optica (NMO), 9, 77, 153
Neuromyelitis optica spectrum disorders (NMOSD)
    AQP4, 153
    disability, 153
    preeclampsia, 153
    relapse prevention in, 153
    rituximab, 153
    women with, 153
Neuronal excitability and seizure susceptibility, 90
Neuro-oncologic diseases
    chemotherapy
        conception, 99
        into semen/other body fluids, 99
    clinical monitoring, 99
    overview and epidemiology, 95
    pregnancy and menopause on brain and CNS tumors, 95, 96
    primary brain/CNS tumors
        gliomas/glioblastoma, 98
        meningiomas, 96, 98
        pituitary tumors, 98
    secondary neiro-oncology conditions
        brain & leptomeningeal metastases, 98
        cancer neurology & CNS complication of paraneoplastic disease, 98
    TTE, 100
Neuroplasticity, 228
Nexplanon, 92
Nicardipine, 135
Non-functional pituitary incidentalomas, 38
Non-hormonal contraceptive methods, 27, 28
NovoTTF device (Optune), 100

O
Obesity, 221, 228, 229
Obsessive compulsive disorder (OCD), 55, 69
    psychosis, 72
    sex differences, 70
    SSRIs, 72
    women with, 71
Obstetrical nerve injuries, 173
    sciatic nerve, 175
Obturator neuropathy, 175
Ocrelizumab, 150
Ocrevus, 150
Olanzapine, 166
Omega-3 fatty acids, 166
Optune, 100
Oral cholestyramine, 149
Oral contraceptives (OC), 152, 206, 207
Oral/infused chemotherapy, 98
Oral pyridostigmine, 179
Oxcarbazepine, 164

P
Panic disorder (PD), 70
Parainfectious conditions, 77
Paraneoplastic disease, neurology and CNS complication of, 98
Paraneoplastic encephalopathy, 99
Parenteral hydrocortisone, 180
Parkinson's disease, gender differences in
    cognition and nonmotor symptoms, 215
    estrogen, effects of, 213, 214
    genetic factors, 213
    motor symptoms, 214–215
    pregnancy, 215, 216
    progressive degenerative disease, 213
Paroxetine, 50, 196
Pasireotide, 40
Patient Health Questionnaire (PHQ), 161
PDPH, *see* Postdural puncture headache (PDPH)
Pelvic organ prolapse (POP), 74
Perimenopause, 191
    period, 96
Perimenstrual phase, 85
Perinatal anxiety disorders, 72
Perinatal depression
    clinical features, 158
    course, 158
    epidemiology, 157
    etiology, 158
    risk factors, 157, 158

Periovulatory phase, 85
Peripartum depression, 151
Peroneal neuropathy, 174
Persistent-hypertension of newborn (PPHN), 163
Pharmacologic therapy, 133
Phenytoin (PHT), 126–128, 180
Phobias, 70
Physiology of pregnancy
    cardiovascular and hemodynamic changes, 121
    hematologic changes, 122
    neurologic conditions, impact of
        cerebral infarctions, 122
        epilepsy, 122, 123
        intracranial hemorrhage, 122
    renal physiology, 121
Pittsburgh Sleep Quality Index (PSQI), 198
Pituitary adenomas, 37
    characterization, 38
    classification, 38
    Cushing's syndrome, 39, 40
    hyperprolactinemia, 39
    imaging, 38
    prolactinomas, 38, 39
Pituitary apoplexy, 41, 42
Pituitary hyperplasia, 37, 42
Pituitary tumors, 37, 98
Plasma exchange (PLEX), 177, 179
Plasmapheresis, 80, 81
Postdural puncture headache (PDPH)
    definition, 136, 137
    epidemiology, 137
    pathophysiology, 137
    treatment, 137
Posterior reversible encephalopathy syndrome (PRES), 135, 140
Postmenopausal hormone therapy, 207
Postmenopause, 191–194
Postnatal adaptation syndrome (PNAS), 163
Postpartum anxiety disorders, 71
Postpartum depression, 161
Postpartum generalized anxiety disorder (PPGAD), 71
Postpartum leg weakness, 176
Postpartum obsessive compulsive disorder (PPOCD), 72
Postpartum psychosis
    clinical course, 160
    epidemiology, 160
    etiology, 160
    evaluation and treatment, 161
    risk factors, 160
Post traumatic stress disorder (PTSD), 69
    fight/flight response, 70
    freeze response, 70
    IPV, 70
    in postpartum period, 71
    risk factors, 70
Prednisolone, 181
Prednisone, 81, 178, 181
Preeclampsia/eclampsia (PEE), 140, 141, 153, 179, 206
    definition, 134
    morbidity and mortality, 134
    pathophysiology, 134, 135
    treatment, 135
Pregnancy
    disease expression, 8
    disease specific, 8
    immunomodulation, 8
Pregnancy-associated ischemic strokes, 140
Pregnancy in Multiple Sclerosis (PRIMS) study, 145

Pregnancy loss
    infertility, 72, 73
    miscarriages, 72
    stillbirth, 72
Premenstrual dysphoric disorder (PMDD), 33, 71–72
Primidone (PRM), 126, 127
Progesterone, 69, 86, 87, 90, 158
Progestin-only oral formulations, 4
Progestin-only pills (POPs), 27
Prolactinomas, 38, 39, 98
Pryridostigmine, 178
Pseudo- Chiari malformation, 137
Pseudoexacerbations, 151
Psychiatric disease, 32–34
Psychogenic Movement Disorders Rating Scale, 55
Psychogenic non-epileptic seizures (PNES), 50–53, 56
    diagnostic levels of certainty, 16
Psychological distress, 73
    definition of, 192, 194
    epidemiology, 192
    risk factors
        demographic risk factors, 192
        lifestyle factors, 193
        medical factors, 193
        psychiatric factors, 193
        psychosocial factors, 193
    treatment, 195
Psychological stress, 73
Psychosis, 72
Psychosocial stressors, 158, 208, 209
Psychotherapy, 50, 52
Pyridostigmine, 177, 181

R
Radiation therapy, 98
Radiculopathy, 174
Raynaud's phenomenon, 10
RCVS, see Reversible Cerebral Vasospasm Syndrome (RCVS)
Receptor activator of nuclear factor kappa-B ligand (RANKL), 79
Receptor-related low-density lipoprotein-4 (LRP-4), 177
Regional anesthesia, 180
Relative infant doses (RID), 152, 162
    antidepressants, 165
    antiphycotics, 166
    mood stabilizers, 165
Repetitive 1Hz transcranial magnetic stimulation (rTMS), 22
Reproductive-aged migraine patients, 29
Retroperitoneal hematoma, 174, 175
Reversible cerebral vasoconstriction syndrome (RCVS), 140
Reversible cerebral vasospasm syndrome (RCVS)
    definition, 135
    epidemiology, 135
    pathophysiology, 135
    treatment, 135
Rheumatoid arthritis (RA), 79
Risk-benefit analysis, 161, 162
Rituxan, see Rituximab
Rituximab, 81, 150, 178, 179, 181
    NMOSD, 153

S
Schizophrenia, 39
Sciatic nerve injury, 174, 175
Secondary pituitary hyperplasia, 38
Second generation antipsychotics (SGAs), 165

Seizures, 85–87, 89–93, 122, 125
   clustering, 85
Selective serotonin reuptake inhibitors (SSRIs), 163, 194, 196
Selegiline, 216
Sellar tumors, 37
Sensory impairment, 175
Sensory loss and anesthesia, 173
Serotonergic agents, 196
Serotonin norepinephrine reuptake inhibitors (SNRI), 163, 194, 196
Serotonin reuptake inhibitors (SSRIs), 72
Sex-based susceptibility to autoimmune diseases, 31
Sex hormones, 31, 85, 86
Sex steroids, 7
Sexual dysfunction, 193
Sheehan syndrome, 42
Short-term Menstrual Migraine Prophylaxis, 4
Sjogren's Syndrome (SS), 10, 11
Sleep deprivation, 230
Sleep disorder, 230
Sleep disturbances, 193
   assessment scale, 198
   clinical presentation, 197
   epidemiology, 197
   nonpharmacological interventions
      CBT, 198
      sleep hygiene, 198
   pharmacological interventions
      antidepressants, 198
      gabapentin, 198
      hypnotic agents, 198
      sedatives, 198
   risk factors
      cultural variations, 197
      depression and anxiety, 197
      metabolic, 197
      vasomotor symptoms, 197
Sleep fragmentation, 197
SLE psychosis, 9
Socialization, 230
Somatic symptom disorder (SSD), 53, 54
   DSM-5 criteria, 47
   epidemiology, 48
   neuropsychologic characteristics, 48
   patterns of distress, 50
   treatment, 48–49
   in women, 56
Somatization, 48
Somatoform disorder
   CD (see Conversion disorder (CD))
   clinical assessment, 54, 55
   clinical care of patients, 57
   differential diagnosis, 55
   factitious disorder, 53
      diagnosis of, 53
      epidemiology, 54
      external motivation, 53
      FD-O, 54
      treatment, 54
   IAD
      diagnosis of, 49
      epidemiology, 49, 50
      neuropsychologic characteristics, 49
      treatment, 50
   sex and gender, influences of, 55–57
      biologic differences, 56
      functional syndromes, 56

      pain, women, 56
      sex-specific biologic influences, 56
      trauma, 57
   SSD (see Somatic symptom disorder (SSD))
   standardized rating scales for, 55
   unexplained symptoms, 47
Somatotrophs, 40
Spinal anesthesia, 175, 176
Stages of Reproductive Aging Workshop (STRAW) Criteria, 191
Steroids, 152
Stevens-Johnson syndrome, 166
Stillbirth, 72
STRAW criteria, 192, 195
Stress dose steroids, 41, 42
Stroke, 30, 31
   acute treatment, 141
   diagnosis, 140–141
   epidemiology, 140
   pathophysiology
      connective tissues/remodeling, alterations in, 140
      hemodynamic changes, 139
      hypercoagulability, 139
      immune-mediated changes, 140
      preeclampsia-eclampsia, 140
      rare causes of, 140
   secondary prevention
      anticoagulation, 142
      antiplatelet agents, 142
      mode of delivery, 142
      pregnancy-associated stroke, 142
   SLE, 9
Stroke risk factors in women, 205
   atrial fibrillation, 208
   depression, 208
   diabetes mellitus, 208
   gestational diabetes mellitus, 206
   hormonal contraceptive use, 206–207
   hypertension, 207, 208
   incidence of, 205
   menopause and menarche, 206
   migraine with aura, 207
   postmenopausal hormone therapy, 207
   pre-eclampsia, 206
   pregnancy, 206
      complications, 206
   psychosocial stress, 208, 209
   sex-specific risk prediction models, 209
Subarachnoid hemorrhage (SAH), 122, 140, 141, 183
Subsyndromal depression, 192, 194
   treatment, 195
Suicidality, 54
Survival bias, 219
Systemic lupus erythematosus (SLE), 8, 9, 77
Systemic vascular resistance (SVR), 121

T
Tecfidera, 148
Teriflunomide, 80, 81, 147, 149
Thin hypothesis, 195
Thrombocytopenia, 122
Thymectomy, 179, 181
TNFα inhibitors, 80
Tocolytic treatment, 166
Topiramate (TPM), 126–128
Transcranial magnetic stimulation (TMS), 52

Transient neonatal myasthenia gravis (TNMG), 180
Tricyclic antidepressant (TCA), 163
TSH deficiency, 41
Tumor treating fields (TTE), 100
Type 2 diabetes, 221, 229
Tysabri, 149–150

U
Unintended pregnancy, 27
United States Medical Eligibility Criteria (USMEC), 27
Unplanned pregnancy, prevention of, 27
Untreated anxiety disorder, 71
Untreated mood disorders, 71
Urinary incontinence, 74
Urinary tract infections (UTIs), 73
U.S. Food and Drug Administration (FDA) drug risk
     categories, 154

V
Vaccination studies in human beings, 7
Valproate, 131, 166
Valproic acid, 73, 123, 125–127, 164
Vasomotor symptoms, 195–197

Venlafaxine, 165, 196
Venous thromboembolism (VTE), 30
Vitamin D, 145, 146
Vulvar pain, 73
Vulvodynia, 73

W
Warfarin, 136
Weight gain, 193
Whitely Index, 55
Window of opportunity hypothesis, 220
Women with epilepsy (WWE)
     best and worst AED choices for, 126–127
     folic acid used in, 127
Worsening headache, 28

X
Xanthomatous hypophysitis, 43

Z
Zinbryta, 149
Zolpidem, 198

Printed by Printforce, the Netherlands